W0105739

ADVANCES IN
PERINATAL
MEDICINE
Volume 5

A Continuation Order Plan is available for this series. A continuation order will bring delivery of each new volume immediately upon publication. Volumes are billed only upon actual shipment. For further information please contact the publisher.

ADVANCES IN
PERINATAL
MEDICINE
Volume 5

Edited by

Aubrey Milunsky, MB.B.Ch., D.Sc., F.R.C.P., D.C.H.

*Boston University School of Medicine
Boston, Massachusetts*

Emanuel A. Friedman, M.D., Sc.D.

*Harvard Medical School
Boston, Massachusetts*

and

Louis Gluck, M.D.

*University of California, Irvine
School of Medicine
Irvine, California*

PLENUM MEDICAL BOOK COMPANY
New York and London

ISBN-13: 978-1-4615-9470-3   e-ISBN-13: 978-1-4615-9468-0
DOI: 10.1007/978-1-4615-9468-0

© 1986 Aubrey Milunsky, Emanuel A. Friedman, and Louis Gluck
Softcover reprint of the hardcover 1st edition 1986

Plenum Publishing Corporation
233 Spring Street, New York, N.Y. 10013

Plenum Medical Book Company is an imprint of Plenum Publishing Corporation

All rights reserved

No part of this book may be reproduced, stored in a retrieval system, or transmitted
in any form or by any means, electronic, mechanical, photocopying, microfilming,
recording, or otherwise, without written permission from the Publisher

Contents of Earlier Volumes

Contributors

Joel J. Alpert, M.D. • Department of Pediatrics, Boston City Hospital, Boston University School of Medicine, Boston, Massachusetts 02118

Robert C. Chantigian, M.D. • Department of Anaesthesia, Harvard Medical School and Brigham and Women's Hospital, Boston, Massachusetts 02115. *Present address:* Department of Anesthesia, Mayo Clinic, Rochester, Minnesota 55905

Valerie Charlton, M.D. • Department of Pediatrics, University of California, San Francisco, California 94143

David A. Eschenbach, M.D. • Department of Obstetrics and Gynecology, University of Washington, Seattle, Washington 98195

K. Hemminki, M.D. • Institute of Occupational Health, SF-00290 Helsinki, Finland

Ralph Hingson, Sc.D. • Section of Social and Behavioral Sciences, Boston University School of Public Health, Boston, Massachusetts 02118

M.-L. Lindbohm • Institute of Occupational Health, SF-00290 Helsinki, Finland

Janet Mitchell, M.D. • Department of Obstetrics and Gynecology, Boston City Hospital, Boston University School of Medicine, Boston, Massachusetts 02118

William Oh, M.D. • Brown University Program in Medicine, Department of Pediatrics, Women and Infants Hospital of Rhode Island, Providence, Rhode Island 02908

Gerard W. Ostheimer, M.D. • Department of Anaesthesia, Harvard Medical School and Brigham and Women's Hospital, Boston, Massachusetts 02115

Steven J. Parker, M.D. • Department of Pediatrics, Boston City Hospital, Boston University School of Medicine, Boston, Massachusetts 02118

Ted S. Rosenkrantz, M.D. • Division of Neonatology, Department of Pediatrics, University of Connecticut Health Center, Farmington, Connecticut 06032

H. Taskinen • Institute of Occupational Health, SF-00290 Helsinki, Finland

Barry S. Zuckerman, M.D. • Department of Pediatrics, Boston City Hospital, Boston University School of Medicine, Boston, Massachusetts 02118

Preface

The state of health care is reflected by perinatal and neonatal morbidity and mortality as well as by the frequencies of long-term neurologic and developmental disorders. Many factors, some without immediately recognizable significance to childbearing and many still unknown, undoubtedly contribute beneficially or adversely to the outcome of pregnancy. Knowledge concerning the impact of such factors on the fetus and surviving infant is critical. Confounding analyses of pregnancy outcome, especially these past two or three decades, are the effects of newly undertaken invasive or inactive therapeutic approaches coupled with the advent of high technology. Many innovations have been introduced without serious efforts to evaluate their impact prospectively and objectively. The consequences of therapeutic misadventures characterized the past; it seems they have been replaced to a degree by some of the complications of applied technology. Examples abound: after overuse of oxygen was recognized to cause retrolental fibroplasia, its restriction led to an increase in both neonatal death rates and neurologic damage in surviving infants. Administration of vitamin K to prevent neonatal hemorrhagic disease, particularly when given in what we now know as excessive dosage, occasionally resulted in kernicterus. Prophylactic sulfonamide use had a similar end result. More recent is the observation of bronchopulmonary dysplasia as a complication of respirator therapy for hyaline membrane disease.

The decade of the eighties opened with the all-time highest rate of cesarean section in the United States. This has come about for reasons that are not entirely clear, although the increased incidence may be attributed to an ostensibly greater astuteness with regard to fetal compromise coupled with a growing reluctance to undertake potentially traumatic vaginal delivery procedures. The method of choice for breech delivery is now being strongly influenced by both early uncontrolled experimental data and intuitive judgment, neither necessarily reliable. Aside from issues related to optimizing delivery practices, intrauterine environmental problems (reflected in fetal growth retardation) and premature labor are matters of exceptionally high priority. In perspective, one recent estimate of the number of low-birth-weight infants born each year around the world is 22 million. The eternal goal is unchanged: to deliver a normal child with unmarred potential. Despite important advances in securing better pregnancy outcome, demanding challenges remain. Recognition of these challenges and the complex approaches required for prevention and treatment have spawned fresh pediatric- and obstetric-team initiatives.

The sharpened focus is exemplified by the interdisciplinary nature of the perinatal health team. In addition to the neonatologist, obstetrician, and hybrid perinatologist, important team members include a host of specialists. Indeed, information culled from many specialties and professions impact directly or indirectly on the burgeoning field of perinatal medicine. This body of knowledge includes contributions from geneticists, teratologists, immunologists, pathologists, endocrinologists, neurodevelopmental and neurobehavioral specialists, physiologists, biochemists, pharmacologists, family practitioners, surgeons, epidemiologists, demographers, toxicologists, intensive care nurses, radiologists and ultrasonographers, psychologists, biomedical and electronic engineers, social workers, health department administrators, public health educators, lawyers, ethicists, theologians, and even psychiatrists. The list is admittedly incomplete and the order is not meant to imply priority of interest or impact.

The progress along the frontiers of perinatal medicine has been and will continue to be made from the individual and collective contributions of representatives of these and other disciplines, each of necessity having limited insights into other tangentially or remotely related specialties. Progress, we believe, can be encouraged and enhanced by insightful interdisciplinary and critically analytical communication. We have, therefore, initiated this new series of *Advances in Perinatal Medicine* to serve as a catalyst and critical forum for the needs of all those interested in optimal pregnancy outcome. We are grateful to those expert contributors who have so graciously shared their time and expertise for this and future volumes. Their papers are meant to evaluate a subject critically and in depth, with special focus on the progress that has thus far been made and the problems that have been encountered in the overlapping and borderland zones of advancing research and clinical application. We hope that this new series will not only serve the interests of those involved in these important pursuits, but, by providing new interdisciplinary insights, will also ultimately benefit future generations.

Aubrey Milunsky
Emanuel A. Friedman
Louis Gluck

Contents

CHAPTER 2

Transplacental Toxicity of Environmental Chemicals: Environmental Causes and Correlates of Spontaneous Abortions, Malformations, and Childhood Cancer

K. HEMMINKI, M.-L. LINDBOHM, and H. TASKINEN

CHAPTER 3

Neonatal Polycythemia and Hyperviscosity

TED S. ROSENKRANTZ and WILLIAM OH

CHAPTER 4

Maternal Psychoactive Substance Use and Its Effect on the Neonate

BARRY S. ZUCKERMAN, STEVEN J. PARKER,
RALPH HINGSON, JOEL J. ALPERT, and JANET MITCHELL

CHAPTER 5

Effect of Maternally Administered Drugs on the Fetus and Newborn

ROBERT C. CHANTIGIAN and GERARD W. OSTHEIMER

CHAPTER 6

Chlamydial Infection

DAVID A. ESCHENBACH

CHAPTER 1

Nutritional Supplementation of the Growth-Retarded Fetus

Rationale, Theoretical Considerations, and *in Vivo* Studies

VALERIE CHARLTON

1. Introduction

In the United States and Great Britain, approximately one-third of all infants born weighing less than 2500 g are not premature but are rather mature infants whose growth has been retarded *in utero*.[1] Even preterm infants may be markedly undergrown for their dates.[2] These intrauterine growth-retarded, or small-for-gestational-age infants, have a higher neonatal death rate than do normally grown infants of the same gestation.[3,4] They have an increased incidence of neonatal problems and long-term adverse sequelae,[1] including a reduction in ultimate stature[5–8] and neurologic abnormalities.[9–11] To avoid these damaging sequelae, means of preventing growth retardation have been sought. One approach that has been suggested, and tried in the human, is intrauterine nutritional supplementation of the poorly growing fetus.[12] It is the purpose of this chapter to present the rationale behind considering nutritional therapy, to discuss the theoretical considerations important in administering nutrients to the fetus, and to review the human and animal studies carried out thus far.

VALERIE CHARLTON ● Department of Pediatrics, University of California, San Francisco, California 94143.

1

2. Rationale for Considering Nutritional Therapy

2.1. Normal Fetal Growth and Nutrition—A Brief Review

2.1.1. Fetal Nutrients

The physiologic alterations that occur in the growth-retarded fetus are more clearly defined when compared with growth and nutrition of the normal fetus. Fetal growth occurs throughout gestation but is most rapid during the second half of pregnancy. It is over this period that demands for nutrients and oxygen are greatest and nutrient deficiencies are most likely to become apparent.[1] By the end of gestation, even the normal fetus appears to outgrow its substrate supply. This results in a slowing of growth and late flattening in fetal growth curves for weight, length, and head circumference.[2]

The macronutrients that cross the placenta into the fetus and make normal growth possible are glucose, amino acids, lactate, fatty acids, and acetate.[13] Our knowledge about the role of these nutrients in fetal nutrition has come from studies in many mammalian species and particularly from investigations on the chronically catheterized fetal lamb.

Glucose, the major source of energy and carbon for the fetus, crosses the placenta by means of facilitated diffusion.[13] Umbilical uptake of glucose is proportional to the glucose concentration gradient between mother and fetus.[14,15] Fetal levels of glucose correlate with maternal levels[14] and are approximately two-thirds to three-fourths of maternal values in the human[16] and one-third of maternal values in the sheep.[14,17] When maternal blood glucose levels are high, fetal levels will be elevated; if maternal glucose levels are low, fetal levels will be depressed.[16,17] Glucose availability is crucial for the developing central nervous system (CNS), as glucose is the primary oxidative substrate for the fetal brain.[18]

Amino acids are the major source of fetal nitrogen and another important source of carbon; they are used to synthesize proteins and build new tissue.[13] In addition, fetal catabolism of amino acids occurs and the resulting nitrogen is excreted as urea.[19] Amino acids enter the fetus by active transport across the placenta, so that fetal levels are higher than maternal.[20,21] In the midtrimester human fetus, the total molar concentration ratio between fetus and mother is 2.4 : 1.0.[20] In the third-trimester fetal lamb, the fetal-to-maternal amino acid concentration ratio is 1.7 : 1.0.[21] If there is an abnormally high level of an amino acid in the mother, such as occurs with phenylalanine in phenylketonuria, the effect is magnified in the fetus.[22,23] This finding has particular relevance for CNS development, as inborn errors of metabolism that elevate amino acid levels can result in marked neurologic impairment.[24,25]

Despite high amino acid levels in the fetus, the margin for adequate availability of some individual amino acids may be small. Lemmons *et al.*[21] compared the umbilical uptake of amino acids by the ovine fetus with carcass accretion of each amino acid. In this initial study, umbilical uptake of the essential amino acids lysine and histidine was found to be close to estimated fetal usage. This study was carried out 4 days after surgical preparation of the animals. A more recent study, performed after a longer, 7-day, recovery period, showed somewhat greater umbilical uptake of lysine but close uptake to usage ratios for histidine, valine, and phenylalanine.[26] If maternal-to-fetal transfer of these essential amino acids should decrease, they might rapidly become growth limiting. In fact, perfusion studies, in the isolated guinea pig placenta, indicate that transport of individual essential amino acids falls rapidly with small decreases in uterine blood flow.[27]

Lactate is the second most important carbohydrate nutrient, after glucose.[13] Fetal lactate is taken up across the umbilical circulation[28,29] and is produced in the fetus from glucose and nonglucose substrates.[30] This results in twofold greater levels of lactate in the fetus than are found in the mother.[28,29] The lactate obtained across the umbilical circulation ultimately derives from maternal glucose, which has been converted to lactate by placental metabolism. Placental lactate is then emptied into both the fetal umbilical and maternal uterine circulations.[28] Lactate is avidly taken up by the fetal liver, where it may be converted into glucose or stored as a carbohydrate reserve.[31]

Lipids and fatty acids are of great structural importance for the developing nervous system. Different animal species show tremendous variation in the extent of fatty acid placental transfer. Animals with a higher percentage of body fat at birth have greater fatty acid transport from mother to fetus.[13,32] Newborn humans and guinea pigs have considerable fat (10–16%), whereas the newborn pig, rat and sheep are leaner (1–2% fat).[13] In all species, transfer of essential fatty acids must occur. Fetal synthesis of nonessential fatty acids must occur as well, since placental transfer is usually insufficient to provide all fetal lipids.[33,34] When maternal lipid levels become elevated, placental transfer of fatty acids is increased.[33,35] In fat species such as the guinea pig, alteration in the type of unsaturated fats fed to mothers during pregnancy is reflected by changes in the proportion of unsaturated fatty acids found in fetal tissues, including the brain.[36]

Acetate, after conversion to acetyl-CoA, is a central building block for synthesis of lipids and steroids.[37] Blood levels of acetate are higher

in herbivores than in other mammals because of microbiologic break-
down of dietary cellulose and other starches in the gastrointestinal (GI)
tract.[37] However, blood acetate turnover rates are as rapid in nonher-
bivores as in herbivores.[37] Studies in the ruminant have shown that
maternal-to-fetal transfer of acetate occurs.[38,39] Fetal blood levels of acetate are proportional to maternal levels and umbilical uptake of acetate
directly correlates with the maternal-to-fetal acetate concentration gradient.[38] Placental transfer of acetate and fetal utilization has been demonstrated in the human. After [^{14}C]acetate was injected into women
during early pregnancy, [^{14}C]cholesterol was found in fetal tissues; labeled cholesterol itself did not cross the placenta.[40]

Other potential fetal macronutrients, such as glycerol,[41] β-hydroxy-
butyrate,[42] acetoacetate,[42] and citrate,[43] have been studied. Under normal conditions, placental transfer of these substrates is minimal.[41–43]
Transfer of ketones is increased, however, when maternal levels are
elevated.[44]

Many micronutrients are also essential for normal fetal growth. Vitamin deficiencies in pregnant experimental animals have long been
known to result in fetal malformations, including CNS defects.[45] Recently, lowered maternal blood cell levels of folate and ascorbic acid,
during the first trimester of pregnancy, have been associated with neural
tube defects in human infants.[46] Smithells *et al.*[47] found multivitamin,
calcium and iron supplementation administered before conception reduced the recurrence rate for having a second infant affected by neural
tube abnormalities. Abnormally high levels of vitamins can also be detrimental to the fetus.[48] Women treated with high doses of vitamin A for
acne have given birth to infants with microcephaly, ventricular dilation,
microphthalmus, and microtia.[48] Both deficiencies and excess amounts
of trace minerals can have an adverse effect on fetal development.[49] In
particular, the role of zinc deficiency in poor fetal growth has received
considerable attention. Pregnant rats fed a zinc-deficient diet have a high
incidence of growth-retarded offspring with gross fetal malformations;
almost one-half of fetuses have brain anomalies.[49] Even transient maternal zinc deficiency, during pregnancy in the rat, leads to fetal CNS
malformation.[49] Recently, in the human, low maternal leukocyte levels
of zinc have been found in women with growth-retarded infants.[50] Lower
plasma zinc levels have also been reported in women giving birth to
congenitally abnormal infants and in the cord blood of the infants themselves.[51]

The discussion thus far has focused on nutrient acquisition, but it
must be remembered that oxygen uptake by the fetus is necessary to
facilitate utilization of these nutrients. It has been variously estimated

that between 20 and 40% of normal fetal oxidative metabolism is used to provide the energy requirements for growth and synthesis of new tissue.[52,53]

2.1.2. Normal Fetal Distribution of Nutrients and Brain Utilization

Like the fetal carcass, the brain undergoes a growth spurt over the second half of gestation,[54] hence the high cerebral demand for nutrients during this period. The peak rate of brain growth, in grams per month, is reached during the last 2 months *in utero*.[54,55]

The developmental processes that occur in the CNS, as part of the brain growth spurt, are listed in Table I. Whereas most cerebral neurons have already been created by the twentieth week, late-maturing neurons of the cerebellum and hippocampus are still forming.[54,56] Neuronal migration, brain organization, massive glial cell proliferation, beginning myelination, and increasing metabolic activity of the brain are also occurring.[54–57] It is important to remember that the cerebellum is the area of the brain that coordinates fine motor activity, whereas the hippocampus, among other functions, is concerned with recent memory and new

Table I. Developmental Processes Occurring in the Central Nervous System over the Second Half of Gestation[a]

Brain growth spurt
  Begins in midpregnancy
  Reaches peak velocity during the last 2 months of gestation
Formation of late-maturing neurons in cerebellum and
      hippocampus
Neuronal migration
  Peaks in midpregnancy
Brain organization
  Peaks in early third trimester
  Continues through a year or more postnatally
  Includes several events
    Alignment of cortical neurons
    Dendrite ramification
    Synapse formation
    Glial cell proliferation
Myelination
  Begins in midpregnancy
  Continues into adult life
Increasing metabolic activity of subcortical pathways and cortex

[a] Compiled from refs. 54–57.

learning.[58] The rapidly forming neuroglial cells are the neuronal support and nurturing cells; some of the glial cells produce myelin sheaths around nerve fibers and tracts in the white matter of the cortex.[58] Although these developmental processes continue after birth, disturbances in brain development during the fetal growth spurt could affect many aspects of brain activity, including motor function, learning, and integration.[55]

The nutrients that reach the fetal brain are used anabolically to produce new tissue and serve as a source of energy for existing tissue. It has been well established that oxygenated blood returning from the placenta is shunted into the left side of the fetal heart and ascending aorta. This results in higher oxygen saturation in arterial blood supplying the fetal upper body than in blood supplying the lower body.[52] We have recently established that nutrients are also not equally distributed throughout the fetus; rather, there is preferential shunting of nutrients to upper body organs, such as the brain and heart.[59] Concentrations of glucose are 10% greater in the carotid artery than in the femoral artery, whereas amino nitrogen levels (total amino acids) are 4% greater. Concentrations of waste products, which are cleared by the placenta (e.g., urea and $[H]^+$) are decreased in blood perfusing the upper body.[59]

Amino acids, glucose, and fatty acids—all initially of maternal origin—have been shown to be avidly taken up by the fetal brain. When a nonmetabolizable, radiolabeled analogue of amino acids (α-aminoisobutyric acid) is injected intravenously into the late-gestation pregnant rat, label is found in the fetal brain at sacrifice 60 min later.[60] When similar studies are performed using a glucose analogue (deoxyglucose), very high concentrations of label accumulate in the fetal brain.[60] In the human, if ^{14}C glucose is injected into a mother, labeled cholesterol appears in the fetal brain within 24 hr.[40] Fatty acids actually appear to concentrate in the fetal CNS. When ^{14}C-labeled essential fatty acids (linoleic and linolenic) are fed to pregnant guinea pigs and humans, the highest concentration of label is found in the fetal brain.[61] In the human fetus, brain radioisotope levels are greater than those measured in either the fetal liver, umbilical plasma, or maternal plasma.[61]

The major oxidative fuel of the brain is glucose.[18,62] The quantity of glucose taken up by the ovine fetal brain is so large that, if all the glucose were oxidized to carbon dioxide and water, glucose oxidation would completely account for brain oxygen consumption; the glucose/oxygen quotient of the fetal brain is, therefore, approximately 1.0.[18] Twenty-four percent of the glucose being taken up across the umbilical circulation is normally consumed by ovine cerebral metabolism, whereas 10% of total fetal oxygen consumption is used by the brain.[18] In the human newborn, which has a larger brain, cerebral uptake of glucose and oxygen is even greater. Brain metabolism is estimated to account for approximately 50% of glucose turnover and 60% of oxygen uptake.[18]

Under normal fed conditions, only glucose is taken up with significant arterio-venous (a–v) difference across the ovine fetal brain; many other metabolites such as lactate, pyruvate, acetoacetate, and β-hydroxy-butyrate have been studied.[18] Brain utilization of ketone bodies has been found in neonatal humans, baboons, cows, and rats under fasting conditions. Only the newborn rat appears to use ketones for cerebral metabolism when well fed.[62]

Local glucose uptake within the fetal brain was studied by Abrams et al.,[57] using [14C]deoxyglucose and quantitative autoradiography. The ovine fetus was studied from 87 days gestation to term, at 145 days. Over this period, average brain glucose utilization rose gradually, almost tripling between 87 days and full term. Close to delivery, the glucose utilization rate averaged approximately 20 μmoles/100 g per min. A further increment of 50% was seen during the first few days postnatally. Glucose utilization was not homogeneous throughout the brain. As gestation advanced, discrete areas were found to become more metabolically active and to take up greater quantities of glucose. In the earliest fetuses studied, glucose utilization rates were low throughout most of the brain but relatively high in the hippocampus, portions of the cerebellum, vestibular nuclei, and oculomotor nuclear complex. By 100 days gestation, augmented glucose uptake rates were also found in the brain stem nuclei of the auditory system. With the approach of full term, uptake increased in the remaining subcortical auditory structures and subcortical areas related to visual function. The rate of glucose utilization varied little throughout the cortical brain regions, but glucose uptake by the entire cortex rose markedly over gestation, with the area of cortical uptake widening as the cortical layers increased in thickness.[57]

Using radiolabeled microspheres to measure blood flow within the fetal brain, Clapp et al.[63] found that specific areas were relatively hyperperfused. In the late-gestation lamb, cortical gray matter contributed 65% of total brain weight and received 60% of total brain blood flow. By contrast, subcortical structures and the cerebellum received a greater percentage of total flow than they contributed to brain weight. This finding is of note, as these latter areas are rapidly developing in late gestation and display increasing metabolic activity.[54,56,57] Flow per gram of tissue was also remarkably high in cortical white matter, relative to flow patterns after birth. This was thought to be related to an elevated metabolic rate in white matter during the period of rapid myelin formation.[63]

The quantity of substrates reaching each region of the brain is determined by regional blood flow. It is therefore not surprising that local brain metabolic activity appears proportional to flow.[63,64] At any given gestation, those brain areas displaying high metabolic activity may be particularly vulnerable to a reduction in substrate availability.

2.2. The Growth-Retarded or Small-for-Gestational-Age Infant

2.2.1. Definition of Intrauterine Growth Retardation

The size achieved by a specific gestational age varies between infants within the same population. Inadequate growth, or intrauterine growth retardation (IUGR), has been defined as fetal weight falling below the tenth percentile on normal growth curves,[1,6] or, more restrictively, as weight less than two standard deviations (2 SD) below the mean (approximately up to the third percentile).[1,8] Researchers have also used definitions based on assessments of body proportions, weight-to-length ratios, or ponderal index.[1,65] Distinctions are often made between symmetrically and asymmetrically growth-retarded neonates.[66] Symmetrically growth-retarded infants show reduced weight, length, and head circumference, whereas those who are asymmetrically growth retarded have relative sparing of head growth.[66]

Placental growth is also affected by the growth retardation process. It is reduced in size compared with placentas from normally grown infants, both in preterm and term, small-for-gestational-age (SGA) infants.[67]

2.2.2. Etiology of Intrauterine Growth Retardation

A number of clinical conditions have been associated with poor intrauterine growth in the human infant,[1,68,69] as summarized in Table II. Apart from the inherently abnormal fetus, most conditions associated with growth retardation result in either (1) decreased availability of nutrients or oxygen in maternal blood; (2) decreased delivery of substrates to the placenta, or (3) decreased transfer of substrates across the placenta into the fetus. The relative role of nutrients versus oxygen in limiting fetal growth is under investigation. Although the severely growth-retarded fetus is often hypoxemic, reduced nutrient availability is a consistent finding in growth retardation of various etiology and even in growth retardation of only a moderate degree.[1,68]

Table II. Conditions Associated with Poor Fetal Growth[a]

Maternal factors
Decreased nutrient availability (e.g., low prepregnancy weight, poor weight gain, malabsorption, grand multiparity, chronic illness, hypoglycemia)
Reduced uteroplacental blood flow (e.g., hypertension, vascular disease, smoking)
Hypoxemia (e.g., hemoglobinopathies, high altitude)
Placental factors
Gross structural changes (e.g., abnormal cord insertion, infarcts, hemangioma, partial separation)
Microscopic changes (e.g., villous necrosis, fibrinosis)
Fetal factors
Chromosomal anomalies (e.g., trisomy, Turner's syndrome)
Dysmorphic syndromes (e.g., Cornelia de Lange, dwarfism)
Intrauterine infection (e.g, rubella, toxoplasmosis, cytomegalovirus, herpes)
Metabolic disorders (e.g., insulin deficiency)
Multiple gestation

[a] Compiled from refs. 1, 68, and 69.

Many investigations have demonstrated a relationship between nutritional deficiency and poor fetal growth. SGA human infants frequently appear wasted and have decreased glycogen and fat stores at birth.[1] At autopsy, findings are similar to those in infants dying of alimentary malnutrition[70]; both show a general decrease in organ size and most marked reductions in size of the liver, spleen, thymus, and adrenals.[70,71]

Mothers delivering growth-retarded infants, as well as the infants themselves, have been found to have reduced blood levels of major nutrients. Low fasting maternal glucose concentrations and unusually rapid maternal glucose utilization are seen in women who give birth to SGA infants.[72] Umbilical venous concentrations of glucose are known to be reduced in growth-retarded neonates as compared with normally grown newborns[73]; growth-retarded infants also have a steeper postnatal drop in blood sugar.[73] Blood concentrations of gluconeogenic precursors (e.g., alanine, glycine, and lactate) are elevated, suggesting a defect in hepatic gluconeogenesis.[73,74]

Amino acid levels were measured by Churchill and Moghissi and co-workers[75,76] in pregnant women and compared with fetal size and fetal amino acid concentration. Women with low total plasma amino acid concentrations between 32 and 36 weeks were found to have smaller infants, with reduced cranial volumes; women with high plasma amino acid concentrations had larger infants, with larger cranial volumes. On more detailed analysis, levels of specific amino acids (e.g., lysine and glycine) in maternal blood appeared to correlate with fetal weight.[76] Maternal levels of other amino acids (e.g., glycine and glutamine) strongly correlated with fetal cranial volume.[76] Several other investigators have also found a relationship between maternal concentration of amino acids and fetal size. However, the specific amino acids that show the strongest correlations with fetal size vary between studies.[76,77] McClain found that total amino acid levels at 20–30 weeks gestation averaged 18% lower in women giving birth to undergrown infants than in women delivering appropriately sized infants[77]; reductions of 15% were seen in levels of essential amino acids and of 20% in nonessential amino acids.

Although fetal concentrations of amino acids are greater than maternal, there is a significant positive correlation between maternal and fetal values for most amino acids.[20] Fetuses born to mothers with low amino acid concentrations, therefore, presumably have decreased amino acid levels. In fact, growth-retarded infants have been found to have decreased umbilical blood levels of several amino acids (isoleucine, cystine, and arginine).[78] Infants born to women wih hypertension and preeclampsia, conditions associated with growth retardation, have lowered umbilical venous concentrations and lowered fetal-to-maternal ratios for several essential amino acids, including phenylalanine and histidine.[79,80]

Investigations in experimental animals also indicate that nutrient deficiency is a major causative factor in growth retardation. Experimental models of growth retardation have been produced in many species,[81] but the model most extensively used for *in vivo* fetal investigations has been the chronically catheterized sheep.

IUGR has been induced in the sheep by multiple methods, including nutritional restriction,[82–85] placental damage,[53,86] limitation of placental implantation,[87] umbilical artery ligation,[88–90] and maternal heating.[91] In these preparations, fetal size and placental weight are reduced.[83,85,87,89,91,92] As in the SGA human, brain growth is relatively spared, and liver, spleen, and thymus are most markedly reduced in size.[83–87,89] Fetal metabolism has been studied in spontaneously growth-retarded lambs[93] and in lambs experimentally growth-retarded by maternal protein-calorie dietary restriction,[85,94,95] by repetitive placental embolization,[53,92] by prepregnancy removal of caruncles (the sites of placental implantation),[87] and by single umbilical artery ligation.[90] In these preparations, fetal levels of major nutrients have been found to be decreased. Total umbilical uptake of nutrients was also seen to be reduced.

Concentrations of metabolites, measured in these studies, are listed in Table III. In fetuses growth retarded by each method, average blood glucose levels are lower than in normal control animals from the same study. The differences achieved statistical significance only in the carunclectomy preparations, however.[53,87,90,93–94] Total amino acids (measured as α-amino nitrogen) were lower in growth-retarded fetuses in both forms of experimental growth retardation in which they were measured.[87,94,95] Interestingly, alanine levels alone were also analyzed in the carunclectomized fetuses and found to be significantly elevated,[87] just as occurs in SGA human neonates.[73,74] Lactate concentrations were found to be lower in growth-retarded animals in two of the three studies in which they were measured[87,95] but were elevated in the severely growth-retarded embolization model.[53] In carunclectomized fetuses, pyruvate was also analyzed and found to be significantly decreased.[87] Carunclectomized animals were noted to have lower concentrations of fatty acids, hydroxybutyrate, and acetate as well, but these differences did not achieve statistical significance.[87] As is indicated in Table III, fetal oxygen tensions were reduced in some forms of growth retardation but not all.[53,87,89,90,93–95] (By definition, oxygen levels would be decreased in the spontaneously

Table III. Comparison of Substrate Levels in Control and Intrauterine
Growth-Retarded Fetal Lambs[a–c]

Substrate IUGR model	Control fetuses	Growth-retarded fetuses
Glucose (mg/dl)		
Spontaneous	17.0 ± 0.9	15.6 ± 1.1
Dietary restriction	15.5 ± 2.0	14.6 ± 1.1
Placental embolization	17.3 ± 1.4	14.2 ± 2.3
Umbilical artery ligation	14.8 ± 2.0	12.1 ± 1.4
Carunclectomy	18.9 ± 1.1	11.7 ± 2.2[e]
Amino nitrogen (mg/dl)		
Dietary restriction	8.3 ± 0.6	6.5 ± 0.3[d]
Carunclectomy	10.4 ± 1.1	9.8 ± 1.3
Lactate (mg/dl)		
Dietary restriction	15.3 ± 1.4	12.7 ± 1.4
Placental embolization	14.7 ± 2.8	18.7 ± 3.0
Carunclectomy	16.5 ± 1.7	8.1 ± 0.9[f]
PaO_2 (mm Hg)		
Spontaneous	20.7 ± 0.4	14.7 ± 0.4[f]
Dietary restriction	19.5 ± 1.7	22.6 ± 1.8
Placental embolization	22.1 ± 0.7	17.5 ± 1.6[d]
Umbilical artery ligation	18.4 ± 2.0	20.0 ± 2.3
Carunclectomy	23.2 ± 0.7	15.0 ± 0.6[f]

[a] Data compiled from refs. 53, 87, 90, 93–95.
[b] Values given are mean ± SEM.
[c] Measurements were made in the femoral artery or descending aorta, except in carunclectomy studies, in which carotid arterial measurements were taken.
[d] $p < 0.05$.
[e] $p < 0.01$.
[f] $p < 0.001$.

growth-retarded group, because these animals were initially chosen for study on the basis of hypoxemia.[93])

Umbilical blood flow and uptake measurements made during the ovine investigations are presented in Table IV. Total umbilical blood flow was lower in all growth-retarded preparations than in control animals from the same studies.[53,85,90,92,93,95,96] Preparations displaying fetal hypoxemia were noted to have the lowest umbilical blood flows.[53,92,93] Blood flow per kilogram of fetal weight was decreased in the embolization model[92] but was the same for growth-retarded and control animals in the other preparations measured.[93,95]

Table IV. Umbilical Blood Flow and Uptake Measurements in Control and Intrauterine Growth-Retarded Fetal Lambs[a-e]

Substrate: IUGR model studied	Control fetuses		Growth-retarded fetuses	
Umbilical flow				
Spontaneous	571	(235 ± 11)	412	(225 ± 26)
Dietary restriction	637 ± 103	(207 ± 37)	547 ± 103	(202 ± 33)
Placental embolization	641 ± 26	(NA)	325 ± 36	(NA)
Placental embolization	717 ± 78	(158 ± 14)	339 ± 28[g]	(109 ± 7)[g]
Umbilical artery ligation	735 ± 70	(NA)	475 ± 24	(NA)
Glucose uptake				
Spontaneous[j]	16.8	(6.9 ± 1.4)	11.9	(6.5 ± 1.4)
Dietary restriction	18.1 ± 2.3	(5.4 ± 0.3)	13.9 ± 1.8	(5.0 ± 0.6)
Placental embolization	18.9 ± 2.0	(6.6 ± 0.6)	9.9 ± 1.7[h]	(4.7 ± 0.6)[g]
Umbilical artery ligation	21.0 ± 1.6	(6.0 ± 0.5)	14.8 ± 1.9[g]	(5.4 ± 0.6)
Amino nitrogen uptake				
Dietary restriction	1.2 ± 0.4	(0.5 ± 1.1)	−0.5 ± 0.7[h]	(−0.2 ± 0.3)
Lactate uptake				
Dietary restriction	3.2 ± 1.1	(1.2 ± 0.4)	5.4 ± 0.9	(1.7 ± 0.3)
Placental embolization	11.0 ± 0.9	(3.7 ± 0.4)	5.6 ± 0.4[i]	(2.7 ± 0.2)[g]
Oxygen uptake				
Spontaneous[j]	17.1	(7.0 ± 0.4)	19.5	(10.7 ± 1.6)[i]
Dietary restriction	23.8 ± 3.9	(7.3 ± 1.2)	15.2 ± 2.2[f]	(5.5 ± 0.7)
Placental embolization	28.1 ± 1.0	(9.5 ± 0.4)	16.0 ± 1.7[i]	(7.8 ± 0.5)[g]

[a] Data compiled from refs. 53, 90, 92–95.
[b] Values given are the mean ± SEM.
[c] NA indicates data not available.
[d] Blood flow and oxygen uptake are in ml/min and (ml/kg per min).
[e] Nutrient uptakes are in mg/min and (mg/kg per min).
[f] $p < 0.10$.
[g] $p < 0.05$.
[h] $p < 0.01$.
[i] $p < 0.001$.
[j] Calculated from mg/kg per min and average fetal weight in reference 93.

Total uptake of glucose was decreased in all growth-retarded groups studied.[53,85,90,93,95] Interestingly, glucose uptake per kilogram of fetal weight was the same in growth-retarded and control animals in all but the placental embolization model.[90,93,95] Even in embolized animals, glucose uptake per kilogram of fetal weight was reduced by only a small margin.[53] These findings suggest that the size achieved by the fetus relates directly to nutrient uptake as well as to umbilical blood flow.

Umbilical gain of total amino acids (α-amino nitrogen) was decreased in the one preparation in which it was measured.[95] Lactate uptake was decreased in one of two studies.[53,95]

Oxygen consumption, both total and per kilogram of fetal weight, was reduced in two of three models studied. The dietary restriction preparation showed no evidence of fetal hypoxemia,[94,95] and the decrease in oxygen consumption was most likely a secondary event, reflecting decreased nutrient availability and slowing of fetal growth. A large drop in oxygen uptake would be expected to accompany a cessation or slowing of growth, as up to 40% of fetal oxygen consumption is utilized in the growth process.[52,53]

Fetuses growth retarded by placental embolization also had decreased oxygen consumption and were hypoxemic.[53] Oxygen transport into these animals may have become limited, as they had a marked reduction—50%—in umbilical blood flow.[53,92,96] In acute experiments, fetal oxygen uptake has been shown to decrease, when umbilical blood flow is reduced below 50% of normal values, i.e., to flow rates ≤120 to 150 ml/kg per min.[97] Studies in which umbilical blood flow has ranged from 390 down to 180 ml/kg per min have shown no change in fetal oxygen consumption.[98] In experiments in which baseline umbilical flow averaged 170 ml/kg per min, however, decreases in umbilical flow of only 20 to 30 ml/kg per min were associated with a fall in oxygen consumption.[99] In the placental embolization model of growth retardation, uteroplacental flow is decreased as well. If uterine blood flow should become reduced by more than 50% in the sheep, fetal oxygen delivery rate and oxygen uptake become compromised.[100]

In the spontaneously growth-retarded and hypoxemic group of animals, oxygen consumption was paradoxically increased.[93] These fetuses appeared to have had a high per-kilogram metabolic rate, but the averaged results were somewhat skewed by an extremely high oxygen uptake in one fetus.[93]

Transfer of substrates into the growth-retarded fetus has also been evaluated in smaller mammalian species. Fetal rats can be growth retarded by ligation of one uterine artery.[101] The resulting pups have a mean average reduction in birth weight of 15–30%.[60,101] As in the human and sheep, placental size is reduced,[102] liver weight is decreased,[60,102] and there is relative sparing of brain growth.[60]

Nitzan et al.[60] injected nonmetabolizable radiolabeled analogues of glucose ([³H]-2-deoxyglucose) and amino acids ([¹⁴C]-α-aminoisobutyric acid) into pregnant rats with litters of growth-retarded and normal fetuses. At sacrifice, 60 min later, the growth-retarded pups had lower glucose and amino acid radioactivity in their plasma and body organs than was found in normally grown fetuses. Maternal-to-fetal transfer of the nutrient analogues was decreased in the growth-retarded animals. Similar studies performed by Saintonge et al.[103] on spontaneously growth-retarded guinea pigs demonstrated reduced maternal-to-fetal transfer of glucose and amino acid analogues, as well as decreased placental blood flow; in guinea pigs, placental transfer of nutrient analogues and fetal weight showed significant correlation.

We have found that even for the chicken, in ovo blood levels of total amino acids correlate with fetal size.[104] Chick brain : body ratios also show an inverse correlation with fetal amino nitrogen; i.e., lower amino nitrogen levels are seen in fetuses with asymmetric growth patterns similar to those of the growth-retarded mammal.[104]

Observations have been made in many different species and experimental models. Reduced nutrient availability and decreased transplacental delivery of nutrients are consistent abnormalities leading to fetal growth retardation. In milder forms of growth retardation, fetal hypoxemia is not present and umbilical blood flow is adequate to maintain normal oxygen uptake.[97] Measured decreases in oxygen consumption therefore appear to be secondary to decreased nutrient availability and slowing of intrauterine growth. If nutrients were made available to the fetus, oxygen uptake could be increased.

In more severe forms of growth retardation, oxygen uptake by the fetus becomes limited. Oxygen availability itself becomes critical for fetal growth and survival. This point appears to have been reached in the ovine placental embolization studies discussed above and is apparent in other severe forms of growth retardation. In pregnant rats with one ligated uterine artery, Vileisis[102] recently found fetal growth retardation to be slightly ameliorated by maintaining the mothers in a 40% oxygen environment. In rats maintained in room air, growth-retarded pups were 67% the size of their normal littermates; in rats raised on 40% oxygen, growth-retarded pups were 74% the size of their control littermates.[102] The mechanism for the increase in fetal weight was not identified. Increased delivery of oxygen to the fetus, improvement in placental blood flow, and correction of placental hypoxemia, with restoration of normal nutrient transport, were all suggested.[102] Marked restriction of oxygen availability is also thought to lead to growth retardation in fetuses of mothers with cyanotic heart disease[68] and in experimental preparations, such as the coated chicken egg, in which there are drastic reductions in respiratory exchange area.[105]

2.2.3. Consequences of Growth Retardation on Fetal Brain Growth and Metabolism

Despite limited availability of substrates, several physiologic mechanisms may act in the growth-retarded fetus in order to maintain fetal brain growth. The preferential distribution of nutrients to the upper body has been discussed.[59] Whether upper and lower body differences in blood nutrient concentration become even more pronounced in the SGA fetus is unknown. However, it has been shown that blood flow per 100 g of brain tissue is higher in fetal lambs growth retarded by placental embolization than in normally grown controls.[92] The ability to sustain substrate delivery to the brain may explain why many growth-retarded infants have an asymmetric pattern of growth, with relative brain sparing.[66]

Even though average brain blood flow per 100 g is increased in growth-retarded animals, pathologic changes do occur in regional flow within the brain.[63] A few specific areas appear to be sacrificed. The percentage of brain blood flow distributed to the cerebellum and corpus callosum is significantly decreased. The corpus callosum is also significantly reduced in weight, and the cerebellum is smaller than in control animals.[63] These changes are particularly striking, because the cerebellum and corpus callosum should be actively developing.[54,56] The white nerve fibers of the corpus callosum are the ones that provide communication between the two hemispheres of the brain.[58]

We know that glucose is the major oxidative fuel used by the fetal brain[18,62] and that glucose levels are reduced in the growth-retarded fetus.[53,85,87,93,94] It is also known that cerebral glucose uptake is proportional to glucose delivery over a wide range of glucose concentrations[106] and that growth-retarded fetal rats have a 26% lower brain uptake of labeled glucose analogues than do normally grown littermates.[60] When a fetal insulin infusion is used to lower ovine fetal glucose levels acutely, cerebral glucose utilization falls 18%.[106] Several investigators have reported that cerebral uptake of oxygen does not change during hypoglycemia.[18] Others have found that cerebral oxygen and glucose uptakes fall proportionally, during ovine fetal insulin infusions; the glucose : oxygen ratio of the fetal brain therefore remains stable and close to 1.0.[107]

If cerebral oxygen uptake is maintained during at least some fetal periods of reduced glucose availability, alternative fuels must be oxidized. Ketone bodies, lactate, and degradation of existing brain substrates have been suggested.[18] Acetoacetate and β-hydroxybutyrate are known to be used by the neonatal brain under fasting conditions.[62] Brain uptake of these metabolites appears proportional to blood ketone levels in newborn baboons, cows, and rats; brain uptake of lactate has been found in fasting baboon neonates and in fetal lambs after an hypoxic episode.[62] In severely hypoglycemic adult rats, there is evidence that cerebral intracellular glycogen stores, citric acid (Krebs) cycle intermediates, and amino acids are depleted; it has even been proposed that endogenous brain lipid is oxidized.[18] Small quantities of amino acids are normally taken up across the fetal and adult ovine brain.[108,109] In the adult, there is a net brain release of amino acids during 6 days of fasting.[108] This release of amino acid is thought to represent degradation of existing brain protein.[108] In the fetus, hypoglycemia induced by maternal insulin infusion also results in decreased brain uptake of most amino acids and net release of several into the fetal circulation.[109] A 46% reduction in brain uptake of radiolabeled amino acid analogues is found in growth-retarded fetal rats as compared with normally grown controls.[60]

In severe fetal growth retardation, brain growth is no longer maintained. Fetal head size as well as length and weight are decreased.[66] Brain size is not uniformly reduced; those areas that should normally be growing rapidly during late gestation are most affected. The changes seen in brain development and cellularity appear similar in the various mammalian species.

Rats born to malnourished mothers have a reduction in overall brain weight and DNA content that is more marked in the cerebellum than in the cerebrum.[110] DNA content is an indicator of tissue cellularity, and microscopic examination of the cerebellum shows a 44% decrease in glial cells and 13% decrease in neurons.[110] Rat pups born to mothers fed a 5% protein and low-calorie diet have a 50% decrease in body size and up to 40% reduction in brain weight.[111] Glial cell number is reduced by 50% in the corpus callosum and in ascending spinal sensory tracts.[111] A deficit in myelination is apparent, with reduced density of myelin fibers and reduced caliber of spinal tracts.[111] When gestational malnutrition is of moderate intensity, the reduction in fetal brain weight can be corrected by enhanced postnatal nutrition in rats.[112] When the prenatal insult is severe, the deficit in brain weight persists, despite a high level of postnatal nutrition.[112]

Fetal monkeys growth retarded by ligation of interplacental blood vessels have a reduction in total brain size.[113] In this study, Hill and co-workers found that weight of the cerebrum was reduced approximately 10%, while cerebellar weight was decreased 20%. A significant decrease in DNA and brain cellularity was also demonstrated in the cerebellum.

Growth-retarded human infants who die during the neonatal period are found to have a reduction in brain weight and cellularity.[114,115] Chase et al.[114] found a 20% decrease in cerebral size and 19% decrease in cerebral DNA and cellularity; cerebellar size was decreased 37% and cerebellar DNA and cellularity were reduced 35%. A deficit of myelin lipids—cerebrosides and sulfatides—was also found. Other studies on growth-retarded infants have verified similar brain abnormalities.[115]

2.2.4. Neurologic Sequelae

What do these changes in brain structure and chemistry mean in terms of neurologic function? Harel et al.[116] observed normal rabbit pups, and those growth retarded by ligation of placental vessels, after birth for eye opening, righting reflex, cessation of falling, circling, and dragging of hindlimbs. At 2 weeks of age, the growth-retarded pups displayed a marked delay in disappearance of falling. This incoordination was considered a result of cerebellar dysfunction,[116] i.e., a behavioral manifestation of abnormalities in cerebellar growth.

At birth, undergrown term human infants may have less muscle tone and activity, but they are often tremulous and easily startled. These infants also score lower on measures of visual fixation and orientation to visual and auditory stimuli.[9]

Follow-up evaluation of growth-retarded infants has yielded conflicting neuromotor results but most studies have reported a less than optimal outcome.[9] Fitzhardinge and Steven[10] studied 96 full-term infants below the third percentile in weight at birth. Neurologic development was followed for up to 8 years. Twenty-five percent of these children were found to have minimal brain dysfunction with hyperactivity, short attention span, poor fine coordination, and learning difficulties. Twenty-six percent of the girls and 33% of the boys had speech defects (immaturity of reception and expression). In other longitudinal studies, term growth-retarded infants were found to have more neurologic abnormalities (38% versus 20%), fidgetiness, and behavioral problems, when tested at age 7, than did children normally grown at birth.[9]

Commey and Fitzhardinge[117] also studied preterm, growth-retarded infants averaging 32 weeks gestational age and a birth weight of 1113 g. All were below the third percentile on normal growth curves. At 2 years of age, 49% had either a major neurologic defect (e.g., recurrent seizures, cerebral palsy) or a low Bayley score for infant development. More recently, Kitchens[118] evaluated very low birth weight infants, with weights less than 1000 grams at birth. When seen at 2 years of age, infants appropriately grown at birth had only a 9% incidence of severe handicap, whereas growth-retarded and/or multiple gestation infants had a 38% incidence of handicap (e.g., motor disabilities, deafness).

Those studies that have found only minor developmental or no differences between growth-retarded and appropriately grown newborns have usually been those with a more liberal definition of growth retardation. Such studies have defined growth retardation as birth weight less than the tenth percentile for gestation, rather than using the stricter criterion of weight below the third percentile (or <2 SD below the mean).[6]

It is, in fact, the severity and duration of insult that determines subsequent handicap. When identical twin pairs have a large difference in birth weight (>300 g), the smaller twin is found to have lower intelligence test scores at long-term follow-up.[11] In a recent study, Harvey et al.[7] followed head size in utero, by serial ultrasound measurements and determined the gestation at which head growth began to lag behind normal curves. Slowing of head growth before 26 weeks gestation was found to be associated with lower scores in perceptual performance, motor skills, and general cognitive index, when the children were tested at 5 years of age.[7] Postnatal catchup growth of the head appears to be a good predictor of ultimate outcome. If catchup in head circumference occurs, developmental test results equal those of children who had been normally grown at birth; if head catchup does not occur, test results remain lower.[55]

In summary, abnormalities in neurologic function are found postnatally in growth-retarded infants and animals. These adverse effects persist during long-term follow-up of severely growth-retarded human infants. The abnormalities noted, such as incoordination and learning difficulties, are consistent with the neuroanatomic deficits found in the brains of growth-retarded infants and experimental animals.

2.2.5. Additional Perinatal and Long-Term Sequelae

Other adverse sequelae of fetal growth retardation have been noted. Perinatal complications include hypoglycemia, polycythemia, asphyxia, and meconium aspiration,[1] all of which, in and of themselves, can compromise neurologic outcome.[1,117] In addition, growth-retarded infants have reduced neonatal and ultimate stature.[5,6,8,11,119]

Infants who are undergrown at birth tend to remain small throughout childhood. Low et al.[6] followed infants who were less than the tenth percentile at birth. At 5 years of age, these children still weighed less than a control group who had been normally grown at birth. The growth-retarded group was also shorter and had smaller head and chest circumferences. Fitzhardinge and Steven[8] followed infants who had been less than the third percentile in weight at birth. At 4 years of age, these children were still small. The mean weight and height for the group was between the tenth and twenty-fifth percentile on normal growth curves, and 35% of the infants were still below the third percentile. Growth in head circumference paralleled linear growth. Faulkner[5] studied identical twin boys who displayed a marked discordance in size at birth (1.46 kg versus 2.81 kg). The smaller twin was still appreciably shorter at 16 years of age; he also lighter and had a slightly smaller head circumference. Babson and Phillips[11] followed nine pairs of identical twins who had an average discordance in birth weight of 36%. The undersized twins remained smaller into adult life.

The insult resulting in short stature appears to be less severe than that required to produce neurologic abnormalities. Growth retardation with slowing of fetal head growth as late as 34 weeks gestation has been associated with small stature on follow-up.[119]

2.3. Summary of Rationale for Supplementation

If the damaging sequelae are to be eliminated, then intrauterine growth retardation needs to be prevented. Since limited availability of nutrients is a major causative factor leading to poor fetal growth and altered brain development, enhanced delivery of nutrients to the fetus might be of therapeutic benefit. Inadequate transport of substrates across the placenta appears to be a major part of the pathologic process; therefore, supplementation of nutrients via paraplacental means has been suggested.[12]

3. Theoretical Considerations in Providing
Nutritional Supplementation

3.1. Potential Toxicity

The aims of supplementation should be to normalize the entry of nutrients into the fetus as well as circulating nutrient concentrations. Restitution of the major substrates, glucose and amino acids, would be of primary importance for fetal growth and brain metabolism.

Augmentation of nutrition to supranormal levels is undesirable. Hyperglycemia to 7- and 10-fold normal glucose concentration is well tolerated by the healthy ovine fetus.[120] However, simply doubling the glucose concentration can result in a fatal acidosis, if fetal oxygenation is compromised.[121] Persistent fetal hyperglycemia can also result in macrosomia, developmental anomalies, and postnatal complications, such as hypoglycemia.[122] Hyperaminoacidemia in the fetus can cause birth defects, growth retardation, and mental retardation, as is seen with phenylalanine.[22,25] Administration of parenteral amino acids to premature infants will lead to azotemia and acidosis, when excessive quantities of amino acids are given.[123,124] Hyperammonemia is seen when a balance of amino acids high in glycine and low in arginine is given.[124] Supplementation of fatty acids in the premature infant can result in lipid deposition in reticuloendothelial cells or along vascular endothelial surfaces, if blood levels are allowed to become elevated.[124]

Although nutritional supplementation is usually discussed in terms of macronutrient needs, micronutrients, such as vitamins and minerals, could also be provided to the fetus. However, accumulation of abnormally high levels of these can also result in fetal malformation and compromised growth.[45,48,49]

Supplementation is most likely to be beneficial in fetuses whose oxygen uptake can be increased to permit metabolism of the nutrients administered. If oxygen uptake itself has become limited, additional nutrients may be toxic, as has been shown for glucose.[121] Early intervention and promotion of placental as well as fetal growth by nutrient supplementation may maintain more normal placental blood flow and prevent development of hypoxemia.

3.2. Routes of Supplementation

Three paraplacental routes are available for fetal supplementation: intra-amniotic, intragastric, and intravascular. Each has potential risks and benefits. Only intragastric supplementation offers the fetus a degree of metabolic regulation, since essentially all portal venous blood perfuses the fetal liver before flowing into the systemic circulation.[125] By contrast, nutrients administered *via* intravascular infusion will enter the fetal systemic circulation directly. The same is true for the major portion of nutrients administered into the amniotic cavity, since these are absorbed through fetal surfaces rather than by swallowing (discussed in Section 4.1).[12]

Because of the unique pattern of the fetal circulation, the partitioning of nutrients within the fetus may be altered by the route of supplementation. Since umbilical venous return is shunted to the upper body,[52] infusion into the umbilical vein might augment the usual upper-body to lower-body nutrient concentration differences.[59] Infusion into a systemic vein could increase nutrient distribution to the lower body and, by raising umbilical artery concentrations, might decrease umbilical uptake of nutrients.[13,15]

4. Fetal Nutritional Supplementation: Human and Animal Studies

Administration of amino acids and glucose has been tried in experimental animals using the amniotic, gastrointestinal, and vascular routes. Intra-amniotic infusion of amino acids has even been carried out in the human.

4.1. Supplementation *via* Intra-amniotic Infusion

4.1.1. Amniotic Fluid Swallowing, Protein Clearance, and Intestinal Transit

Fetal swallowing of amniotic fluid has been well documented. Swallowing has been found in the early second-trimester human fetus,[126] and by the end of the third trimester the fetal human and sheep ingest up to 750 ml/day (average 400–500 ml/day).[127,128–130] Many substances, such as proteins and thyroxine, are cleared from amniotic fluid mainly by swallowing.[127,128,130] The average half-time for amniotic clearance of proteins has been found to be 29 hr in the late third-trimester human fetus.[127] Ingested material passes down the GI tract, and within 20 hr substances injected into the amniotic cavity are found in the colon of the third-trimester human fetus.[126] In the guinea pig, progressively faster times from injection of marker in the amniotic cavity to appearance in the fetal stomach, intestines, and colon have been documented as the third-trimester advances.[131] In the presence of hypoxia, the fetal guinea pig shows enhanced swallowing of amniotic fluid, but intestinal motility is decreased with slower transit time of marker.[131] Fetal swallowing of amniotic fluid also appears more rapid in human patients in labor than in women not in labor.[127]

4.1.2. Amniotic Injections in the Human

Fetal swallowing of nutrients injected into the amniotic cavity would appear to provide a straightforward route for supplementation. However, when Renaud and colleagues injected a casein hydrolysate into the amniotic cavity of patients preparing to undergo a repeat cesarean section, the concentration of amino acids in amniotic fluid decreased rapidly.[78] The half-time of amino acid clearance was close to 1 hr, a rate too fast to have occurred by fetal swallowing alone. Heller also injected amino acids into the amniotic cavity in the human and found the same rapid disappearance of amino acids; amniotic amino acid levels were close to pretreatment values within 24 hr.[132] Interestingly, disappearance of amino acids from the amniotic cavity was not uniform: 45 min after intra-amniotic injection, more than 80% of the lysine, valine, isoleucine, aspartic acid, and methionine had left the amniotic fluid, but only 43% of the proline had been removed.[78] Renaud investigated uptake of these administered amino acids by measuring fetal, maternal, and placental amino acid profiles in normal women: 45 min after intra-amniotic injection of 5 g of an amino acid mixture (10% Aminosol, Vitrum Laboratories), only small increases in the concentration of a few amino acids were noted in umbilical and maternal blood samples.[78] However, the placenta demonstrated large increases in tissue amino acid concentrations for 16 of the 18 amino acids measured. The ultimate fate of the amino acids accumulating in the placenta was not determined.

In an attempt to define the time course of appearance of administered amino acids in fetal blood, Saling et al.[133] measured samples of maternal blood, umbilical blood, and amniotic fluid for three essential amino acids (valine, leucine, and threonine) at normal control deliveries and at deliveries occurring at various times, after intra-amniotic infusion of approximately 20 g of amino acids. Umbilical venous levels of amino acids were increased by 1 hr after infusion. However, marked elevations were noted 1½ to 2 hr after administration of amino acids—later than the sampling time used in Renaud's study. Even with these high doses, however, maternal levels still showed little change. To evaluate how the amino acids were entering the fetus, Saling et al.[133] immersed the umbilical vein in an 8% amino acid solution containing valine. These investigators found that concentrations of valine increased rapidly in umbilical blood, indicating that absorption was occurring through the umbilical surface.

In addition to conducting these basic investigations with intra-amniotic injection, these same investigators have used amino acid injections therapeutically. In gestations with fetal growth retardation, Renaud et al.[78] administered up to 14 injections between 30 and 38 weeks gestation. Each 50-ml injection provided 5 g of amino acids from a protein hydrolysate solution (10% Aminosol). Maternal 24-hr urinary estriol excretion rose to normal in four of five pregnancies in which it was measured. Pretreatment human chorionic somatomammotropin levels were low in one of two patients in which it was measured; with treatment, levels returned to normal. Fetal head growth was claimed to improve in one fetus who had shown a plateauing of biparietal diameter.[78] At delivery, placental concentration of amino acids was found to be markedly elevated for 15 of 17 amino acids analyzed, including seven of the essential amino acids (tryptophan was not measured).

Heller[132] administered 8–12 g of an amino acid solution created to meet fetal needs; the volume infused was approximately 200 ml. He reported that estriol excretion normalized in women with growth-retarded fetuses when repetitive intra-amniotic injections were given.[132]

Massobrio et al.[134] found that amniotic injections of amino acids improved estriol levels and growth in two of five fetuses in whom this therapy was tried. No other factor in the prenatal course could explain the change in fetal status. A third fetus also showed improvement, but a decrease in maternal blood pressure attributable to concomitant medical therapy may have been responsible.

As a whole, investigations in the human fetus demonstrate that (1) nutrients injected into amniotic fluid will enter the fetus, (2) the routes of fetal entry are different for proteins and amino acids, (3) the amino acid uptake rate is different for individual amino acids, (4) placental uptake of amino acids is appreciable and occurs rapidly, and (5) intermittent intra-amniotic administration of amino acids is not overtly harmful. Indeed, some hormonal indices of fetal well-being and of fetal growth appear to improve. However, these investigations do not define (1) the time course for appearance and disappearance of exogenous nutrients in an individual fetus, (2) the metabolic effects of nutrient administration, (3) whether these metabolic effects are the same for different routes of absorption, (4) the percentage of injected nutrients that enter the fetus, and (5) whether the administered nutrients are utilized. Human studies cannot currently be done to answer these questions. These issues have, therefore, been studied using animal models.

4.1.3. Amniotic Injections in Animal Models

In our laboratory, we used healthy third-trimester chronically catheterized sheep to study the appearance of amino acids and glucose in fetal and maternal blood after intra-amniotic injection.[135] A dose of 20 g of either amino acids or glucose was injected into the amniotic cavity of 128–138-day-gestation fetal sheep. Fetal blood metabolite levels were followed for 4 hr. The fetal carotid arterial concentrations of total amino acids (measured as α-amino nitrogen) and glucose are listed in Table V.

Amino acids were administered as a 200-ml infusion of an L-crystalline, amino acid solution (10% Aminosyn, Abbott Laboratories, North Chicago, Ill.). An equal volume of amniotic fluid was removed immediately before the dose was given. As is seen in Table V, α-amino nitrogen concentrations rose quickly after the amino acid injection and continued to rise for 4 hr. Urea nitrogen concentration also increased significantly ($+3.6$ mg/dl), as did blood ammonia ($+123$ μg/dl) (values given are the mean). Fetal carotid arterial blood showed highly significant decreases in oxygen saturation (-8.4%), oxygen content (-1.2 ml/dl), and pH (-0.05). Fluid shifts within fetal compartments were implied by an increase in fetal hemoglobin ($+1.0$ g/dl).

Glucose was administered as a 40-ml bolus of a 50% dextrose so-

Table V. Fetal Carotid Arterial Nutrient Concentrations after Intra-amniotic Bolus Injection[a,b]

Nutrient	Time (min)							
	-15	0	15	30	60	120	180	240
Glucose (mg/dl)	24.1	23.4	42.7[c]	49.2[d]	48.7[e]	49.7[f]	48.8[d]	41.7[e]
	±4.1	±4.1	±4.6	±7.2	±7.0	±6.5	±7.5	±6.3
Amino nitrogen (mg/dl)	8.0	8.1	11.9[d]	13.5[d]	16.5[e]	19.3[e]	21.3[d]	22.3[e]
	±0.3	±0.4	±0.8	±1.3	±1.7	±2.5	±3.2	±3.1

[a] Data compiled from ref. 135.
[b] Values given are mean ±SEM for amino acid injections $N = 7$ and for glucose studies $N = 6$. All p values are compared with time 0.
[c] $p < 0.05$.
[d] $p < 0.025$.
[e] $p < 0.01$.
[f] $p < 0.005$.

lution. An equal volume of amniotic fluid was removed immediately before the injection. Fetal blood glucose concentration rose rapidly and peaked by 2 hr. Lactate concentration also increased significantly (+8.1 mg/dl), while decreases were found in oxygen saturation (−5.7%) and pH (−0.04).

Three of the lambs used in these studies had both carotid and femoral arterial catheters in place. Intra-amniotic glucose administration produced a trend toward widening of the carotid and femoral arterial concentration difference for glucose.[135]

These amniotic injection studies used large pharmacologic doses of nutrients in an attempt to elicit possible noxious effects of supplementation. The instantaneous bolus injected was equal to the quantity of amino acids or glucose taken up across the umbilical circulation over an entire day by a 3-kg fetus.[13,21,93] Adverse effects on fetal metabolism were, in fact, seen. Fetal urea synthesis, which normally proceeds at a high rate,[19] was still unable to keep pace with the ammonia generated by amino acid catabolism. Much of the glucose load ended up being metabolized anaerobically to lactate.[30] The resultant decline in oxygen levels may have been caused by increased substrate usage leading to increased oxygen utilization and extraction. This type of augmented substrate use leading to hypoxemia has been found during fetal insulin infusions.[136] As in the insulin studies, distribution of cardiac output may have also changed, resulting in a decrease in umbilical blood flow.[136]

It should be noted that the 20-g dose of amino acids used in our amniotic studies was only two- to four-fold greater than the 5 to 12 g of amino acids administered in human supplementation trials.[78,132,134] The safety of intra-amniotic amino acid injections of the slightly lower 5–10-g doses still remains to be evaluated in an animal model.

Continuous intra-amniotic infusion of amino acids and glucose has been carried out for 8 days in the third-trimester lamb. Infusion rates ranged from 120 to 250 ml/day using a 6.8% amino acid solution (diluted from 8.5% Travasol, Travenol Laboratories, Deerfield, Ill.) with 4% glucose. Small elevations in blood amino nitrogen, glucose, and urea levels were noted, but there was no change in fetal pH, blood gases, or oxygen saturation (V. Charlton, personal observation). These intra-amniotic supplements were administered at rates equal to, or less than, normal umbilical uptake. At these rates, supplements appeared well tolerated.

Although metabolic studies have not been carried out on smaller mammals, continuous intra-amniotic infusion models have been attempted in the rabbit, guinea pig, and rat[137,138]; the rabbit model appears to be the least fragile and most promising.[138]

4.2. Supplementation *via* Gastrointestinal Administration of Nutrients

Using healthy third-trimester fetal lambs, we have investigated the fetal response to both small intestinal and intragastric administration of nutrients.[99,139–141]

4.2.1. Intestinal Injections

Table VI presents the rise in blood levels of α-amino nitrogen, after intraduodenal administration of 1.2 g/kg of amino acids (3.0–4.3 g total dose). An 8.5% amino acid solution (Travasol), buffered to pH 7.0, was used.[139] Amino nitrogen concentrations peaked by 2 hr. Proof that the rise in fetal amino nitrogen was due to intestinal absorption of amino acids was provided by simultaneous sampling from fetal femoral arterial and mesenteric venous catheters.[140] Paired amino nitrogen measurements were obtained in six studies, both before and 1 hr after the intraduodenal bolus. Values are presented in Table VII.

After intestinal administration of amino acids, no changes in fetal blood gases or ammonia were found during a 4-hr observation period. Significant increases were seen in fetal levels of urea ($+1.7$ mg/dl), glucose ($+2.8$ mg/dl), and lactate ($+4.2$ mg/dl). A nonsignificant drop in ammonia concentration also occurred (-17 μg/dl).[139]

During these studies, the administered amino acids were apparently largely catabolized, and the ammonia generated was adequately handled by enhanced urea production. The increase in glucose and lactate levels may have been due to production of these metabolites from amino acids[142] or to decreased utilization of carbohydrates, while the excess amino acids were utilized.

Table VI. Fetal Femoral Arterial Amino Nitrogen Concentrations after Intraduodenal Administration of Amino Acids[a]

Nutrient	Time (min)					
	0	30	60	120	180	240
Amino nitrogen (mg/dl)	7.7 ±0.6	8.7[c] ±0.7	9.4[d] ±0.8	9.8[d] ±0.8	9.0[d] ±0.7	8.9[d] ±0.8

[a] Data from ref. 139.
[b] Values given are the mean ±SEM; $N = 13$; amino acid dose was 1.2 g/kg. All p values are compared with time 0.
[c] $p < 0.005$.
[d] $p < 0.001$.

Table VII. Paired Simultaneous Measurements of Femoral Arterial and Cranial
Mesenteric Venous Amino Nitrogen Concentrations
before and after Intraduodenal Amino Acid Administration[a,b]

	Before		60 min after	
	FA	CMV	FA	CMV
	10.1	9.8	11.5	12.8
	10.8	11.3	12.5	12.8
	10.7	9.3	13.7	15.5
	3.1	4.6	5.7	6.4
	6.7	6.6	7.6	8.3
	7.1	6.9	7.0	7.4
Mean	8.1	8.1	9.7	10.5
± SEM	1.2	1.0	1.4	1.5
Difference	N.S.		$p < 0.025$	

[a] Data drawn from ref. 139.
[b] Values are of α-amino nitrogen.
[c] FA, femoral arterial; CMV, cranial mesenteric venous.

Table VIII presents the rise in fetal femoral arterial levels of glucose after intraduodenal administration of 2 g/kg of glucose (3.5–8 g total dose). Glucose concentration rose quickly and peaked within 30 min.[141] Simultaneous measurement of glucose concentration in the fetal femoral artery and cranial mesenteric vein[140] demonstrated that absorption of glucose was occurring through the intestine.[12]

During the glucose studies, a significant increase in fetal lactate concentration was seen (+ 2.7 mg/dl), which was proportional to the increase in glucose level. A small but significant decrease in pH (−0.03) was also noted.[141]

The quantities of amino acids and glucose provided to the fetal intestine were lower than the amounts used in the amniotic fluid injection

Table VIII. Fetal Femoral Arterial Glucose Concentration after Intraduodenal
Administration of Glucose[a,b]

	Time (min)					
	0	15	30	60	90	120
Glucose (mg/dl)	16.3	29.4[c]	32.9[c]	31.5[c]	26.3[c]	22.5[c]
	± 1.4	± 1.2	± 1.9	± 1.7	± 2.0	± 1.7

[a] Data from ref. 141.
[b] Values given are the mean ± SEM; $N = 12$; glucose dose was 2 g/kg.
[c] $p < 0.001$, compared with time 0.

experiments (see Section 4.1). Although the intestinal doses were still excessive, they appeared better tolerated than those given intra-amniotically.

4.2.2. Intragastric Infusions

Amino acids and glucose have also been infused, to excess, into the ovine fetal stomach and enteral uptake rates measured.[99] We found GI uptake of amino acids to average 45% of normal umbilical amino acid uptake and GI uptake of glucose to average 42% of normal umbilical glucose uptake.[99] Individual enteral uptake rates as high as 9.8 mg/min for amino acids and 7.4 mg/min for glucose were observed.[99]

Whether GI supplementation actually increases the quantity of nutrients reaching the fetus or merely substitutes one route of acquisition for another was investigated by assessing the effects of intragastric infusion on fetal umbilical uptake of nutrients.[99] Umbilical nutrient uptake measurements in fetuses receiving intragastric amino acids are given in Table IX. Comparison of the control period and 60–120-min infusion period showed no differences in uptake.

During the amino acid infusions, there was a significant increase in fetal blood concentrations of amino nitrogen ($+1.3$ mg/dl), urea ($+1.0$ mg/dl), and lactate ($+5.2$ mg/dl). There was also a slight decrease in oxygen uptake (-0.7 ml/kg/min) due to rerouting of aortic blood flow to the intestine. Supplementation appeared to result in an increase in the total quantity of amino acids entering the fetus.[99]

During intragastric glucose infusions, fetal femoral arterial glucose concentration increased significantly ($+5.9$ mg/dl); lactate levels rose as well ($+5.7$ mg/dl). Umbilical uptake measurements in fetuses receiving

Table IX. Umbilical Uptake Measurements in Fetuses Receiving Intragastric Infusions[a,b]

	Amino N uptake		Glucose uptake		Lactate uptake	
	C	I	C	I	C	I
Amino acid infusions						
Mean	0.43	0.52	4.4	3.9	1.9	1.4
±SEM	0.19	0.08	0.5	0.4	0.6	0.3
Glucose infusions						
Mean	0.50	0.34	3.9	1.7	1.6	2.5
±SEM	0.13	0.19	1.3	0.5	0.5	1.5

[a] Data compiled from ref. 99.
[b] Values given are in mg/kg per min. $N = 7$ for both amino acid and glucose studies.
[c] C, control period; I, infusion period.

Table X. Change in Umbilical Uptake of Glucose Accompanying Intragastric Infusion
of Glucose[a-c]

Gastric infusion rate (mg/kg per min)	Increase in fetal femoral arterial glucose (mg/dl)	Change in umbilical glucose uptake (mg/kg per min)
14	+2.2	+1.1
14	+2.6	-0.4
15	+2.4	+0.7
26	+4.9	-1.6
27	+7.3	-1.9
30	+11.3	-4.0
38	+10.6	-9.2

[a] Data adapted from ref. 99.
[b] The correlation between the gastric infusion rate and the decrease in umbilical uptake was $r = -0.922$, $p < 0.005$.
[c] The correlation between the increase in fetal glucose concentration and the decrease in umbilical uptake was $r = -0.859$, $p < 0.025$.

intragastric glucose are presented in Table IX. No differences in mean amino nitrogen and lactate uptake were found between the control and infusion periods. Umbilical uptake of glucose decreased, however, in inverse proportion to both the infusion rate of glucose and the rise in fetal blood glucose concentration. These highly significant relationships are apparent in the data from individual animals in Table X. The quantity of glucose actually gained by the fetus, through supplementation, appeared to be limited by the decrease in placental uptake that accompanied any increase in glucose concentration.[99]

4.3. Supplementation *via* Intravascular Administration of Nutrients

Intravenous administration of nutrients was evaluated by Young *et al.*[143] These investigators infused a 3.3% casein hydrolysate solution with 5% glucose into normally growing fetal lambs for up to 14 days after surgical preparation. Administration was through the fetal jugular vein at rates approximating one-third of normal fetal nitrogen uptake. No consistent or marked changes in fetal concentrations of either individual amino acids or glucose were found.[143]

We have infused a 6.8% amino acid solution (diluted from 8.5% Travasol) with 4–5% glucose into the femoral vessels in 3 healthy fetal lambs for up to 21 days. Daily infusion rates approximated one-third to one-fourth of normal fetal uptake. There were no changes in fetal amino nitrogen concentration, glucose concentration, pH value, or oxygen saturation (V. Charlton, personal observation, 1985). Birth weights of all lambs receiving prolonged intravascular and intra-amniotic infusions (see Section 4.1) were greater than 4 kg and high for chronically catheterized animals in our studies (V. Charlton, personal observation, 1985; reference 95).

At these low physiologic rates of supplementation, intravascular administration of nutrients appears to be well tolerated. Long-term infusions may also augment the growth of normal fetuses.

4.4. Utilization of Administered Nutrients

Whether the administered nutrients are actually utilized has been specifically evaluated in several animal studies. Dudenhausen et al.[144] showed that amino acids injected into the amniotic cavity are taken up by fetal organs. Labeled valine injected into the amniotic cavity of pregnant rats resulted in high concentrations of radioactivity in the fetal liver and intestines within $2\frac{1}{2}$ hr.

Pitkin and Reynolds[145] showed that administered proteins can be digested and the resulting amino acids used. Labeled pig protein was injected into the amniotic cavity of pregnant rhesus monkeys. As expected, the administered proteins were cleared slowly from the amniotic fluid, at a rate consistent with fetal swallowing. Proteolysis was found along the fetal digestive tract and maximal concentration of labeled amino acids occurred in fetal plasma 3 days after protein administration. Maximal concentration of labeled protein was present in fetal plasma 1 day later, on the fourth day, indicating protein synthesis from the labeled amino acids.

Al-Murrani[146] injected the yolk sac of 8-day-old chicken embryos with an amino acid mixture chosen to replenish the amino acids consumed during the first week of development. Fetuses in these injected eggs and control noninjected eggs were randomly sacrificed. Injected fetuses weighed more at 20 days gestation and at hatching on day 21 than did chickens from control eggs. Furthermore, hatchlings from supplemented eggs continued to be larger during the 56-day period of investigation after birth.

Mulvihill infused the amniotic cavity in fetal rabbits with solutions containing either 5%, 10%, or 15% glucose or 10% glucose plus 2.25% amino acids.[138] Infusions were carried out continuously for a 5-day period close to term. When delivered at 28-days gestation, infused fetuses were significantly larger than sham operated and nonoperated control animals. Controls were from the same litter and matched for uterine position but were located in the opposite uterine horn. Infused fetuses were heavier, had a longer crown–rump length, and had larger livers and brains. Furthermore, the size of fetuses within the treated group was proportional to the average number of nonprotein calories administered each day.[138] In the few fetuses given both amino acids and glucose, the small quantity of amino acids in the infusate did not further augment fetal size.

The supplementation studies described so far, have been carried out on healthy animals. Using the fetal sheep, we have shown that experimentally-induced growth retardation can actually be prevented by intrauterine nutritional supplementation. The first model of growth retardation used was that produced by maternal protein-calorie malnutrition.[94,95] Early third-trimester pregnant sheep with singleton gestations were randomly assigned to one of three treatment groups:

R   Maternal dietary restriction
RS   Maternal dietary restriction and fetal supplementation
C   *Ad libitum*-fed controls

The mothers were weighed before surgical preparation at a mean of 116 days gestation. After surgery, the animals were fed *ad libitum* for a mean of 6 days before baseline metabolic and blood flow studies were performed. After the baseline studies, animals in the R group were diet restricted; protein intake was limited to one-half and caloric intake to one-third that recommended for late third-trimester ewes.[147] RS ewes were similarly protein–calorie restricted, but their fetuses were supplemented with continuous intragastric infusions of 6.8% essential and nonessential amino acids and 4% glucose. The infusions were gradually increased and estimated to provide one-half of fetal nitrogen and one-third of fetal glucose needs.[13,93,99] Control ewes were allowed to feed *ad libitum*. Maternal weight, blood chemistries, and umbilical flow were measured weekly.

Over the study period, no change in weight was seen in the diet-restricted maternal groups, whereas control mothers showed a normal increase in weight ($+4.1$ kg). R mothers showed evidence of malnutrition and increased protein catabolism; they had significant decreases in glucose (-9.9 mg/dl) and α-amino nitrogen (-1.5 mg/dl) and a significant increase in urea ($+4.0$ mg/dl). RS mothers also experienced a large decrease in glucose (-11.2 mg/dl) but seemed to have less of a fetal drain on their amino acid stores; they showed a nonsignificant decrease in amino nitrogen, and urea levels showed a decrease rather than an increase. Control mothers had stable nutrient levels. R fetuses, like their mothers, were found to display a malnutrition pattern, with a large decrease in glucose (-5.8 mg/dl) and an increase in urea ($+3.9$ mg/dl). A small decrease in α-amino nitrogen resulted in significantly lower amino nitrogen levels near term than in the other groups. RS fetuses also had a large decrease in glucose concentration (-4.2 mg/dl) but, unlike the R group, RS amino nitrogen concentration rose and urea fell. There were no significant changes in nutrient levels in the control group. There were no changes in other fetal chemistries or blood gases except for an increase in hemoglobin concentration in the RS group ($+2.0$ g/dl).

Delivery occurred at 142 ± 2, 142 ± 1, and 143 ± 2 days gestation in groups R, RS, and C, respectively. As shown in Table XI, the combined weights of the fetus, placenta, and fetal membranes were significantly lower in the restricted group. Fetal weights alone and crown–rump lengths were also lower in R. R fetuses were markedly smaller in relationship to their mothers' size and brain-to-body weight ratios were elevated, indicating asymmetric growth retardation.[66] By contrast, supplemented fetuses were close to controls in size and brain-to-body ratios. Placental size was also reduced 28% in R fetuses compared with controls, whereas RS placental size was intermediate.

The disparity in fetal size was explained by differences in nutrient acquisition between groups. Umbilical uptake measurements were available in five animals in each group. Measurements made near delivery are presented in Table XII. Over the experimental period, caloric intake

Table XI. Fetal Size at Delivery in Maternal Dietary Restriction/Fetal Supplementation Studies

	Restricted ($N = 8$)	Restricted/fetus supplemented ($N = 7$)	Controls ($N = 8$)
Uterine contents (g)	$2933 \pm 199^{b,e}$	3519 ± 123 (6)	3611 ± 283
Fetal weight (g)	$2702 \pm 182^{a,d}$	3235 ± 121	3290 ± 297
Crown–rump length (cm)	$42.0 \pm 1.7^{b,c}$	46.5 ± 1.1	46.6 ± 1.4
Fetal/maternal weight (%)	$5.2 \pm 0.3^{b,f}$	6.8 ± 0.3	6.8 ± 0.6
Brain/body weight (%)	$1.9 \pm 0.1(6)^{b,f}$	1.5 ± 0.04	1.5 ± 0.1
Placenta weight (g)	231 ± 26^{b}	$265 \pm 54(6)$	320 ± 29

[a] Data compiled from refs. 12, 94 and 95.
[b] Values given are the mean $\pm$ SEM; measurements are for all animals except where indicated by parentheses. *Note:* footnotes c and d represent restricted compared with controls, e–h restricted compared with restricted/fetus supplemented group.
[c] $p < 0.10$.
[d] $p < 0.05$.
[e] $p < 0.10$.
[f] $p < 0.025$.
[g] $p < 0.05$.
[h] $p < 0.01$.

Table XII. Substrate Uptakes Close to Delivery in Maternal Dietary Restriction/Fetal Supplementation Studies[a,b]

| Substrate uptake | Restricted: umbilical | Restricted/fetus supplemented | | | Controls: umbilical |
		Umbilical	Gastrointestinal	Total	
CHO (glucose + lactate)	17.1 ± 2.4	18.1 ± 4.5	3.9 ± 0.3	22.0 ± 4.3	23.5 ± 3.0
Amino nitrogen	-0.5 ± 0.7^c	-0.3 ± 1.1	0.8 ± 0.1	0.5 ± 1.1	1.2 ± 0.4
Oxygen	15.2 ± 2.2	17.3 ± 3.5	—	17.3 ± 3.5	23.8 ± 3.9

[a] Data from ref. 95.
[b] Values given are the mean $\pm$ SEM; uptakes are in mg/min for carbohydrates and amino nitrogen and in ml/min for oxygen.
[c] $p < 0.10$; restricted compared with controls.

increased 24% in C fetuses, which had the highest umbilical uptakes of carbohydrate and total amino acids (α-amino nitrogen) at the end of gestation. After regulation of maternal diet, R and RS fetuses showed dramatic decreases in umbilical uptake of amino nitrogen; umbilical uptake of carbohydrate in these groups remained static, rather than increasing as it did in controls. Caloric intake fell 42% in R and, as can be seen in Table XII, late-gestation nutrient uptake was lowest in R fetuses. RS fetuses also had low umbilical uptakes of carbohydrates and amino nitrogen, but they were receiving additional intragastric supplements. In RS fetuses, combined umbilical plus GI carbohydrate uptake equaled that of controls, and total entry of amino nitrogen and calories was intermediate between that of groups R and C. Interestingly, RS fetuses were able to maintain sufficient oxygen uptake to utilize the administered nutrients.

In these studies, fetal supplementation appeared to decrease the impact of maternal malnutrition on the fetus. Fetal nutrient levels were normalized, and supplemented fetuses achieved more normal growth.[94,95] Placental growth may also have been augmented.

Studies evaluating the effects of nutritional supplements on growth retardation produced by placental embolization are nearing completion.[148] As fetuses in this experimental model frequently become hypoxemic,[92] nutrient administration might be expected to be toxic. Three groups of animals have been studied: (1) E, placental embolization; (2) ES, placental embolization with fetal supplementation; and (3) C, normal controls. The experimental design is similar to that of the dietary-restriction investigations with placental embolization alone or placental embolization and fetal supplementation begun after six days of postoperative recovery. Supplements of 6.8% amino acids and 5% glucose are being provided at rates similar to those in the dietary restriction studies but nutrients are being infused directly into the fetal femoral vein.

At delivery near term, the E group fetuses have been reduced in size, with a mean birth weight of 2986 ± 419 SEM g ($n = 7$) versus weights of 3623 ± 223 g ($n = 6$) in ES and 3756 ± 290 g ($n = 7$) in C. Embolized-nonsupplemented animals also have lower fetal/maternal weight ratios and ponderal indices than the other groups.[148] The duration of placental embolization and the mean number of microspheres used for embolization has been the same in groups E (16×10^6) and ES (15×10^6).

What has been most striking in these studies has been the marked increase in placental size found in the ES animals. Placental weight has averaged 299 ± 50 g in E, 558 ± 98 g in ES, and 459 ± 5 g in C ($p < 0.05$ E versus ES; $p < 0.10$ ES versus C).[148] We have, in fact, found a strong correlation between placental weight (wet and dry) and the quantity of nutrients infused during the first half of the third trimester ($r = 0.925$, $p < 0.01$). In the singleton ovine fetus, placental weight continues to increase over the third trimester,[82] so that the large placental size we are finding may be due to both nutritionally enhanced growth and amelioration of the damage produced by embolization. Since 40% of venous return from the fetal inferior vena cava is directed out toward the placenta,[149] a large quantity of the administered nutrients may be reaching the placenta directly in these infusion studies.

5. Conclusions

The major nutrients used by the fetus for normal growth and development have been defined. The demands for these nutrients are great over the second half of gestation when total fetal growth and brain growth are rapid.

Intrauterine growth retardation appears to be caused by decreased transfer of nutrients into the fetus and decreased circulating blood concentration of nutrients. In some situations, availability of oxygen becomes limited and may adversely affect the ability of the fetus to utilize nutrients.

The effects of growth retardation on the fetus include a reduction in stature and brain growth. Areas of the brain that should normally be rapidly developing, such as the cerebellum, are sacrificed. With severe growth retardation, the deficits in brain size and biochemistry cannot be made up after birth and are permanent. Persistent neurologic abnormalities and learning disabilities are found.

To prevent growth retardation from developing or progressing, intrauterine supplementation of fetal nutrition has been investigated. In both human and animal studies, nutritional supplementation for treatment of IUGR appears promising. The major nutrients, amino acids and glucose, have been shown to enter the fetus when given by the intraamniotic, GI, or intravascular routes. However, the proportion of these nutrients actually entering the fetus has not been quantitated for amniotic injection, where placental uptake is known to occur. The nutrients that do enter the fetus can be utilized to synthesize new tissue and prevent the development of fetal growth retardation. With some routes of supplementation, placental growth appears to be enhanced. Nutrient administration appears safe when kept within the physiologic range, i.e., at or below rates of normal umbilical uptake. At higher rates of supplementation, fetal metabolic capabilities are exceeded.

Most acute animal studies have been carried out using normal fetuses. More extensive studies are therefore needed to define the margin of safety with exogenous nutrients and the severity of growth retardation that can be safely treated. Supplementation may be most beneficial if used to prevent progression of early growth retardation rather than as therapy for an already markedly stunted and hypoxemic fetus. Although the risks and benefits of fetal nutrient administration are still being defined, animal studies in progress are providing new insights into fetal and placental growth and nutrient needs.

References

1. Cassady, G., 1981, The small-for date infant, in: *Neonatology*, 2nd ed. (G. Avery, ed.), p. 262, J. B. Lippincott, Philadelphia.
2. Lubchenco, L., 1981, Assessment of weight and gestational age, in: *Neonatology*, 2nd ed. (G. Avery, ed.), p. 205, J. B. Lippincott, Philadelphia.
3. Cunningham, G., Hawes, W., Madore, C., *et al.*, 1976, *Intrauterine Growth and Neonatal Risk in California*, Infant Health Section, Maternal and Child Health, State of California, Department of Health.
4. Lubchenco, L., Searls, D., and Brazie, J., 1972, Neonatal mortality rate: Relationship to birth weight and gestational age, *J. Pediatr.* **81**:814.
5. Faulkner, F., 1981, Maternal nutrition and fetal growth. *Am. J. Clin. Nutr.* 34(suppl):769.
6. Low, J., Galbraith, R., Muir, D., *et al.*, 1982, Intrauterine growth retardation: A study of long term morbidity, *Am. J. Obstet. Gynecol.* **142**:670.
7. Harvey, D., Prince, J., Bunton, T., *et al.*, 1982, Abilities of children who were small for gestational age babies, *Pediatrics* **69**:296.
8. Fitzhardinge, P., and Steven, E., 1972, The small for date infant. I. Later growth patterns, *Pediatrics* **49**:671.

9. Allen, M., 1984, Developmental outcome and followup of the small for gestational age infant, *Semin. Perinatol.* **8**:123.
10. Fitzhardinge, P., and Steven, E., 1972, The small for date infant. II. Neurological and intellectual sequelae, *Pediatrics* **50**:50.
11. Babson, S. G., and Phillips, D., 1973, Growth and development of twins dissimilar in size at birth, *N. Engl. J. Med.* **289**:937.
12. Charlton, V., 1984, Fetal nutritional supplementation. *Semin. Perinatol.* **8**:25.
13. Battaglia, F., and Meschia, G., 1978, Principal substrates of fetal metabolism, *Physiol. Rev.* **58**:499.
14. James, E., Raye, J., Gresham, E., *et al.*, 1972, Fetal oxygen consumption, carbon dioxide production and glucose uptake in a chronic sheep preparation, *Pediatrics* **50**:361.
15. Simmons, M., Battaglia, F., and Meschia, G., 1979, Placental transfer of glucose, *J. Dev. Physiol.* **1**:227.
16. Morriss, F., Makowski, E., Meschia, G., *et al.*, 1975, The glucose/oxygen quotient of the term human fetus, *Biol. Neonate* **25**:44.
17. Schreiner, R., Burd, L., Jones, M. D., *et al.*, 1978, Fetal metabolism in fasting sheep, in: *Fetal and Newborn Cardiovascular Physiology*, Vol. 2 (L. Longo and D. Reneau, eds.), p. 197, Garland Press, New York.
18. Jones, M., 1979, Energy metabolism in the developing brain, *Semin. Perinatol.* **3**:121.
19. Gresham, E., James, E., Raye, J., *et al.*, 1972, Production and excretion of urea by the fetal lamb, *Pediatrics* **50**:372.
20. Soltesz, G., Harris, D., Mackenzie, I., *et al.*, 1985, The metabolic and endocrine milieu of the human fetus and mother at 18–21 weeks of gestation. I. Plasma amino acid concentrations, *Pediatr. Res.* **19**:91.
21. Lemons, J., Adcock, E., Jones, M. D., *et al.*, 1976, Umbilical uptake of amino acids in the unstressed fetal lamb, *J. Clin. Invest.* **58**:1428.
22. Levy, H., Lenke, R., and Koch, R., 1984, Lack of fetal effect on blood phenylalanine concentration in maternal phenylketonuria, *J. Pediatr.* **104**:245.
23. Kerr, G., Chamove, A., Harlow, H., *et al.*, 1968, Fetal PKU: The effect of maternal hyperphenylalaninemia during pregnancy in the rhesus monkey, *Pediatrics* **42**:27.
24. Nicholson, J., 1983, Inborn errors of metabolism, in: *Neonatal–Perinatal Medicine* (A. Fanaroff and R. Martin, ed.), p. 815, C. V. Mosby, St. Louis.
25. Lipson, A., Beuhler, B., Bartley, J., *et al.*, 1984, Maternal hyperphenylalaninemia, Fetal effects, *J. Pediatr.* **104**:216.
26. Lemons, J., and Schreiner, R., 1983, Amino acid metabolism in the ovine fetus. *Am. J. Physiol.* **244**:E459.
27. Young, M., 1974, The influence of a reduction in maternal, placental blood flow on the placental transfer of glucose, total amino nitrogen, leucine, and lysine, in: *Size at Birth, Ciba Symposium 27* (G. Dawes, ed.), p. 22, Elsevier, Amsterdam.
28. Burd, L., Jones, M. D., Simmons, M., *et al.*, 1975, Placental production and foetal utilization of lactate and pyruvate, *Nature (Lond.)* **254**:710.
29. Charlton Char, V., and Creasy, R., 1976, Lactate and pyruvate as fetal metabolic substrates, *Pediatr. Res.* **10**:231.
30. Sparks, J., Hay, W., Bonds, D., *et al.*, 1982, Simultaneous measurements of lactate turnover rate and umbilical lactate uptake in the fetal lamb, *J. Clin. Invest.* **70**:179.
31. Gleason, C., Rudolph, C., Bristow, J., *et al.*, 1985, Lactate uptake by the fetal sheep liver, *J. Dev. Physiol.* **7**:177.
32. Hull, D., 1975, Storage and supply of fatty acids before and after birth, *Br. Med. Bull.* **31**:32.

33. Dancis, J., Jansen, V., Kayden, H., *et al.*, 1973, Transfer across the perfused human placenta. II. Free fatty acids, *Pediatr. Res.* **7**:192.
34. Hummel, L., Schirrmeister, W., and Wagner, H., 1975, Quantitative evaluation of the maternal–fetal transfer of free fatty acids in the rat, *Biol. Neonate* **26**:263.
35. Edson, J., Hudson, D., and Hull, D., 1975, Evidence for increased fatty acid transfer across the placenta during a maternal fast in rabbits, *Biol. Neonate* **27**:50.
36. Pavey, D., and Widdowson, E., 1980, Body lipids of guinea pigs exposed to different dietary fats from mid-gestation to three months of age. V. The fatty acid composition of the brain lipids at birth, *Nutr. Metab.* **24**:357.
37. Ballard, F., 1972, Supply and utilization of acetate in mammals, *Am. J. Clin. Nutr.* **25**:773.
38. Charlton Char, V., and Creasy, R., 1976, Acetate as a metabolic substrate in the fetal lamb. *Am. J. Physiol.* **230**:357.
39. Comline, R., and Silver, M., 1976, Some aspects of foetal and uteroplacental metabolism in cows with indwelling umbilical, uterine, vascular catheters, *J. Physiol. (Lond.)* **260**:571.
40. Plotz, E., Kabara, J., Davis, M., *et al.*, 1968, Studies on the synthesis of cholesterol in the brain of the human fetus, *Am. J. Obstet. Gynecol.* **101**:534.
41. James, E., Meschia, G., and Battaglia, F., 1971, A–V differences of free fatty acids and glycerol in the ovine umbilical circulation, *Proc. Soc. Exp. Biol. Med.* **138**:823.
42. Morriss, F., Boyd, R., Makowski, E., *et al.*, 1974, Umbilical V–A differences of acetocetate and betahydroxybutyrate in fed and starved ewes, *Proc. Soc. Exp. Biol. Med.* **145**:879.
43. Charlton Char, V., and Creasy, R., 1977, Fetal umbilical venous–arterial differences in citrate in the chronically catherised sheep, *Res. Vet. Sci.* **23**:130.
44. Miodovnik, M., Lavin, J., Harrington, D., *et al.*, 1982, Effect of maternal ketoacidemia on the pregnant ewe and fetus, *Am. J. Obstet. Gynecol.* **144**:585.
45. Hurley, L., 1980, Fat soluble vitamins and water soluble vitamins, in: *Developmental Nutrition*, p. 125, Prentice-Hall, Englewood Cliffs, N.J.
46. Smithells, R., Sheppard, S., and Schorah, C., 1976, Vitamin deficiencies and neural tube defects, *Arch. Dis. Child.* **51**:944.
47. Smithells, R., Sheppard, S., Schorah, C., *et al.*, 1981, Apparent prevention of neural tube defects by periconceptual vitamin supplementation, *Arch Dis. Child.* **56**:911.
48. Editorial, 1985, Vitamin A and teratogenesis, *Lancet* **i**:319.
49. Hurley, L., 1980, Trace elements. I. Iron, copper, iodine. II. Manganese and zinc, in: *Developmental Nutrition*, p. 183, Prentice-Hall, Englewood Cliffs, N.J.
50. Meadows, N., Smith, M., Keeling, P., *et al.*, 1981, Zinc and small babies, *Lancet* **ii**:1135.
51. Soltan, M., and Jenkins, D., 1982, Maternal and fetal plasma zinc concentration and fetal abnormality, *Br. J. Obstet. Gynaecol.* **89**:56.
52. Rudolph, A., 1984, Oxygenation in the fetus and neonate—A perspective, *Semin. Perinatol.* **8**:158.
53. Clapp, J., Szeto, H., Larrow, R., *et al.*, 1981, Fetal metabolic response to experimental, placental, vascular damage, *Am. J. Obstet. Gynecol.* **40**:446.
54. Dobbing, J., 1984, Infant nutrition and later achievement, *Nutr. Rev.* **42**:1.
55. Brandt, I., 1981, Brain growth, fetal malnutrition and clinical consequences, *J. Perinatol. Med.* **9**:3.
56. Volpe, J., 1977, Normal and abnormal human brain development, *Clin. Perinatol.* **4**:3.
57. Abrams, R., Ito, M., Frisinger, J., *et al.*, 1984, Local cerebral glucose utilization in fetal and neonatal sheep, *Am. J. Physiol.* **246**:R608.

58. Somjen, G., 1983, *Neurophysiology—The Essentials*, Williams & Wilkins, Baltimore.
59. Charlton, V., and Johengen, M., 1984, Nutrient and waste product concentration differences in upper and lower body arteries of fetal sheep, *J. Dev. Physiol.* **6:**431.
60. Nitzan, M., Orloff, S., and Schulman, J., 1979, Placental transfer of analogs of glucose and amino acids in experimental intrauterine growth retardation, *Pediatr. Res.* **13:**100.
61. Crawford, M., Williams, G., and Hassam, A., 1976, Essential fatty acids and fetal brain growth, *Lancet* **i:**452.
62. Cremer, J., 1982, Substrate utilization and brain development, *J. Cerebral Blood Flow Metab.* **2:**394.
63. Clapp, J., McLaughlin, M., Gellis, J., *et al.*, 1984, Regional distribution of cerebral blood flow in experimental intrauterine growth retardation, *Am. J. Obstet. Gynecol.* **150:**843.
64. Furlow, T., Martin, R., and Harrison, L., 1983, Simultaneous measurement of local glucose utilization and blood flow in the rat brain: An autoradiographic method using two tracers labeled with carbon-14, *J. Cereb. Blood Flow Metab.* **3:**62.
65. Miller, H., and Merritt, A., 1979, Objectives, in: *Fetal Growth in Humans*, p. 1, Yearbook Medical Publishers, Chicago.
66. Gaston, A., 1982, Small for gestational age infants, in: *Pediatrics* Seventeenth edition (A. Rudolph, ed.), p. 154, Appleton-Century-Crofts, East Norwalk, Conn.
67. Molteni, R., Stys, S., and Battaglia, F., 1978, Relationship of fetal and placental weight in human beings: Fetal/placental weight ratios at various gestational ages and birth weight distributions, *J. Reprod. Med.* **21:**327.
68. Kliegman, R., and King, K., 1983, Intrauterine growth retardation: Determinants of abnormal fetal growth, in: *Neonatal–Perinatal Medicine*, 3rd ed. (A. Fanaroff and R. Martin, eds.), p. 49, C. V. Mosby, St. Louis.
69. Miller, H., and Merritt, A., 1979, Abnormal factors affecting fetal growth, in: *Fetal Growth in Humans*, p. 25, Yearbook Medical Publishers, Chicago.
70. Naeye, R., 1965, Malnutrition—Probable cause of fetal growth retardation, *Arch. Pathol.* **79:**284.
71. Naeye, R., and Kelly, J., 1966, Judgement of fetal age, *Pediatr. Clin. North Am.* **13:**849.
72. Sokol, R., Kazzi, G., Kalhan, S., *et al.*, 1982, Identifying the pregnancy at risk for intrauterine growth retardation: Possible usefulness of the intravenous glucose tolerance test, *Am. J. Obstet. Gynecol.* **143:**220.
73. Haymond, M., Karl, I., and Pagliara, A., 1974, Increased gluconeogenic substrates in the small-for-gestational age infant, *N. Engl. J. Med.* **291:**322.
74. Mestyan, J., Soltesz, G., Schultz, K., *et al.*, 1975, Hyperaminoacidemias due to the accumulation of gluconeogenic amino acid precursors in hypoglycemic small-for-gestational age infants, *J. Pediatr.* **87:**409.
75. Churchill, J., Moghissi, K., Evans, T., *et al.*, 1969, Relationships of maternal amino acid blood levels to fetal development, *Obstet. Gynecol.* **33:**492.
76. Moghissi, K., Churchill, J., and Kurrie, D., 1975, Relationship of maternal amino acids and proteins to fetal growth and mental development, *Am. J. Obstet. Gynecol.* **123:**398.
77. McClain, P., Metcoff, J., Crosby, W., *et al.*, 1978, Relationship of maternal amino acid profiles at 25 weeks gestation to fetal growth, *Am. J. Clin. Nutr.* **31:**401.
78. Renaud, R., Kirschtetter, L., Koehl, C., *et al.*, 1974, Amino acid intraamniotic injection, in: *Recent Progress in Obstetrics and Gynecology, Proceedings of the Seventh World Congress of Obstetrics and Gynecology* (L. Persianinov, T. Chervakova, and J. Presl, eds.), p. 234, Excerpta Medica, Prague.

79. Lindblad, B., 1971, The plasma aminogram in small for dates newborn infants, in: *Metabolic Processes in the Newborn Infant* (J. Jonxis, H. Visser, and J. Troelstra, eds.), p. 191, S. Karger, Basel.
80. Butterfield, J., and O'Brien, D., 1963, The effect of maternal toxemia and diabetes on transplacental gradients of free amino acids, *Arch. Dis. Child.* **38:**326.
81. Evans, M., Mukherjee, A., and Schulman, J., 1983, Animal models of intrauterine growth retardation, *Obstet. Gynecol. Surv.* **38:**183.
82. Wallace, L., 1948, The growth of lambs before and after birth in relation to the level of nutrition. II and III, *J. Agric. Sci.* **38:**243.
83. Wallace, L., 1948, The growth of lambs before and after birth in relation to the level of nutrition. III, *J. Agric. Sci.* **38:**367.
84. Koritnik, D., Humphrey, W., Kaltenbach, C., *et al.*, 1981, Effects of maternal undernutrition on the development of the ovine fetus and the associated changes in growth hormone and prolactin, *Biol. Reprod.* **24:**125.
85. Charlton, V., and Johengen, M., 1982, Metabolism of the fetal lamb growth retarded by maternal malnutrition, *Pediatr. Res.* **16:**109A (abs.).
86. Creasy, R., Barrett, C., DeSwiet, M., *et al.*, 1972, Experimental intrauterine growth retardation in the sheep, *Am. J. Obstet. Gynecol.* **112:**566.
87. Robinson, J., Kingston, E., Jones, C., *et al.*, 1979, Studies in experimental growth retardation in sheep. The effect of removal of endometrial caruncles on fetal size and metabolism, *J. Dev. Physiol.* **1:**379.
88. Emmanouilides, G., Townsend, D., and Bauer, R., 1968, Effects of simple umbilical artery ligation in the lamb fetus, *Pediatrics* **42:**919.
89. Hobel, C., Emmanouilides, G., Townsend, D., *et al.*, 1970, Ligation of one umbilical artery in the fetal lamb, *Obstet. Gynecol.* **36:**582.
90. Oh, W., Omori, K., Hobel, C., *et al.*, 1975, Umbilical blood flow and glucose uptake in the lamb fetus following simple umbilical artery ligation, *Biol. Neonate* **26:**291.
91. Alexander, G., 1974, Birth weight of lambs: Influences and consequences, in: *Size at Birth, Ciba Symposium 27* (G. Dawes, ed.), p. 215, Elsevier, Amsterdam.
92. Creasy, R., DeSwiet, M., Kahanpaa, K., *et al.*, 1973, Pathophysiological changes in the fetal lamb with growth retardation, in: *Foetal and Neonatal Physiology, Proceedings of the Sir Joseph Barcroft Centenary Symposium* (K. Cross, ed.), p. 398, Cambridge University Press, Cambridge.
93. Charlton Char, V., and Creasy, R., 1977, Glucose and oxygen metabolism in normally oxygenated and spontaneously hypoxemic fetal lambs, *Am. J. Obstet. Gynecol.* **127:**499.
94. Charlton, V., and Johengen, M., 1983, Effects of fetal nutritional supplements on growth retardation, in: *Program of the Society for Gynecologic Investigation, Thirtieth Annual Meeting, Washington, D.C.*, p. 114 (abs.).
95. Charlton, V., and Johengen, M., 1985, Effects of intrauterine nutritional supplementation on fetal growth retardation, *Biol. Neonate* **48:**125.
96. Clapp, J., Szeto, H., Larrow, R., *et al.*, 1980, Umbilical blood flow response to embolization of the uterine circulation, *Am. J. Obstet. Gynecol.* **138:**60.
97. Itskovitz, J., LaGamma, E., and Rudolph, A., 1983, The effect of reducing umbilical blood flow on fetal oxygenation, *Am. J. Obstet. Gynecol.* **145:**813.
98. Clapp, J., 1978, The relationship between blood flow and oxygen uptake in the uterine and umbilical circulations, *Am. J. Obstet. Gynecol.* **132:**410.
99. Charlton, V., and Reis, B., 1981, Effects of gastric nutritional supplementation on fetal umbilical uptake of nutrients, *Am. J. Physiol.* **241:**E178.
100. Wilkening, R., and Meschia, G., 1983, Fetal oxygen uptake, oxygenation and acid–base balance as a function of uterine blood flow. *Am. J. Physiol.* **244:**H749.

101. Wigglesworth, J., 1974, Animal model: Uterine vessel ligation in the pregnant rat, *Am. J. Pathol.* **77:**347.
102. Vileisis, R., 1985, Effect of maternal oxygen inhalation on the fetus with growth retardation, *Pediatr. Res.* **19:**324.
103. Saintonge, J., and Rosso, P., 1981, Placental blood flow and transfer of nutrient analogs in large, average and small guinea pig litter mates, *Pediatr. Res.* **15:**152.
104. Charlton, V., and Johengen, M., 1985, Blood substrate levels in ovo: relationship to fetal size, *Pediatr. Res.* **19:**152A.
105. McCutcheon, I., Metcalfe, J., Metzenberg, A., *et al.,* 1982, Organ growth in hyperoxic and hypoxic chick embryos, *Respir. Physiol.* **50:**153.
106. Bissonette, J., Holzimer, A., Richardson, B., *et al.,* 1983, Fetal cerebral glucose uptake is limited by blood brain barrier transport, in: *Program of the Society for Gynecologic Investigation, Thirtieth Annual Meeting, Washington, D.C.,* p. 111 (abs.).
107. Richardson, B., Hohimer, A., Bissonette, J., *et al.,* 1983, Effect of insulin induced hypoglycemia on cerebral metabolism in the fetal lamb, in: *Program of the Society for Gynecologic Investigation, Thirtieth Annual Meeting, Washington, D.C.,* p. 299 (abs.).
108. Pell, J., and Bergman, E., 1983, Cerebral metabolism of amino acids and glucose in fed and fasted sheep, *Am. J. Physiol.* **244:**E282.
109. Schulman, J., Mann, L., Doores, L., *et al.,* 1975, Amino acid metabolism by the fetal brain during normal and hypoglycemic conditions, *Biol. Neonate* **25:**57.
110. Clos, J., Favre, C., Selme-Matrat, M., *et al.,* 1977, Effects of undernutrition on cell formation in the rat brain and especially on cellular composition of the cerebellum, *Brain Res.* **123:**13.
111. Robain, O., and Ponset, G., 1978, Effects of undernutrition on glial maturation, *Brain Res.,* **149:**379.
112. Resnik, O., and Morgane, P., 1983, Animal models for small for gestational age neonates and infants at risk, *Brain Res.* **312:**221.
113. Hill, D., Myers, R., Holt, A., *et al.,* 1971, Fetal growth retardation produced by experimental placental insufficiency in the rhesus monkey, *Biol. Neonate* **19:**68.
114. Chase, P., Welch, N., Dabiere, C., *et al.,* 1972, Alterations in human brain biochemistry following IUGR, *Pediatrics* **50:**403.
115. Gonzalez-Sastre, F., Rodes, M., Sabater, J., *et al.,* 1978, Intrauterine growth retardation: Biochemical changes in human central nervous system, *An. Esp. Pediatr.* **11:**13.
116. Harel, S., Shapira, Y., Hartzler, J., *et al.,* 1978, Neuromotor development in relation to birth weight in rabbits, *Biol. Neonate* **33:**1.
117. Commey, J., and Fitzhardinge, P., 1979, Handicap in the preterm, small for gestational age infant, *J. Pediatr.* **94:**779.
118. Kitchen, W., Ford, G., Orgill, A., *et al.,* 1984, Outcome in infants wih birthweight 500 to 999 gm, *J. Pediatr.* **104:**921.
119. Fancourt, R., Campbell, S., Harvey, D., *et al.,* 1976, Followup of small-for-dates babies, *Br. Med. J.* **1:**1435.
120. Robillard, J., Sessions, C., Kennedy, R., *et al.,* 1978, Metabolic effects of constant hypertonic glucose infusion in well-oxygenated fetuses, *Am. J. Obstet. Gynecol.* **130:**199.
121. Shelly, H., Bassett, J., and Millner, R., 1975, Control of carbohydrate metabolism in the fetus and newborn, *Br. Med. Bull.* **31:**37.
122. Fletcher, A., 1981, The infant of the diabetic mother, in: *Neonatology,* 2nd ed. (G. Avery, ed.), p. 287, J. B. Lippincott, Philadelphia.
123. Heird, W., and Winters, R., 1975, Total parenteral nutrition, *J. Pediatr.* **86:**2.
124. Mauer, A., Collipp, P., Dweck, H., *et al.,* 1983, Commentary on parenteral nutrition, *Pediatrics* **71:**547.

125. Edelstone, D., Rudolph, A., Heymann, M., 1978, Liver and ductus venosus blood flows in fetal lambs in utero, *Circ. Res.* **42**:426.
126. Davis, E., and Potter, E., 1946, Intrauterine respiration of the human fetus, *J.A.M.A.* **131**:1194.
127. Gitlin, D., Kumate, J., Morales, C., *et al.*, 1972, The turnover of amniotic fluid protein in the human conceptus, *Am. J. Obstet. Gynecol.* **113**:632.
128. Pritchard, J., 1965, Deglutition by normal and anencephalic fetuses, *Obstet. Gynecol.* **25**:289.
129. Mistretta, C., and Bradley, R., 1975, Taste and swallowing in utero, *Br. Med. Bull.* **31**:80.
130. Riddick, D., Maslar, I., Luciano, A., *et al.*, 1979, Thyroxine uptake and metabolism by fetal sheep after intraamniotic thyroxine injection. *Am. J. Obstet. Gynecol.* **133**:618.
131. Becker, R., Windle, W., Barth, E., *et al.*, 1940, Fetal swallowing, gastro-intestinal activity and defecation in amnio, *Surg. Gynecol. Obstet.* **70**:603.
132. Heller, L., 1974, Intrauterine amino acid feeding of the fetus, in: *Parenteral Nutrition in Infancy and Childhood* (H. Bode and J. Warshaw, eds.), p. 206, Plenum Press, New York.
133. Saling, E., Dudenhausen, J., and Kynast, G., 1974, Basic investigations about compensatory nutrition of the malnourished fetus, in: *Recent Progress in Obstetrics and Gynecology, Proceedings of the VII World Congress of Obstetrics and Gynecology* (L. Persianinov, T. Chervakova, and J. Presl, eds.), p. 227, Excerpta Medica, Prague.
134. Massobrio, M., Margaria, E., Campogravide, M., *et al.*, 1975, Treatment of severe feto-placental insufficiency by means of intraamniotic injection of amino acids, in: *Therapy of Feto-Placental Insufficiency* (B. Salvadori, ed.), p. 296, Springer-Verlag, Berlin.
135. Charlton, V., and Johengen, M., 1984, Intraamniotic administration of nutrients, *Pediatr. Res.* **18**:136A (abs.).
136. Milley, J. R., Rosenberg, A., Phillips, A., *et al.*, 1984, The effect of insulin on fetal oxygen extraction. *Am. J. Obstet. Gynecol.* **149**;673.
137. Harrison, M., and Villa, R., 1982, Trans-amniotic fetal feeding I. Development of an animal model: Continuous amniotic infusion in rabbits, *J. Pediatr. Surg.* **17**:376.
138. Mulvihill, S., Albert, A., Synn, A., *et al.*, 1985, In utero supplemental fetal feeding in an animal model: Effects on fetal growth and development, *Surgery* **98**:500.
139. Charlton, V., and Reis, B., 1980, Response of the chronically catheterized fetal lamb to intestinal administration of amino acids, *Clin. Res.* **28**:121A (abs.).
140. Charlton, V., 1984, Nutrient administration to the fetus via gastrointestinal, vascular and intraamniotic routes, in: *Animal Models in Fetal Medicine*, Vol. IV (P. Nathianelsz, ed.), p. 59, Perinatology Press, Ithaca, N.Y.
141. Charlton, V., and Rudolph, A., 1979, Digestion and absorption of carbohydrates by the fetal lamb in utero, *Pediatr. Res.* **13**:1018.
142. Prior, R., and Christensen, R., 1977, Gluconeogenesis from alanine in vivo by the ovine fetus and lamb, *Am. J. Physiol.* **233**:E462.
143. Young, M., Soltesz, G., Noakes, D., *et al.*, 1975, The influence of intrauterine surgery and of fetal intravenous nutritional supplements (in utero) on plasma free amino acid homeostasis in the pregnant ewe, *J. Perinat. Med.* **3**:180.
144. Dudenhausen, J. W., Gutsche, H. V., and Koch, M., 1973, Zur intrauterinen ernahrung des mangelversorgten feten, *Fortschr. Med.* **91**:1264.
145. Pitkin, R., and Reynolds, W. A., 1975, Fetal ingestion and metabolism of amniotic fluid protein, *Am. J. Obstet. Gynecol.* **123**:356.

146. Al-Murrani, W., 1982, Effect of injecting amino acids into the egg on embryonic and subsequent growth in the domestic fowl, *Br. Poult. Sci.* **23:**171.
147. National Academy of Sciences, 1975, *Nutrient Requirements of Sheep*, 5th ed. p. 42, National Academy of Sciences, Washington, D.C.
148. Charlton, V., and Johengen, M., 1986, Nutrient supplementation of fetuses growth retarded by placental embolization, *Pediatr. Res.* **20:**185A (abs.).
149. Edelstone, D., and Rudolph, A., 1979, Preferential streaming of ductus venosus blood to the brain and heart in fetal lambs, *Am. J. Physiol.* **237:**H724.

CHAPTER 2

Transplacental Toxicity of Environmental Chemicals

Environmental Causes and Correlates of Spontaneous Abortions, Malformations, and Childhood Cancer

K. HEMMINKI, M.-L. LINDBOHM, and H. TASKINEN

1. Introduction

The mechanisms of reproductive ill effects are complex because both maternal and paternal factors can operate.[1-3] It is clear that maternal factors have an important role in spontaneous abortion and malformations. Increasing attention has recently been paid to the possibility that paternal effects may cause spontaneous abortions and childhood cancer in the offspring.[4] This review is restricted to human transplacental effects that interact with the embryo or fetus during pregnancy only.

Reproductive and childhood cancer epidemiology is a new field, particularly in relationship to environmental chemicals. Three important events stimulated research in this field. First was the thalidomide episode, which launched studies on malformations because it was believed that environmental chemicals as well as pharmaceutical drugs may cause malformations. Research on spontaneous abortions was intensified after work with anesthetics was reported to involve an increased risk of spontaneous abortions. Research activities were subsequently widened to include other chemical exposures, and today the literature on spontaneous abortions

K. HEMMINKI, M. -L. LINDBOHM, and H. TASKINEN • Institute of Occupational Health, SF-00290 Helsinki, Finland.

is as extensive as the studies on malformations. Studies on environmental chemicals and childhood cancer were set off by a report in which the father's exposure to hydrocarbons was associated with an increased risk of malignancies in the offspring.[5] Although this area of research is hampered by the rarity of the events studied, research reports have been forthcoming from a number of countries.

As a result of reproductive and childhood cancer studies, several methodologic problems have been recognized and many solutions have been found, as described elsewhere.[6-9] The most severe problem in the studies of all these outcomes is the bias of reporting or response, or both. Bias should and can be tackled. It is comforting to note that most recent studies address the possibility of bias. Proven risk factors can be undoubtedly accepted once such methodologic principles are applied in the field. For the time being, there are still some reservations, as this chapter will show.

2. Environmental Chemicals and Spontaneous Abortions

2.1. Occupational and Social Correlates of Spontaneous Abortions

Analysis according to social class provides some information about the effects of environmental factors on spontaneous abortions. A Finnish investigation[10] found that the age-standardized rate of spontaneous abortion increased from 5.9% in the highest social group (higher-level officials, employers) to 8.5% in the lowest social group (unskilled workers). The study population comprised all spontaneous abortions treated in Finnish hospitals (Table I). A Danish study used interviews to obtain data on abortions. No association was observed between the proportion of women with one or more spontaneous abortions and social class, education, or net family income.[11]

One of the basic problems in studies on spontaneous abortions is how to get valid information on abortions and exposures. Interview data entail the danger of reporting bias and response bias; i.e., both reporting and response may depend on pregnancy outcome and exposure. Studies that use medical records may be biased by spontaneous abortion patients' selection of medical services.

Different data sources may explain why the above-mentioned studies on social class and spontaneous abortions have yielded conflicting

Table I. Age-Standardized Rates of Spontaneous Abortions by Social Class
in Finland in 1973–1975

Social class	Number of spontaneous abortions[a]	Rate of spontaneous abortions	Standardized rate ratio[b]
Higher-level officials, enterprisers, employers	1,826	5.88[d]	0.79
Lower-level officials, small entrepreneurs	5,546	7.27	0.97
Skilled workers	6,873	7.65[c]	1.02
Unskilled workers	1,458	8.47[d]	1.13
Farmers	999	7.56	1.01
Students	862	8.28[c]	1.11
All women	18,733	7.43	1.00

[a] Women aged 15–44.
[b] Age-standardized rate of the social class over the rate of all women.
[c] $p < 0.05$.
[d] $p < 0.001$, normal distribution.

results. Especially comparisons between social groups may be invalidated by differences in reporting and response or differences in care-seeking behavior. Furthermore, studies have measured the prevalence of abortions in different ways. The absence or presence of differences between social classes should be confirmed by other studies.

A few comparisons have also been made between working women and homemakers. The above-mentioned Finnish study found a small but significant difference between these two groups. The age-standardized rates were 7.4 and 6.9, respectively.[10] When the data were analyzed for occupational information retrieved from the population census the difference became even smaller.[12] One drawback was that parity, which may be an important confounding factor in comparisons between working women and homemakers, was not controlled.

A case-control study performed by Kline et al.[13] compared the frequency of maternal work before or during pregnancy between women who had experienced spontaneous abortions with different fetal karyotypes and women who had delivered a child. Maternal work during pregnancy was not associated with the abortion of a chromosomally normal fetus.

Two other studies compared industrial work to homework. An Italian questionnaire study reported a higher age-standardized spontaneous abortion rate among women who were factory workers than among homemakers.[14] An interview study carried out in Iran also found a clear difference in the rates for working women (12%) and nonworking women (8%).[15] The Iranian workers were employed by two textile factories, and obviously most of them had also been working there during pregnancy.

Factory workers have been found to have a higher risk of spontaneous abortions than other workers. The analysis of age-standardized rates of hospitalized abortions by occupation showed that industrial and construction workers and also agricultural workers had higher rates than other occupational groups.[10] Another study compared factory workers in the rubber, plastics, machine, and tin industries with shop assistants and packers. After age, pregnancy order, and gravidity (the total number of pregnancies) had been controlled for, the odds ratio among factory workers was significantly increased—1.7 when analyzed for self-reported data on pregnancies and 1.4 when analyzed for hospital records.[16]

The results of these studies suggest that environmental factors affect the risk of spontaneous abortions. They also appear to show that factory workers are exposed to some risk factors of abortions.

2.2. Health Care Personnel

2.2.1. Anesthesia Personnel

A considerable portion of all epidemiologic investigations on occupational reproductive hazards have dealt with the effects of anesthetic gases in operating theaters or dental clinics (see Table II). Most studies have indicated increased rates of spontaneous abortions among exposed women,[17-26] but some negative results have been published as well.[27-29] Several reviewers of the available literature conclude that there is reasonably convincing evidence that the exposed women have a moderately increased risk of spontaneous abortions.[30-32] High concentrations of nitrous oxide have been suggested to be the primary causative factor.[33] A study carried out among dental chairside assistants found a positive relationship between dose and response.[26]

Lately the validity of these studies has been questioned. It has been suspected that the results are attributable to either recall or response bias, or both. All the studies have obtained information on pregnancies and exposures through questionnaires. The response rates have been fairly low, and the exposed and the nonexposed have had different response rates. Axelsson and Rylander[34] observed that the inclusion also of nonrespondents' pregnancies collected from the medical records reduced the difference in the rates of spontaneous abortions between the

Table II. Effects of Exposure to Ethylene Oxide, Glutaraldehyde, and Formaldehyde on the Rate of Spontaneous Abortions According to Interview Data and Hospital Register Data

	Interview data		Register data	
Chemical sterilizing agent	Pregnancies (N)	Adjusted[a] rate of abortions	Pregnancies (N)	Rate of[b] abortions
Ethylene oxide (alone or with other agents)	146	12.7[c]	61	19.7[c]
Glutaraldehyde (alone or with other agents)	440	9.3	219	13.7
Formaldehyde (alone or with other agents)	50	8.4	20	10.0
Ethylene oxide alone	82	16.1[d]	32	25.0[d]
Glutaraldehyde alone	364	9.4	254	13.5
Controls working	—	—	332	9.6

[a] Adjusted for age, parity, decade of pregnancy, smoking habits, and alcohol and coffee consumption using the logistic regression model; tested against not exposed during pregancy.
[b] Age-stratified (under 30 years, at or over 30 years) rates tested with the Mantel-Haenszel method.
[c] $p < 0.05$.
[d] $p < 0.01$.

exposed and nonexposed women (15.1 versus 11.0, relative risk 1.19, not significant).

In order to avoid response and reporting bias, a Finnish study[35] used only registered data on pregnancies, and the exposure data were obtained from questionnaires sent to the leading head nurses of the hospitals. No significant association was observed between spontaneous abortions and exposure to anesthetic gases (odds ratio 1.2, confidence interval 0.7–2.4). A Danish study that used hospital registers as a data source for pregnancies also found no increased risk of abortions among dental assistants exposed to nitrous oxide.[16]

Although many of the previous investigations among operating theater staff are open to bias, it is certainly difficult to say whether such bias accounts for all the differences in spontaneous abortions. One factor that may have made the results susceptible to differences is that the concentrations of anesthetic gases varied and may have been very much higher in the past. Both the anesthetic agents used and ventilation have varied as well. Thus, the possibility of a causal relationship between exposure to anesthetic gases and increased risk of spontaneous abortions cannot be excluded. The latest studies with improved study designs have, however, failed to detect a significant increase in the spontaneous abortions of anesthesia staff, providing evidence that the occupational risks have been largely overcome.

2.2.2. Other Hospital Exposures

Ethylene oxide, glutaraldehyde, and formaldehyde are widely used to sterilize hospital equipment, pharmaceutical preparations, and foodstuffs. In Finland a study was conducted among hospital staff engaged in sterilizing instruments with ethylene oxide, glutaraldehyde, and formaldehyde.[36–37] The information on exposure was obtained from supervising nurses, and the data on pregnancies were collected both from women *via* postal questionnaire and through a separate analysis of hospital registers. The data from both sources, analyzed separately, suggested an association between exposure to ethylene oxide in early pregnancy and the risk of spontaneous abortions (Table II). The data had been adjusted for a number of possible confounding factors.

An association between exposure to ethylene oxide and an increased frequency of spontaneous abortions was also reported in an earlier investigation among ethylene oxide production workers.[38] However, insufficient information on the workers' age distribution and the work histories makes it difficult to interpret the results. Another Russian study found that threatened abortions were more common among textile workers exposed to formaldehyde than among nonexposed industrial sales personnel.[39]

The investigation among Finnish hospital staff was the first reproductive study considered as the basis for an occupational health standard by the U.S. Occupational Safety and Health Administration (OSHA), and so it was a subject to extensive review by officials and industry-sponsored scientists.[40] Several types of reanalysis have been carried out to date, and there has been no indication that any demonstrated study design or analytic factor can refute the association between exposure to ethylene oxide and risk of spontaneous abortions.[40]

Many antineoplastic agents have been reported to be teratogenic when given to pregnant cancer patients (see Chapter 3, Section 3.2.2). Aminopterin, an antimetabolite, has been used as an abortifacient. An increase in the rate of spontaneous abortions has also been reported in women previously treated with chemotherapy.[41,42] However, the treated women had had trophoplastic tumors, and the high rates of abortions may have been caused by tumor-induced damage to the genital tract.

Hospital and pharmacy personnel may be occupationally exposed to antineoplastic drugs. The relationship between nurses' spontaneous abortions and their exposure to antineoplastic drugs has been investigated in a case-referent study conducted in Finland.[43] The nurses' pregnancies were identified from the hospital discharge register, and exposure data were obtained *via* questionnaires to the nurses. A statistically significant association for spontaneous abortions and exposure during the first trimester of pregnancy was found (odds ratio 2.30, $p = 0.01$). Differential bias by pregnancy outcome in the recall of pregnancy-related exposure was probably minor in this study, as the odds ratio for anesthetic gases was low (odds ratio 0.96), even though several reports have linked this exposure to spontaneous abortions.

The effects of nurses' occupational exposure to antineoplastic drugs were also analyzed in another Finnish study.[35] Here information of exposure was requested from the head nurses of the hospitals. No association was detected between exposure and abortions, but the study did not include nurses working in the departments where cancer chemotherapy is the most extensive (e.g., oncology wards) and where exposure may have been higher.

Since these two studies covered partially overlapping populations, it was possible to compare the consistency of the reporting of exposure by the nurses themselves and by the head nurses. Although the final results are not yet available, both the nurses' and their supervisors' reports agree to a large extent and thereby corroborate the above findings.

2.3. Laboratory Workers and Solvents

Laboratory workers are another occupational group that has been the object of several studies (see Table III). Unlike health care personnel, they may be exposed to many potentially embryotoxic chemicals, such as solvents, heavy metals, and carcinogens. Two Swedish investigations based on questionnaire data found increased occurrences of spontaneous abortions among women at work in hospital laboratories.[44,45] The number of pregnancies was small in both studies. An increased rate of spontaneous abortions (18%, not statistically significant) was also found among women employed in chemical laboratories in the pharmaceuticals industry compared with women employed in nonchemical laboratories (10%).[46] A study concerning the workers of a virologic laboratory found a tendency toward increased rates of miscarriage and perinatal death among women exposed to airborne viruses and a specific disinfectant.[47] A slightly increased risk of spontaneous abortions (odds ratio = 1.3, $p < 0.01$) has also been observed among Finnish laboratory assistants in a nationwide study based on registered pregnancy data.[12]

Table III. Studies on the Association between Spontaneous Abortions and Hospital Exposures, Laboratory Exposures, and Solvents[a]

Occupation or exposure	Association with exposure	Reference
Health care personnel		
Anesthetic gases	Ten positive and six negative studies	See text
Sterilizing staff (ethylene oxide)	+	Hemminki *et al.*[36,37]
Antineoplastic agents	+	Selevan *et al.*[43]
	−	Hemminki *et al.*[35]
Laboratory work		
Hospital laboratory	(+)	Strandberg *et al.*[45]
	(+)	Kolmodin-Hedman *et al.*[44]
	−	Heidam[49]
University laboratory (solvents)	−	Axelsson *et al.*[48]
	−	Heidam[49]
Pharmaceuticals industry laboratory	(−)	Hansson *et al.*[46]
Industrial laboratory	−	Heidam[49]
Virologic laboratory	(+)	Axelsson *et al.*[47]
Laboratory assistants	+	Lindbohm *et al.*[12]
Solvents		
Painters	(+)	Heidam[16]
Laundry workers	+	Lindbohm *et al.*[12]
Occupations involving solvent exposure	−	Lindbohm *et al.*[12]
Cleaning service worker	+	Kline *et al.*[13]
Pharmaceuticals workers solvent (methylene chloride) exposure	(+)	Taskinen *et al.*[64]

[a] +, Positive association; −, no association; the parentheses indicate limitations such as standardization of confounding factors, lack of a control group, borderline significance, or small sample size.

Many of these investigations have suggested exposure to solvents as one of the potential etiologic factors. Two other occupational groups with solvent exposure have also been found to be at excess risk, namely painters[16] and laundry workers.[12] A recent study using pregnancy data verified from hospital records found that the miscarriage rate was slightly, but not significantly, increased (relative risk 1.3) among the solvent-exposed workers of a university laboratory.[48] If miscarriages reported by the women had also been included in the analysis, the difference between the nonexposed and the exposed would have attained statistical significance, as exposure to solvents was reported more frequently for miscarriages not medically verified. The latter finding seems to indicate reporting bias.

Two sources of data on pregnancies, i.e., a postal questionnaire and hospital records, were also available in a Danish study on spontaneous abortions among women at work in hospital, university, and industrial laboratories.[49] Pregnancy outcome was not associated with laboratory work or alleged exposure to organic solvents or any other single chemical. In this study both data sources showed reasonable agreement. Contrary to the results of Axelsson *et al.*,[48] however, the reference group had more self-reported unverified abortions than the exposed group. The laboratory workers' smaller proportion of self-reported abortions may also be due to better medical insight which prompted them to seek care more frequently than the reference group (physiotherapists, occupational therapists, office workers, and technical assistants and designers).

The observations of these investigations illustrate the methodologic problems incurred in studies on spontaneous abortions, i.e., the danger of reporting bias to questionnaire studies and potential selection in abortion patients' use of medical services when medical records serve as data sources (see Section 2.1).

The results for laboratory workers are conflicting. Questionnaire studies done in individual laboratories suggest an increased risk of spontaneous abortions, but studies based on larger populations and medical records indicate no increase or only a slightly increased risk. Because the nature and degree of exposure vary in different type of laboratories, no final conclusions can be made for all laboratory workers. The research results now available suggest that laboratory workers may be exposed to chemicals harmful to the embryo, but this observation probably concerns limited subgroups only.

2.4. Workers in the Metals Industry

Reports written in the nineteenth century suggest that women exposed to lead have had many different kinds of reproductive failures. Rom[50] cited many older reports according to which women working with lead have experienced exceptionally high numbers of spontaneous abortions. More recent investigations of how exposure to lead affects pregnancy outcome are lacking, however.

A Swedish work group has carried out a study on pregnancy outcome among smelter workers, who may be exposed to lead, arsenic, sulfur dioxide, and mercury.[51] Women working in close connection with smelting processes had a significantly increased frequency of spontaneous abortions (28.0%) as compared with administration, laboratory, and restaurant workers (13.6%). Women employed during pregnancy or employed before pregnancy and still living close to the smelter also had an increased abortion frequency. The analysis was based on pregnancy data collected from medical records that covered several decades, but the reliability of the data was not clarified. Neither age nor calendar year was controlled, however; these flaws weaken any conclusions.

Another Swedish work group analyzed spontaneous abortions among the workers of a steel plant.[52] Data on pregnancies and occupations were obtained through interviews performed by a nurse. Steel workers who could have been exposed to carbon monoxide, nitrous oxides, sulfur dioxide, lime and ferrous/ferric oxides, and solvents had a slightly higher rate of spontaneous abortions (10.8%) than did nonexposed factory and clerical workers (8.5%). After stratification for age and smoking, the relative risk of spontaneous abortions (1.18%) was not statistically significant.

In Finland the occurrence of hospitalized spontaneous abortions has been investigated among the members of the Metal Workers' Union. In the first analysis for 1973–1976, the age-standardized frequency of abortions was significantly higher for pregnancies that occurred during Union membership than for pregnancies that occurred before it.[53] The production of radio and television sets, and particularly soldering work, appeared to involve a high risk. Information for the second analysis[54] was acquired for 3 more years and for women who had resigned from the Union during the study period. In every 5-year age group, the rates of spontaneous abortions were still higher for pregnancies conceived during membership than for pregnancies conceived before or after membership, but the difference was very small (7.8 and 7.1%, respectively).

Further analysis has concentrated on industrial branches in which exposure to metals was possible (i.e., the manufacture of metal products, shipbuilding, the manufacture of iron and steel, mining, and foundry work). No significant differences were found between the "exposed" and "nonexposed" pregnancies. Spontaneous abortions have also been analyzed by occupation, which was obtained from the census. The rates for smelter workers, foundry workers, or welders did not differ from those for other industrial workers.[54] The number of women employed as smelters or foundry workers, however, was very small.

Two Russian studies have reported high numbers of spontaneous abortions for women exposed to mercury.[55,56] The former study was performed among women employed in the preparation of mercury ore, the latter among women exposed in dentistry. The absence of detailed information on data sources and confounding factors makes it difficult to base conclusions on these studies. A third Russian study found an increased spontaneous abortion rate among machine tool operators exposed to a number of chemicals. Their controls, however, had an exceptionally low rate of abortions.[57]

An American study,[58] based on birth records, analyzed fetal deaths for the most recent pregnancy among multigravid women. Fetal death risk adjusted for age and gravidity was significantly elevated among women exmployed in the metal industry. A Finnish study using hospital registers and census data found no association between spontaneous abortions and employment in metal industry occupations.[12]

Many types of reproductive ill effects have been elicited by metals in experimental animals.[59,60] The evidence of their effects in human population, however, is limited. The above results suggest that further studies are needed at least among smelter workers and among workers exposed to lead or mercury (see Table IV).

Table IV. Studies on the Assocation between Spontaneous Abortions and Metals or the Metals Industry[a]

Occupation or exposure	Association with exposure	Reference
Metals and the metals industry		
Lead (historical reports)	(+)	Rom[50]
Mercury		
In dentistry	(+)	Marinova et al.[56]
In the preparation of mercury ore	(+)	Goncaruk[55]
Smelter workers	(+)	Nordström et al.[51]
Members of the Union of Metal Workers	(+)	Hemminki et al.[53,54]
Steel workers	(−)	Kolmodin-Hedman et al.[52]
Machine tool operators	(+)	Pavlova[57]
Metals industry	+	Vaughan et al.[58]
Occupations involving metal exposure	−	Lindbohm et al.[12]
Textile industry		
Formaldehyde-exposed workers	(+)	Shumlina[39]
Textile industry	(+)	Kline et al.[13]
	+	Vaughan et al.[58]
Textile occupations	−	Lindbohm et al.[12]
Weavers	+	Lindbohm et al.[12]
Spinners, fabric inspectors, nonspecific occupations related to cutting and sewing	(+)	Lindbohm et al.[12]

[a] See Table III for explanation of symbols.

2.5. Workers in the Chemicals and Plastics Industry

Hospitalized spontaneous abortions have been analyzed among the members of the Union of Chemical Workers in Finland.[61,62] The first study showed that, compared with all Finnish women, workers in the plastics industry and particularly those employed in styrene-manufacturing workplaces, the viscose rayon industry, and the pharmaceuticals industry had significantly higher abortion rates. According to the latter Finnish study, for which more complete data were available, younger women (under 30 years old) had higher rates and older women (over 30 years old) had lower rates of spontaneous abortions for pregnancies that occurred during membership when compared with the frequencies for periods before or after membership. Women employed in the pharmaceuticals industry and in the viscose rayon industry were again found to be at excess risk. Also, an earlier report has suggested that exposure to carbon disulfide in the viscose rayon industry may increase the risk of spontaneous abortions.[63]

The observations of pharmaceutical workers' high risk of abortions prompted a more specific examination. A case-control study was conducted in eight Finnish pharmaceuticals factories.[64] Data on the workers' pregnancies were collected from the hospital register, and exposure data were requested from the occupational health services of the factories. Workers exposed to estrogens had a significantly ($p = 0.05$) elevated abortion risk. The results also indicated some association between abortions and exposure to several solvents, as the odds ratio for exposure to more than three solvents was 3.5 ($p = 0.05$). Of specific solvents methylene chloride seemed to be associated with abortion risk. The small numbers of exposed cases and controls, however, restricted the analysis of abortions and different types of solvents.

Although the overall rate of spontaneous abortions was not increased among Finnish plastics workers, the heterogeneity of plastic work warranted also a detailed study on the individual exposures.[65] The results suggested that neither the processing of polyvinyl chloride or styrene plastics nor exposure to thermal degradation products were associated with spontaneous abortions. Because the samples were small, only strong effects could be ruled out. A significant difference between the cases and the controls was found for the frequency of employment in the polyurethane processing industry. Aldyreva *et al.*[66] reported high rates of spontaneous abortions among women exposed to phthalate plasticizers, which are used as additives in plastics.

An interview study has been carried out on the pregnancy outcome of female lamination workers exposed to styrene.[67] The proportion of spontaneous abortions for all pregnancies was 25% (4 of 16) in the exposed group and 18% (4 of 20) in the referent group. The small number of pregnancies and a marked difference in the occurrence of induced abortions between the exposed and nonexposed groups make it difficult to interpret these results.

A questionnaire study conducted among Italian factory workers showed that women in the plastics and rubber production industry experienced significantly more spontaneous abortions than all factory workers or homemakers.[14] The rates were increased in every age group and among both smokers and nonsmokers. No detailed information, however, is given on the workers' specific exposures.

All the above results indicate that the plastics, viscose rayon, and pharmaceuticals industries involve some risk factors (see Table V). The available evidence cannot, however, be used to draw final conclusions but provides the basis for further study.

2.6. Workers in the Rubber Industry

Rubber workers may be exposed to many agents suspected of being mutagenic or carcinogenic. The earliest reports on an increased frequency of spontaneous abortion among rubber workers were published by Russian investigators (Table V). Glueing operators in a mechanical rubber product factory, where exposure to petroleum—a major source of benzene—and chlorinated hydrocarbons was common, were found to have an increased number of abortions.[68] A high occurrence of abortions has also been reported among rubber workers exposed to gasoline.[69] No detailed information on the comparability of exposed women and their controls was given in these two studies.

Rubber workers have been the object of a few studies also in Sweden and Finland. A register-based Swedish study found no difference in the observed and expected numbers of miscarriages among workers of a rubber factory.[70] A Swedish interview study, based on a cluster of spontaneous abortions, found an increase in pregnancy complications (miscarriages, threatened abortions, and malformations) among tire builders. The result persisted after age, smoking, pregnancy order, and calendar year had been taken into account.[71]

Spontaneous abortions treated in hospitals have been analyzed for members of the Union of Rubber and Leather Workers in Finland. The rubber workers' abortion frequencies did not appreciably differ when the pregnancy occurred during Union membership compared with pregnancies that occurred before or after membership.[72] The same results

Table V. Studies on the Association between Spontaneous Abortions and Employment
in the Chemicals, Plastics, or Rubber Industry[a]

Occupation or exposure	Association with exposure	Reference
Chemicals industry		
Carbon disulfide (viscose rayon industry)	(+)	Ehrhardt[63]
Ethylene oxide production workers	(+)	Jakubova et al.[38]
Pharmaceuticals workers in the Union of Chemical Workers	(+)	Hemminki et al[61,62]
Pharmaceuticals workers exposed to estrogens and many solvents	(+)	Taskinen et al.[64]
Chemicals industry	+	Vaughan et al.[58]
Plastics industry		
Phthalates	(+)	Aldyreva et al.[66]
Styrene (lamination workers)	(−)	Härkönen et al.[67]
Plastics and rubber production industry	+	Figa-Talamanca[14]
Polyurethane-processing industry	(+)	Lindbohm et al.[675]
Rubber industry		
Gluers in a rubber factory (petroleum, hydrocarbons)	(+)	Muhametova et al.[68]
Rubber workers (gasoline)	(+)	Beskrovnaja[69]
Rubber workers	(−)	Kestrup et al.[70]
Tire builders	(+)	Axelson et al.[71]
Footwearworkers (rubber chemicals)	(+)	Lindbohm et al.[73]
Members of the Union of Rubber and Leather Workers	−	Hemminki et al.[72]
2,4,5-T and TCDD	(+)	Smith[76], Longo[77], Santi et al.[78]

[a] See Table III for definition of symbols.

were observed among the workers of a Finnish rubber factory. A case-control study was done to investigate the effects of more specific exposures at the factory. A significantly increased odds ratio of abortions was observed among the workers exposed to rubber chemicals in the footwear department but not among those in the tire department.[73] These findings may be explained by the footwear workers' concomitant exposure to solvents, which could have aggravated the exposure to rubber chemicals.

In the studies cited, the numbers of pregnancies have often been small, potentially confounding factors have seldom been controlled, and spontaneous abortions have not been analyzed for more specific exposures or work processes. Possibly for these reasons, the results of the studies are conflicting. The need for further studies is obvious.

2.7. 2,4,5-T and TCDD

Animal studies have shown that dioxin 2,3,7,8-tetrachlorodibenzo-p-dioxin (TCDD) is teratogenic.[74,75] A significant increase in the number of spontaneous abortions has been reported among women in Oregon, an area where large quantities of 2,4,5-trichlorophenoxyacetic acid (2,4,5-T), an herbicide with low levels of TCDD, have been sprayed. Most of the abortions occurred during June and July, just after the peak spraying period.[76] Reports from Vietnam have also appeared that suggest increased abortion rates following spraying of the countryside with the herbicide called Agent Orange.[77] In Seveso, Italy, TCDD was dispersed over a wide area after an explosion in a chemicals factory. Significant upward trends in the number of spontaneous abortions have been reported in the more heavily contaminated areas for at least 18 months after the explosion.[78]

The observations on the effects of TCDD are based on a cluster of adverse effects or observations made on anticipated adverse effects that follow a hazardous exposure. More systematic studies on the effects of TCDD are needed to confirm these findings.

2.8. Other Occupational Groups

Two studies have used registered records to analyze simultaneously multiple associations between spontaneous abortions and a variety of occupations. Vaughan et al.[58] examined the birth records of multigravid women in the state of Washington. Statistically significant elevations in fetal death risk for the most recent pregnancy were found for chemical, metal, textile, wood, and farm workers and medical technicians. Flight attendants, therapists, pet store workers and veterinarians, hairdressers, and electronic technicians were also found to be at excess risk.

A Finnish study[12] grouped occupations into seven categories according to presumed exposure: solvents, metals, exhaust fumes, polycyclic aromatic hydrocarbons, other chemicals, textile dust, and animal microorganisms. The relative risks of spontaneous abortions were not significantly increased in any exposure group. As the womens' exposure was deduced from their occupations, it is possible that the heterogeneity of occupations with respect to exposure intensity diluted any possible effects. Analysis of detailed occupational categories showed some female occupations with an increased risk. After age, number of children, and place of residence had been controlled, spinners, fabric inspectors, and women in nonspecific occupations related to cutting and sewing had an increased abortion risk ($p < 0.10$) and weavers had a significantly increased risk ($p < 0.01$). In addition, butchers and sausagemakers, laboratory assistants, and workers caring for fur-bearing animals had significantly elevated risk.

A wide range of occupations has been explored also in a case-control study conducted among the patients of three New York City hospitals.[13] The investigators examined the association between occupation and the chromosomal characteristics of the aborted conceptus. Data on occupation were obtained by interview. Because of the small sample size, adjustment for potentially confounding factors was possible only when the data for the largest occupational groups were analyzed. Maternal employment as a cleaning service worker was associated with the abortion risk of a chromosomally normal conceptus (odds ratio adjusted for age and payment status 2.28; 95% CI 1.10, 4.75). No association was observed after adjustment between employment in a factory before pregnancy and any type of abortions. Bivariate analysis showed, however, that the unadjusted risk of abortions was significantly increased among women employed in the jewelry industry, the textile industry, and in other industry. Increased unadjusted risks were also found for several other occupations: transportation worker; food service worker; radiologic technician; wholesale representative and business salesperson; professional, administrator, owner, and manager; machine operator and physical laborer.

In all these studies, textile work was positively associated with spontaneous abortions. Vaughan *et al.*[58] reported a significantly increased risk for all textile workers, Kline *et al.*[13] for employment in the textile industry; in the Finnish study[12] the risk was increased in some separate textile occupations. Working with animals seemed to influence the risk in two studies, as pet store workers and veterinarians as well as workers caring for fur-bearing animals had an increased risk.

One weakness of all these studies is the nature of the "exposure" data. The analyses were based on occupational information; no details on the exposure were available. Another weakness is the multiple comparisons made. Statistically significant results may have been found by chance even if there had been no real associations between occupation and spontaneous abortions. The findings initially detected in these studies provide clues for future studies.

2.9. Air Pollution

Surveillance of the effects of environmental exposures affecting the general population has been carried out only in a few cases. Nordström et al.[79] examined the frequency of spontaneous abortions in populations located at different distances from a smelter in northern Sweden. The smelter emits a number of potentially genotoxic agents (e.g., lead, arsenic, and sulfur dioxide) into the environment. A statistically significant increase in the abortion rate was found in the population living within a distance of a few kilometers from the smelter when compared with a more distant population. The study did not control for employment in the smelter, however, making it impossible to distinguish the effects of inner and outer air pollution.

The association between the quality of ambient air and spontaneous abortions has also been analyzed in an industrialized Finnish community.[80] Maps provided by the Institute of Metereological Sciences were used to divide the community residents into groups according to the level of pollution in their residential area. The study provided no clear evidence that ambient air sulfur dioxide, hydrogen sulfide, or carbon disulfide could be associated with the risk of spontaneous abortion.

Investigations of the effects of chemicals in the ambient air face many problems. It is especially difficult to acquire valid exposure data that cover the entire study period and all the populations residing in different areas. It may also be hard to find a stable population large enough for a pregnancy outcome study. To date, epidemiologic evidence on the effects of air pollution on spontaneous abortions is deficient.

3. Environmental Chemicals and Malformations

3.1. Occupational and Social Correlates of Malformations

Several studies in different countries have suggested an association between socioeconomic factors and congenital malformations.[81-83] In Finland an analysis based on the data of the Finnish Register of Congenital Malformations[84] yielded an association between maternal occu-

Table VI. Studies on the Association between Congenital Malformations and
Occupation in Industry

Type of industry	Association with exposure[a]	Types of malformations	Reference
Reinforced plastics	(+)	CNS malformations	Holmberg[114]
Printing	+	Gatroschisis, omphalocele	Erickson[105]
Work in copper smelter	(+)		Nordström et al.[118]
Industrial and construction workers	+	CNS malformations, oral clefts	Hemminki et al.[84]

[a] +, Positive association. Signs are in parentheses (+) if the statistical test revealed only borderline significance, the sample size was small, or the study lacked a control group.

pation in industry and an increased risk of central nervous system (CNS) malformations in the offspring (OR 1,8, $p < 0.05$) (see Table VI). Multivariate analysis was used to control a number of confounding factors (e.g., maternal illnesses, medication, obstetric history, smoking, drinking, social factors). Occupation can be one of the factors underlying the social class gradient noted in the prevalence of malformations in some countries.

3.2. Health Care Personnel

3.2.1. Anesthesia Personnel

Many published studies have concerned the reproductive outcome of people exposed to anesthetic gases. Most investigations have been based on the selection of the exposed and nonexposed groups from professional or employment records, but exposure status has generally been defined according to the information obtained from the study subjects *via* questionnaires. The pregnancy outcome was determined from postal questionnaires in most studies. One study used a national delivery register,[85] the others hospital records.[34,35] The questionnaire response rates have ranged from 40 to 92%.

Many of the studies have found a correlation between maternal exposure and malformations in the offspring. Knill-Jones *et al.*,[20] Corbett *et al.*,[86] Cohen *et al.*,[22] Knill-Jones *et al.*[23] (in comparison with one control group only), Göthe and Hoffman[87] (for nonsmokers only), Pharoah *et al.*[27] (heart-great vessels defects), and Cohen *et al.*[26] (for light users of anesthetics only) showed statistically significant different prevalence rates between exposed and nonexposed subjects. Four of these studies controlled for potential confounders. In one investigation only a single agent, nitrous oxide, was associated with malformations.[26] The other studies showed no statistically significant differences.[19,21,29,34,87,88] The negative results obtained by Ericson and Källen[85] and by Hemminki *et al.*[35] are relevant, since outcome was assessed through objective sources. The risk ratio in the study conducted by Hemminki *et al.*[35] was 1.2 (95% confidence interval 0.3–4.6, *p* value 0.8), and it covered pregnancies between 1973 and 1979 in Finland.

The excesses of specific malformations were not systematic, as Corbett *et al.*[86] reported hemangiomas and inguinal hernias, Knill-Jones *et al.*[23] minor defects, Pharoah *et al.*[27] heart-great vessels defects, Rosenberg and Vänttinen[28] luxation of the hip and inguinal hernias, Tomlin[25] CNS and musculoskeletal defects, and Cohen *et al.*[26] musculoskeletal defects. Minor malformations are more susceptible to information bias[34]; i.e., an apparent excess may be attributable to higher participation and more accurate reporting by the exposed subjects. Taken together, most of the positive studies on anesthetic gases suffer from weaknesses in study design and execution that reduce the strength of the evidence on teratogenicity. The studies with improved design have had negative results, but they have also been recent and probably only surveyed populations exposed to relatively low levels of anesthetic gases (see Table VII).

Table VII. Studies on Congenital Malformations among the Offspring of Health Care Personnel[a]

Occupation or exposure	Association with exposure	Types of malformations	Reference
Anesthesia personnel	(±)		See text
Nurses using	(+)		Halling *et al.*[89]
hexachlorophene	(−)		Baltzar *et al.*[90,91]
Health personnel (registered nurses mainly)	+	Oral clefts	Erickson *et al.*[105]
Women employed in medical occupations	−		Baltzar *et al.*[90]
Nurses handling cytostatic drugs	+		Hemminki *et al.*[35]

[a] +, Positive association; −, no association. Signs are in parentheses (+) if the statistical test revealed only borderline significance, the sample size was small, or the study lacked a control group.

3.2.2. Other Hospital Exposures

Halling[89] compared the occurrence of malformations in six groups of nurses using 1% hexachlorophene soap and in six hospital-matched groups not using the soap. Pregnancy outcomes were retrieved from the records of obstetric departments. The exposure comprised 20–60 daily washings, both before and during the first trimester of pregnancy. No major malformations were found in 233 control births (versus four to five major malformations expected on the basis of national figures); 25 were found in 460 exposed births.

Baltzar *et al.*[90,91] published two separate studies done in order to reinvestigate such findings. In the first study, 63 hospitals were asked to provide lists of women employed in medical occupations who had left work because of childbirth in 1965–1975. At the same time the hospitals were asked whether hexachlorophene soap was used. Only 31 hospitals replied and provided data on approximately 1,500 women. They had all worked at least during late pregnancy. Malformed children were identified through registers that showed an excess in one area (Gothenburg) only, the area from which the cases described by Halling[89] also came. The second study[91] reported the outcome of 29,806 pregnancies among women employed in medical occupations during 1973–1975 as retrieved from the Medical Birth Record Register. A total of 1,551 defective children were born in the study group versus 1,491 expected; an excess in one area (Gothenburg) was detected again (42 observed, 29 expected; $p < 0.01$). No association was revealed between malformations and the use of hexachlorophene soaps in the particular hospitals (see Table VII).

The possible adverse effects of occupational exposure to antineoplastic drugs has been studied recently among hospital personnel preparing and administering them to the patients. Those studies have detected increased frequencies of sister chromatid exchanges,[92–94] chromosomal gaps,[94] and mutagenic agents in the urine.[95–98] After hygienic improvements (protective clothing and vertical-laminar flow hoods), the mutagenicity in the urine of those nurses was on the same level as that of the nonexposed controls.[99] There are also studies that did not find increased mutagenic activity in the urine[100] or increased frequencies of sister chromatid exchanges.[101]

Most common antineoplastic drugs have been found to be teratogenic and embryotoxic in animal tests at doses of 1–10 mg/kg. These results indicate moderate teratogenic potency (see Table VIII). Vinblastine, vincristine, and for one animal species (rat) also methotrexate have caused those effects at doses of 0.1–0.5 mg/kg, findings show high teratogenic and embryotoxic potency.[102] The doses used in human cancer therapy are mostly of about the former level, except vinblastine and chlorambucil, which are used in 0.05–0.2 mg/kg daily doses. The doses derived from occupational exposure are smaller than the therapeutic doses, but traces of antineoplastic drugs have been found in the urine of hospital personnel preparing the drugs for patients.[103,104]

The data on human teratogenicity consist of case reports and small series of patients treated with cytostatic drugs during or before pregnancy (see Table IX). An IARC working group considered methotrexate a human teratogen because of two similar malformation cases (deformities of the bones of the skull, hypertelorism, and limb-reduction defects) and cyclophosphamide to be a suspected teratogen because of two case reports of limb reductions.[102] Patient materials show evidence that many types of antineoplastic drug therapy during the first trimester of pregnancy increase the risk of malformations in the offspring. The studies on patients treated with antineoplastic drugs have some drawbacks, such as the small numbers of cases and the use of many different drugs or radiation, or both. The types of "abnormality" reported have also varied in different studies.

Very few reproductive studies have been done on personnel occupationally exposed to antineoplastic drugs. A case-control study has been carried out among hospital nurses collected from a central register on health personnel in Finland.[35] The case nurses, each of whom had a malformed child, were selected from the Register of Congenital Malformations; the controls for each case nurse were three nurses with a normal birth. Data on exposure were gathered through the head nurses of the hospitals. Handling of antineoplastic drugs at least once a week or more was associated with malformations in the offspring (eight cases, odds ratio 4.7, $p = 0.02$, 95% confidence limits 1,2–18,1). There were two malformations of the ear, face and neck, one of the heart, one of the urinary organs, and four of the limbs.

A study based on the Metropolitan Atlanta Congenital Defects Surveillance Program of the Centers for Disease Control (CDC) detected an increased risk of delivering an infant with cleft lip among women working in the health field, mainly registered nurses.[105] This finding conflicts with the Swedish study, described above, which did not find any increased risk of congenital malformations among women employed in medical occupations.[90]

3.3. Laboratory Work and Solvents

Many epidemiologic studies have suggested that exposure to solvents is associated with teratogenic risks; some studies have not dem-

Table VIII. Teratogenicity of Antineoplastic Agents According to an IARC (1981) Working Group

Agent	Animal tests	Doses used in therapy	Level of human evidence
5-Azacytidine	Teratogenic (mice 1–1.5 mg/kg) at doses nontoxic to the dam; embryolethal	3.7–4.9 mg/kg per day	No data
Azathioprine	Embryolethal at doses nontoxic to the dam (1–20 mg/kg); severe teratogenic effects in several animal species (doses 10–30 mg/kg or a single dose of 50 mg/kg)	1–3 to 2–5 mg/kg per day	Crosses the placenta; reduces birth weight; data insufficient to evaluate teratogenic potential
BCNU (bis-chloroethyl nitrosourea)	Teratogenic at doses 1–4 mg/kg to rats, 0.4–4 mg/kg to rabbits; embryolethal and fetolethal	100–250 mg/m² body surface	No data
Bleomycins	No data	10–20 mg/m², total dose 300–400 mg (~200 mg/m²)	No data
Chlorambucil	Teratogenic to several animal species (to rat at doses 6–12 mg/kg; to mice at 5–6 mg/kg); embryolethal at doses nontoxic to the dam	0.1–0.2 mg/kg per day or 10–20 mg/day for 2-week courses	Insufficient data
CCNU [1-(2-chloroethyl)-3-cyclohexyl-1-nitrosourea]	Teratogenic to rats at doses of 2–8 mg/kg (during organogenesis)	130 mg/m² as a single dose every 6 weeks	No data
Cisplatin	Embryolethal to mice at doses 3–13 mg/kg; data on teratogenicity limited—not evaluated	50–120 mg/m² as a single dose every 4 weeks	No data
Cyclophosphamide	Teratogenic in several species (to rhesus monkey at doses 2.5–20 mg/kg); embryolethal at doses nontoxic to the dam	10–15 mg/kg thrice weekly or 1–5 mg/kg per day	Two cases of limb-reduction defects reported
Dacarbazine	Teratogenic to rats at a single dose 200–1000 mg/kg or 30–70 mg/kg per day; to rabbits at dose 10 mg/kg per day	2.4–5 mg/kg daily for 10 days, repeated after intervals of 4 weeks	No data

Drug	Animal data	Human dose	Human risk
5-Fluorouracil	Teratogenic to several animal species (golden hamster at doses 3–9 mg per day per animal; mice at a single dose of 20–30 mg/kg); embryotoxic to rhesus monkey at doses of 20–40 mg/kg	500 mg/m² per day for 5 days of a 4–6 weeks cycle or 12–15 mg/kg per day for 5–6 days, then 12–15 mg once a week	Insufficient
Isophosphamide	Teratogenic to mice at 20 mg/kg		No data
6-Mercaptopurine	Teratogenic to several animal species (rat at doses of 50–75 mg/kg; mice 0.5–1 mg/kg; rabbit 1 mg/kg); embryolethal at doses nontoxic to the dam	2.5 mg/kg per day	Insufficient
Methotrexate	Teratogenic to several species (mice at a single dose of 25 or 50 mg/kg; rabbit 19.2 mg/kg; rat 0.2–0.3 mg/kg); embryolethal at doses nontoxic to the dam	5 mg/day for 10 days	Teratogen (case report 1: dose 2.5 mg/day for 5 days at 9th week; case report 2: 5 mg/day during first 2 months: abnormalities in the bones of the skull, limb reduction defects, and hypertelorism in both cases)
Treosulphan	No data	1–1.25 g/day for 4 weeks; then 500 mg/day	No data
Vinblastine sulfate	Teratogenic to several animal species (mice 0.35 mg/kg; rat: 0.025 mg single dose and 0.25 mg/kg per day); embryolethal at doses nontoxic to the dam	0.05 mg/kg per week	Insufficient
Vincristine sulfate	Teratogenic in several animal species (mice: 0.25–0.35 mg/kg single dose; golden hamster 0.1–0.5 mg/kg; single dose; rhesus monkey: 0.15–0.20 mg/kg single dose); embryolethal in doses nontoxic to the dam	Adults 1.4 mg/m², children 2.0 mg/m² once a week (or children 0.05–0.15 mg/kg once a week)	Insufficient

Table IX. Studies on Pregnancy Outcome in Patients Treated with Cytostatic Drugs

Reference	Medication	Findings
Cote *et al.*[186]	Prednisone and azathioprine *during* pregnancy (case report)	Transient (in 15 weeks) immunosuppression of the offspring
Holmes and Holmes[187]	Chemotherapy alone, radiotherapy alone or in combination in treatment for Hodgkin's disease *before* pregnancy	5 of 9 abnormal offspring in the group treated with chemotherapy and irradiation ($p < 0.047$)
McKeen *et al.*[188]	Chemotherapy or radiotherapy *during* pregnancy (Hodgkin's disease)	Chemotherapy during first trimester: 2 of 4 malformations; chemotherapy during second or third trimester: 2 of 2 normal offspring; radiotherapy during first trimester: 2 of 2 abnormal offspring (inner ear deafness; learning difficulties)
	Chemotherapy *before* pregnancy	3 of 23 (7.5%) malformed offspring of live births
	Pregnancies *before* therapy	1 of 17 (6%) malformed offspring of live births
Horning *et al.*[189]	Chemotherapy, radiotherapy, or both (Hodgkin's disease) *before* pregnancy	No malformations among 24 pregnancies
Rusting *et al.*[190]	Chemotherapy *before* pregnancy (gestational tumours)	Slight excess of congenital abnormality—not significant

onstrated any special risk (see Table X). A possible relationship between the syndrome of caudal regression, or sacrococcygeal agenesis, and exposure to organic solvents during pregnancy was reported by Kucera.[106] Six of nine mothers who had a child with sacral agenesis had been exposed to chemicals during pregnancy; five of these women had been exposed to organic solvents, such as acetone, trichloroethylene, methyl chloride, xylene, and petrol. One mother had also been exposed to tanning agents. One had only been exposed to aniline dyes, but her exposure had been constant. One of the exposed mothers had diabetes mellitus, as did one of the nonexposed mothers. One of the nine mothers had neither a known exposure to chemicals nor a reported disease. Maternal age (mean 23.4 years) was unrelated to the syndrome. The

Table X. Studies on the Association between Congenital Malformations and Maternal Occupation in Laboratory Work or Occupational Solvent Exposure

Occupation or exposure	Association with exposure[a]	Type of malformations	Reference
Hospital laboratory	−		Baltzar et al.[91]
University laboratory	+	Intestinal atresias or stenosis	Meirik et al.[107]
Laboratories in the pharmaceuticals industry	(+)		Hansson et al.[46]
Laboratories in the pulp and paper industry	+		Blomqvist et al.[108]
Laboratory work	+	Gastrointestinal atresias	Ericson et al.[109]
Laboratory work	(−)		Olsen[116]
Laboratory work	+		Ericson et al.[110]
University laboratories	−		Axelsson et al.[48]
Solvents	(+)	Sacral agenesis	Kucera[106]
Styrene, acetone	(+)		Holmberg[114]
Solvents	+	Central nervous system malformations	Holmberg[111]
Solvents	+	Oral clefts	Holmberg et al.[113]

[a] +, Positive association; −, no association. Signs are in parentheses (+) and (−) if the statistical test revealed only borderline significance, the sample size was small, or the study lacked a control group.

cases had occurred randomly in time, from 1959 to 1966, in Czechoslovakia. The major drawback of the study was that no control group had been used.

Several studies on women working in laboratories have been conducted by a Swedish group. A study on female laboratory staff of Uppsala University found a significant increase in the malformation rate, which mainly referred to serious malformations (among 245 pregnancies, 11 observed malformation cases versus 4 expected, $p < 0.01$).[107] Malformations included four cases of intestinal atresia or stenosis (less than 1 per 1000 expected) and three cases of clubfoot. The information on malformations was checked against the Swedish Malformation Register or against hospital records. Data on laboratory work during pregnancy were gathered from employer files and partly by interviews. Control mothers had worked in the same laboratories but not during their pregnancies. Although the cohort was small, the authors concluded that the results suggest the existence of unidentified hazards to the embryo in laboratory work.

In another Swedish cohort study, women working in chemical laboratories in the pharmaceuticals industry had more children with major malformations (5.6%) than did the control group (0.7%). Malformations included two oral clefts and one gut atresia.[46] The age distributions of the study and control groups were similar. The cluster of abnormal births (including two major malformations in the total of 35 infants) that initiated the study was included. Their inclusion probably did not bias the study, as the rate is still high after these cases are eliminated.

Women working in laboratories of the Swedish pulp and paper industry were studied by Blomqvist *et al.*,[108] who found an excess of serious malformations (6 versus 2.9 expected, standardized for age, parity, and hospital of delivery). Malformations included two gut atresias, two heart defects, one anencephaly, and one cleft palate. This study also included two women from the original cluster of abnormal pregnancies that initiated the study. Their inclusion may have biased the result. Blomqvist and co-workers summarized the data from this paper and some earlier studies done with the same design by the same group,[107,46] concluding that there is a total increase in malformation rate among the infants of female laboratory workers for the incidence of two types of malformation: cleft lip/palate and gut atresia.

The same Swedish group further investigated the possible relationship between gastrointestinal (GI) atresia and maternal work during pregnancy in laboratories.[109] Laboratory work was reported to occur more often (7 of 164, 4.3%) among case mothers than among controls (5 of 364, 1.4%). Although this study confirmed the prior findings, the investigators concluded that the excess risk is probably not very great.

Ericson *et al.*[110] studied the delivery outcome of female laboratory workers from the Swedish census. In that cohort of 1161 women, there was a significant increase in the number of infants with major malformations, but only two children had GI atresia, and only three had cleft lip or palate. The cohort was too small to study the possible relation between gut atresia or facial clefts and maternal laboratory work. Within the cohort, a case-control study was done on type of work and possible exposures. No specific type of laboratory or laboratory work was more common among cases than among controls. The case group stated more specific exposures per woman than did the control group, but no difference in exposure to specific agents (e.g., organic solvents) could be demonstrated. According to Ericson and colleagues, it is possible that the multiple and complex chemical exposures, rather than exposure to one specific chemical, during laboratory work may be harmful to the offspring during pregnancy. Table XI summarizes the results of the Swedish studies.

In a Finnish case-control study on CNS malformations, exposure to

Table XI. Summary of the Studies of the Swedish Group on Infants Born to Women
Working in Chemicals Laboratories during Pregnancy

Type of laboratory	Infants (N)	Major malformations (N)	Major malformations (%)	Oral cleft (N)	Gut atresia (N)	Reference
Pharmaceuticals industry	103	6	(5.8)	2	1	Hansson et al.[46]
Uppsala University	245	11	(4.5)	1	4	Meirik et al.[107]
Pulp and paper industry	162	6	(3.7)	1	2	Blomqvist et al.[108]
Laboratory workers from the census	1161	28	(2.4)	3	2	Ericson et al.[110]
Total	1671	51	(3.1)	7	9	

various organic solvents was found to be overrepresented: 14 case mothers versus 3 control mothers; after reanalysis, when the data on exposure were reevaluated, 12 versus 6.[111,112] Another case-control study on mothers of children born with oral clefts showed that significantly more case mothers than control mothers had been exposed to organic solvents during the first trimester of pregnancy.[113] The information on exposures in these studies was collected retrospectively by personal interview, and the exposure classes were formed according to an industrial hygienist's estimation.

Exposure to solvents is one common factor in some industrial areas for which an increased risk of malformations among the offspring of women workers has been reported. In Finland a case-control study revealed two cases of CNS defects in children of mothers working in the reinforced plastic industry; less than one was expected.[114] The women had been exposed at work to a combination of styrene, polyester resin, organic peroxides, and acetone. However, no new cases exposed to styrene have been noted since.

A report from Atlanta,[105] based on the Congenital Defects Surveillance Program of the Metropolitam Area, noted an increased risk of gastroschisis and omphalocele in the offspring of mothers employed in the printing industry. This increase was not found in a Finnish study.[115]

No excess risk of malformations in the offspring of female hospital laboratory staff was found in a wide survey of women employed in medical occupations in Sweden.[90] A recent study among personnel employed in laboratory work at Gothenburg University did not reveal an excess risk of congenital malformations in the 1027 deliveries of 745 women.[48] In Denmark, Olsen[116] did not find a statistically significant excess risk in his study on malformations among the offspring of women employed in laboratory occupations.

In some studies organic solvents have been suspected of being the harmful agents present in laboratory environments. The complex and multiple exposures involved in laboratory work may contribute to the hazardous effects on the offspring of pregnant workers. Although the specific harmful agents have not been identified, the WHO meeting on Women and Occupational Health Risks[117] concluded that there is evidence of a likely association between laboratory work during pregnancy and malformations in the offspring.

3.4. Metals Industry

Nordström *et al.*[118] studied the incidence of malformations among the offspring of Swedish copper smelter workers. The possible exposures were lead, arsenic, cadmium, and sulfur dioxide. Information on employment (1955–1976) was obtained from the company, the information on pregnancy outcome from the local hospital records. The paper does not describe the completeness of the follow-up study. The women who had been working at the smelter during their pregnancies had more malformed children (17 of 291, 5.8%) than did women not employed at the smelter (22 of 1000, 2.2%); the difference was statistically significant ($p < 0.0005$). Multiple malformations in particular contributed to this difference (see Table VI).

3.5. Methylmercury

The embryotoxicity of methylmercury was confirmed in studies that examined the effects of food poisoning.[119–121] These studies include the well-known epidemic in Minamata, Japan,[121] describing disorders in adults who had ingested fish contaminated with methylmercury. A few years later, affected children were found who had symptoms resembling those of cerebral palsy. Between 1953 and 1971, at least 25 children were born with brain damage. After systematic research, a syndrome was delineated and linked to the mothers' ingestion of fish contaminated with alkylmercury. Maternal intake of about 1 mg methylmercury per day resulted in a risk of about 6% of offspring being affected by cerebral palsy.[119,121]

A similar epidemic of microcephaly and other neurologic disorders occurred in Iraq in 1972, as the result of the ingestion of grain treated

with methylmercury.[122,123] Of 32 infants exposed *in utero,* 10 showed
cerebral palsy at the age of 1 year. In Iraq as well as in Minamata, mercury
was found in biologic samples from the affected mothers and children,
thereby confirming the exposure. Dose–response relationships have been
established (e.g., daily maternal exposure to 1–1.2 mg/kg conveyed a
50% risk of neurologic symptoms in the offspring).[124] The observations
from Minamata and Iraq have also been confirmed in other small series
of cases from the U.S.S.R., Sweden, and the United States[119,118,125] (see
Table XII).

**Table XII. Studies on the Association between Congenital Malformations and
Occupational and Environmental Exposures**

Exposure	Association with exposure[a]	Types of malformations	Reference
Methylmercury	+		Snyder[125]
	+	Microcephaly neurologic disorders,	Amin-Zaki et al.[122,123]
	+	cerebral palsy, brain damage	Reviewed by Koos and Longo,[119] Harada[121]
	+		Chang et al.[118]
Polychlorinated biphenyls	+		Miller[127]
(Kanechlor)	+		Kuratsune[128]
	+		Yamashita[129]
2,4,5-T and TCDD	(+)	Down's syndrome	Tung et al.,[153] Rose and Rose,[154] Honoroff[155]
		Two malformed infants	Advisory Committee[156]
		Spina bifida (2 cases)	Sare and Forbes[157]
	(+)	Anencephaly, oral clefts, clubfoot, and hydrocephaly	Cutting et al.[158]
	(+)	Oral clefts	Brogan et al.[165]
	(+)		Bruzzi et al.[166]
	−		Roan and Morgan[160]
	−		McQueen et al.[161]
	(−)		Hanify et al.[162]
	−		Field and Kerr[163]
	−		Thomas[164]

(continued)

Table XII. (*Continued*)

Exposure	Association with exposure[a]	Types of malformations	Reference
Vinyl chloride	(+)		Infante[167]
	−		Edmonds[168]
	(+)		Edmonds[169]
Potato blight	(+)	Anencephaly,	Renwick[131,132]
	−	spina bifida	Several studies (see text)[133–141]
	−		Roberts *et al.*[142]
	−		Clarke *et al.*[143]
	−		Spiers *et al.*[144]
	−		Nevin and Merret[145]
Soft water	+		Fedrick[146]
	−		Several studies (see text)[147–150]
	−		St. Leger *et al.*[151]
	−		Elwood and Goldman[152]
Water fluoridation	+	Down's syndrome	Berry[171]
	−		Rapaport[170]
	−		Needleman *et al.*[173]
	−		Erickson *et al.*[172]
	−		Knox *et al.*[174]
	−		Erickson[175]

[a] +, Positive association; −, no association. Signs are in parentheses (+) and (−) if the statistical test revealed only borderline significance, the sample size was small, or the study lacked a control group.

3.6. Kanechlor (Polychlorinated Biphenyls)

A PCB-induced fetopathy (Yusho) was detected as a feature of food poisoning that had occurred in 1968 in Japan. Some 1000 persons of all ages were accidentally intoxicated by rice oil contaminated with Kanechlor 400, a technical tetrachlorobiphenyl product. The Yusho oil contained about 1000 ppm of PCBs and 5 ppm of polychlorinated dibenzofurans, and it is impossible to ascribe the effects found specifically to any one component.[126] The etiologic role of the ingestion of this oil was ascertained for intoxicated persons through (1) examination of oil containers, the shipping records of the producing company, and the records of oil dealers; (2) analysis of biologic samples; and (3) a case-control study of 121 adult patients and 121 adult controls on their use of oil and fats.[127]

The fetotoxic effect of Kanechlor was first recognized when 11 intoxicated mothers and two unaffected wives of patients delivered 13 infants with a syndrome that included dark brown pigmentation of the skin and mucous membranes, retarded growth, gingival hyperplasia, and spotted calcification of the skull.[127-129] Hyperkeratosis, atrophy of the skin, and cystic dilatation of hair follicles were described in stillborn babies delivered by exposed mothers.[127,128] PCBs were detected in the skin by chromatography. The intake of PCBs were estimated at 65–839 μg/day[130] (see Table XII).

3.7. Potato Blight

Renwick[131,132] reported a positive geographic correlation between the ingestion of spoiled potato (potato blight) and the prevalence of anencephaly–spina bifida, but more recent correlation studies have failed to support the finding.[133-141]

Analytic epidemiologic studies have been published as well. Roberts et al.[142] interviewed the mothers of 336 malformed babies (neural tube defects) and as many normal controls in Glamorghan, South Wales. They found no difference in the consumption of home-grown potatoes between the cases and the controls. In another case-control study that estimated potato consumption during pregnancy,[143] 83 children with spina bifida were compared with 85 children chosen from the general population and matched for sex, month and year of birth, residence, and social class. No difference in maternal potato consumption during pregnancy was found between cases and controls.

Negative results were also reported in a case-control study from New York City,[144] in which 265 mothers of infants with anencephaly–spina bifida and 549 control mothers were interviewed by telephone on their current potato consumption. An intervention study by Nevin and Merret[145] on 88 pregnant women who had a previous infant with anencephaly–spina bifida and who were advised to avoid eating potatoes in subsequent pregnancies also had negative results.

Thus, studies on potato blight or the consumption of potato do not support a potato-related etiology of anencephaly–spina bifida (see Table XII).

3.8. Soft Water

Fedrick[146] reported an inverse correlation between water hardness and the prevalence of anencephaly in 10 areas in the United Kingdom, but this finding conflicts with the results of many subsequent correlation studies.[147-150]

Two case-control studies have also been negative. The one in Cardiff included 108 cases of neural tube defects and as many controls matched for sex, age, and social class. The determination of eleven elements in the drinking water failed to reveal any difference between the cases and the controls.[151] Another case-control study in Canada included 468 deaths from anencephaly and a random sample of 4129 live births.[152] The mothers lived in 142 localities for which the water concentration of 14 elements was known. No association was found for any of the 14 elements. The risk estimates had been adjusted for potential confounding factors (parity, season and year of birth, maternal age, and others).

In summary, the suggestion that soft water is a causal factor of malformations has been proved incorrect by subsequent negative studies (Table XII).

3.9. 2,4,5-T and TCDD

The pesticide 2,4,5-T contains other chlorination products such as dioxins, of which TCDD is the best known super toxin. It is not possible to discern exposure to 2,4,5-T from exposure to contaminant chlorination products. Some publications on the effects of 2,4,5-T are case reports (Table XII). Tung *et al.*[153] described four pregnant women who had been hit by herbicide sprays in Vietnam: Two mothers had children with Down's syndrome. Other anecdotal reports about Vietnam have been published by Rose and Rose[154] and Honoroff.[155] Two cases of malformed infants were described in Lapland; their malformation was attributed to phenoxy herbicide spraying.[156] In New Zealand a report by Sare and Forbes[157] described two infants with spina bifida born to mothers exposed to 2,4,5-T spraying during pregnancy.

The other publications described more formal epidemiologic studies. Cutting *et al.*[158] surveyed malformations retrospectively in 22 hospitals in South Vietnam, as reported on the Daily Summaries prepared by midwives. Private clinics were not surveyed, some hospital records had been destroyed, home deliveries were excluded, as was the Chinese minority of the population. The prevalence rates were 5.5 per 1000 in 1960–1965 (light spraying of Agent Orange) and 4.5 per 1000 in 1966–1969 (heavy spraying). Overall, 2355 defects in 488,852 births were identified. Anencephaly, cleft lip or palate, clubfoot, and hydrocephaly accounted for 80% of all malformations. Heavily sprayed areas were apparently underrepresented, however, and there was no precise knowledge of the pregnant women's exposure.[159]

Roan and Morgan[160] carried out an epidemiologic study based on the hospital records in the areas near Globe, Arizona, where 2,4,5-T had been massively sprayed. The analytic measurements of tissues and fluids were all negative. The authors found no trends in perinatal mortality that could be attributed to the herbicide.

In a geographic correlation study on 2,4,5-T spraying in New Zealand, McQueen et al.[161] collected cases of anencephaly and spina bifida in three areas where clusters of cases had allegedly occurred. The authors found no connection between 2,4,5-T and the birth defects. Hanify et al.[162] compared the prevalence rates of malformations in seven New Zealand areas during 1960–1966, when no exposure to 2,4,5-T occurred, and during 1972–1976, when 2,4,5-T spraying was common. The quantity, dates, and places of spraying were determined from data supplied by the companies. No geographic or temporal correlation could be found, with the possible exceptions of the cases of talipes and hypospadias/ epispadias. Other studies found no evidence of a correlation between birth defects and 2,4,5-T spraying in Australia[163] or Hungary.[164] A further correlation study in western Australia suggested a role of "insecticides" and "herbicides" in the occurrence of cleft lip palate but provided no firm evidence.[165]

A Birth Defect Registry survey in the Seveso area in Italy, which was highly polluted by TCDD in 1976, collects data on malformations in 11 towns (222,000 residents) from the lists of live births and stillbirths seen by pediatricians.[166] The Registry area was divided into four zones according to the TCDD concentrations in the soil: A (most polluted), B, R, and Out (least or not polluted). The rates were compared with regional Lombardy hospital records and other birth defect registries. In comparison with the Lombardy hospital records, elevated rate ratios (RR) were found for spina bifida (RR = 2, $p = 0.1$) and hypospadias (RR = 13.5, $p < 0.0001$). In addition, the rate ratio for other anomalies in the zones A + B versus R + Out was 6.6. These findings have been reported as preliminary results. It remains to be seen whether the working group can exclude the contribution of detection bias due to greater diagnostic accuracy and reporting in the highly polluted areas.

3.10. Vinyl Chloride

Infante[167] analyzed the birth certificates for 1970–1973 in Ohio communities in an investigation of whether the local vinyl chloride polymerization (PCV) industry increased the prevalence of birth defects. The prevalence rates of birth defects (per 1000 live births) were 10.14 for the entire state of Ohio, 17.37 for Asthabula, 18.10 for Painesville, and 20.33 for Avon Lake (the three communities with vinyl chloride polymerization plants). The excess in the three communities was statistically significant ($p < 0.01$). However, similar prevalence rates were found also in two other cities without vinyl chloride polymerization plants. The excess cases of central nervous system defects came mainly from Painesville (with vinyl chloride polymerization facilities) and from North Ridgeville (without such facilities).

A case-control study was subsequently conducted by Edmonds *et al.*[168] in Ohio. All infants born with CNS malformations in the Painesville hospital in 1970–1974 (six with anencephaly and nine with spina bifida) were compared with a group of 30 control infants (the first infant born immediately before and the first immediately after the case). The parents of the cases were interviewed, whereas information for the controls was collected from the clinical records. None of the 15 case parents and two of the 30 control parents worked in vinyl chloride polymerization plants; more control mothers than cases mothers worked within 10 miles of the Painesville polymerization plant.

Another case-control study was conducted by Edmonds *et al.*[169] in Kanawna County, Ohio. Incident cases of CNS malformations were compared with a group of control infants identified as in the previous study and matched for paternal education, maternal age, month of birth, race, and social status. The parents were interviewed by telephone about their work in vinyl chloride polymerization plants and place of residence. Two of 41 case fathers and two of 41 control fathers worked in such plants at the time of conception; none of 41 case fathers and three of 41 control fathers worked in polymerization plants with a contract work before conception. More cases than controls lived within 3 miles of the polymerization facilities ($p < 0.02$) (see Table XII).

Studies on communities with vinyl chloride polymerization plants are somewhat contradictory. For unexplained reasons, however, residence close to a vinyl chloride polymerization plant may correlate with the likelihood of bearing a malformed child.

3.11. Water Fluoridation

Rapaport[170] assessed the prevalence rates of Down's syndrome in Illinois towns divided into three categories of fluoridation levels and reported a positive correlation, but two other investigations failed to show such correlations.[171,172] Only Erickson's paper number took maternal age into account. In another study,[173] the prevalence rates of Down's syndrome were very similar in 30 towns before fluoridation and after fluoridation. Maternal age and temporal trends of Down's syndrome were taken into account in the prefluoridation–postfluoridation comparison.

A further study dealt with congenital malformation patterns before and after the introduction of fluoride in Birmingham, England.[174] The minor changes in the prevalence of malformations were attributed to demographic changes or to modified ascertainment and classification. The authors' conclusion is that there was no evidence of an association. Similarly, an American study that adjusted for maternal age found no difference in the prevalence rates of birth defects in cities with and without fluoridated water suppliers.[175] In summary, there is no epidemiologic evidence to support that water fluoridation is a cause of congenital malformations (Table XII).

4. Parental Occupation and Cancer in the Offspring

Malignancies constitute one of the leading causes of childhood mortality in industrialized countries. They include leukemias, brain tumors, neuroblastomas, kidney tumors, lymphomas, and tumors at other sites. The incidence is usually the highest in the first year of life and declines thereafter.[176] The age-specific incidence rate in the first year is 22.3 in a population of 10^5 for boys and 17.6 in 10^5 for girls in Finland. Compared with other industrialized countries, the incidence is also relatively high in the Scandinavian countries in the young age groups (under 5 years). The incidence is 18.8 in 10^5 for boys and 12.8 in 10^5 for girls under 5 years of age in the Connecticut cancer register, quite similar to the incidence figures in Utah, Birmingham, England, and the German Democratic Republic.[176]

The incidence of all childhood cancer has increased slightly over the two past decades in Finland. This increase is almost entirely attributable to an increased incidence in the youngest age groups (under 5 years). The change in incidence in the youngest age group (under 1 year) is particularly striking—more than double for boys and less than double for girls in two decades.[176] During 1966–1977, the increased incidence of childhood cancer is mainly due to an increase in brain tumors in very young children (under 1 year). The apparent increase in brain tumors can also be confirmed by comparison with earlier incidence data from Finland. We cannot exclude the possibility that the increased incidence is partly due to improved diagnosis for very young patients. An increased incidence of childhood cancer has been noted also in Sweden, Denmark, and England over the past three decades, but the sites of increase have not been confined to brain tumors.

Epidemiologic studies suggest a number of risk factors for childhood cancer. They include factors associated with the child and his or her environment, with the mother during pregnancy, and with the father or the mother before conception. The nonoccupational risk factors include the ingestion of diethylstilbestrol (DES), X-ray irradiation, viral infections during pregnancy, the mother's history of abortions, Down's syndrome in the child, cancer in the sibs, and low social class.[176]

Parental occupations have recently attracted a number of studies, stimulated by the study of Fabia and Thuy,[5] who reported that paternal exposure to hydrocarbons was associated with a cancer process in the offspring. Most subsequent studies have only investigated paternal occupations and/or exposures, thus searching for an effect mediated by germ cells. It is unfortunate that most studies have merely tested the hypothesis on hydrocarbon-related risks and have overlooked all other types of exposures that their data may have shown. *Hydrocarbon* is an extremely broad term chemically: It encompasses compounds and classes of compounds the biologic effects of which are dissimilar. It should be a requirement that the search for germ cell mediated effects considers mutagenic compounds only. As the term hydrocarbon includes both mutagens and nonmutagens, it is not an appropriate class of chemicals for consideration.

The 11 studies that analyze parental effects are listed in Table XIII. Five of these studies have detected some association with hydrocarbon-related paternal occupations, whereas six have not. The odds ratios have generally been small, 2–3, thereby showing that any risk at the level of such broad occupational definitions is relatively small. Such nonspecific occupational classification may miss truly exposed individuals. If these individuals, who probably represent a small subgroup of the occupational categories used, contribute to the excess, their risk may be substantial. Studies relating to specific exposure would help to resolve these controversies.

Maternal exposures directly relevant to this review as transplacental effects may also be noted in such studies. Only three studies, however, addressed the question of maternal occupational exposure and cancer in offspring (Table XIII). The studies have been exploratory and have not identified uniform maternal risk occupations. It is curious that our study[177] and the recent Dutch study[178] identified some occupational categories where true chemical exposures may have taken place.

The field of childhood cancer and occupation has many methodologic difficulties, as reviewed by Gold *et al.*,[6] who list the essential diffi-

Table XIII. Parental Occupation and Cancer in the Offspring

Cancer data	Source of occupational data	Findings	Reference
(N = 386) Fathers of Quebec children under 5 years of age who died from cancer in 1965–1970	Birth certificates (paternal occupations at time of birth)	Excess of cases with fathers in hydrocarbon-related occupations (motor vehicle mechanics, machinists, miners, and painters) compared with controls (OR = 2.1)	Fabia and Thuy[5]
(N = 852) Fathers of incident cancer cases, Finland Cancer Registry, 1959–1986	Records of maternity welfare centers (paternal occupation at time of conception)	No significant associations between childhood cancer and hydrocarbon-related occupations	Hakulinen et al.[172]
(N = 149) Fathers of incident Wilms' tumor cases from the Connecticut Tumor Registry, 1935–1973	Birth certificates	Significant excess of cases with fathers in lead-related occupations (OR = 5.0); no significant excess of cases with fathers in hydrocarbon-related occupations	Kantor et al.[180]
(N = 692) Fathers of children born in Massachusetts in 1947–1957 and 1963–1967 who died of cancer before age 15	Birth certificates	Significant excess of paternal employment as paper or pulp mill worker and children with tumors of the brain and nervous system (OR = 2.8); significant excess of paternal exposure as mechanic or machinist and children with urinary tract tumors (OR = 2.5); no significant association between hydrocarbon-related occupations and childhood cancer	Kwa and Fine[181]

(continued)

Table XIII. (*Continued*)

Cancer data	Source of occupational data	Findings	Reference
(N = 296) Fathers and mothers of children with cancer at Texas Children's Hospital Research Hematology Clinic in 1976–1977	Interviews including inquiries about occupation in the interval from the year before the birth of the child through the year of diagnosis	No association between hydrocarbon-related occupations and childhood cancer for any case-control comparison	Zack et al.[182]
(N = 92) Parents of patients with brain tumors under 10 years of age identified from 1972 to 1977 by the Los Angeles County Cancer Surveillance Program	Telephone interviews inquiring about occupation during the interval from a year before pregnancy through lactation and time of diagnosis of the case	Significant excess of maternal exposure to chemicals and childhood cancer (OR = 2.8); significant excess of paternal exposure to solvents (OR = 2.8) or paternal occupation in the aircraft industry and childhood cancer (OR = ∞)	Peters et al.[183]
(N = 1730 mothers, fathers) Parents of incident cancer patients in children under 15 years of age from the Finland Cancer Registry, 1959–1975	Pregnancy records of maternity welfare centers (parental occupation at the time of pregnancy)	Significant positive associations between childhood cancer and maternal occupation as pharmacist (OR = 3.2), factory worker (OR = 2.3), or baker (OR = 2.4); significant positive associations between childhood cancer and paternal occupation as farmer (OR = 1.2), motor vehicle driver (OR = 1.3), or painter (OR = 2.8)	Hemminki et al.[177]

(N = 4395) Fathers of all children dying from neoplasms in England and Wales in 1959–1963	Child's death certificate (paternal occupation at the time of the child's death)	Suggestive association between kidney tumors and hydrocarbon-related occupations (PMR = 119); significant excess of cancer among children of fathers with professional occupations (PMR = 132)	Sanders *et al.*[184]
(N = 2525) Fathers of all children dying from neoplasms in England and Wales in 1970–1972	Child's death certificate (paternal occupation at time of the child's death)	Suggestive association between kidney tumors and hydrocarbon-related occupations, (PMR = 114); significant excess of cancer among children of fathers with professional occupations (PMR = 125)	Sanders *et al.*[184]
(N = 113) Fathers of Baltimore Area children under 20 years of age with diagnosed leukemia in 1969–1974 or with brain tumors in 1965–1974	Personal view of the mothers; father's occupation before and after birth	More motor vehicle and hydrocarbon-related occupations as compared with controls with cancer but not as compared with normal controls	Gold *et al.*[6]
(N = 60) Fathers of children with leukemia diagnosed under 1 year of age and reported to the New York State Tumor Registry	Personal interview of the mothers; father's exposure to gasoline exhaust fumes for at least a year before the birth	High-exposure occupations (gas station attendants, car repairmen, aircraft maintenance) in excess (OR = 2.4–2.5)	Vianna *et al.*[185]
(N = 519) Parents of children with acute leukemia diagnosed in Holland in 1973–1980 based on a register	Postal questionnaire	During pregnancy more mothers, but not fathers, worked in hydrocarbon-related occupations (OR = 2.5)	van Steewsel-Moe *et al.*[178]

[a] OR, odds ratio; PMR, proportional mortality ratio.

culties as "small sample size, lack of validation of employment history, lack of detail and validation of occupational exposure, inadequate information regarding critical time of exposure and latency, lack of detailed information on the role of maternal occupational exposure, multiple comparisons resulting in statistical significance, and insufficient information regarding whether specific cell types of malignancies are particularly associated with increased risk." With such formidable methodologic problems, we must not be too optimistic in using childhood cancer as an indicator of a specific chemical exposure. Incidence trends should still be monitored, however, and studies on environmental factors should be conducted with large population samples.

5. Conclusions

Reproductive and childhood cancer epidemiology has only recently attracted concentrated research effort. The field is now at the stage where relevant outcomes have been investigated and study designs validated. It had become apparent that these studies pose a number of special problems in epidemiology, such as the rarity, recurrence, and sensitivity of events, voluntary decisions involved, and the precise timing of reproductive processes. The acquisition of data on exposure is particularly demanding in environmental studies, and the common inaccuracies and misclassifications are likely to weaken any associations. As the associations are likely to be relatively weak anyway (because the levels of environmental exposures are relatively low), misclassifications may lead to unwarranted conclusions about the absence of risk. For such reasons, it is difficult critically to evaluate the results obtained, and, for that matter, it is easy to use superficial criticism to play down positive associations. Food poisoning episodes have shown that the ingestion of alkylmercury and food oil contaminated by technical polychlorinated biphenyls leads to congenital defects in the offspring. It also appears to be relatively well proved that laboratory work poses reproductive problems, possibly because of exposure to many types of solvents. Although exposure to anesthetic gases at the levels now used probably does not entail detectable hazard, other exposures that occur in hospitals, such as exposure to antineoplastic agents or ethylene oxide, may pose risk, unless well controlled. By this time there should be sufficient understanding and agreement on methods and data bases large enough for case retrieval in order to assess further the role of occupational and other environmental factors in reproduction.

Acknowledgment

We wish to thank Sheryl Hinkkanen for the linguistic revision of the text.

References

1. Strobino, B. R., Kline, J., and Stein, Z., 1978, Chemical and physical exposures of parents: Effects on human reproduction and offspring, *Early Hum. Dev.* **1:**371.
2. Sullivan, F. M., and Barlow, S. M., 1979, Congenital malformations and other reproductive hazards from environmental chemicals, *Proc. R. Soc. Lond. (Biol)* **205:**91.
3. Hemminki, K., Sorsa, M., and Vainio, H., 1979, Genetic risks caused by occupational chemicals, *Scand. J. Work Environ. Health* **5:**307.
4. Haas, J. F., and Schottenfeld, D., 1979, Risks to the offspring from parental occupational exposures, *J. Occup. Med.* **21:**607.
5. Fabia, J., and Thuy, T. D., 1974, Occupation of father at time of birth of children dying of malignant diseases, *Br. J. Prev. Soc. Med.* **28:**98.
6. Gold, E. B., Diener, M. D., and Szklo, M., 1982, Parental occupations and cancer in children, *J. Occup. Med.* **24:**578.
7. Hemminki, K., Axelsson, O., and Niemi, M. -L., *et al.,* 1983, Assessment of methods and results of reproductive occupational epidemiology: Spontaneous abortions and malformations in the offspring of working women, *Am. J. Ind. Med.* **4:**293.
8. Hemminki, K., and Vainio, H., 1984, Occupational epidemiology and reproduction, in: *Recent Advances in Occupation Health,* Vol. 2 (J. M. Harrington, ed.), p. 117, Churchill Livingstone, Edinburgh.
9. Lindbohm, M.-L., Taskinen, H., and Hemminki, K., 1985, Reproductive health of working women, *Public Health Rev.* **13:**55.
10. Hemminki, K., Niemi, M.-L., Saloniemi, I., *et al.,* 1980, Spontaneous abortions by occupation and social class in Finland, *Int. J. Epidemiol.* **9:**149.
11. Rachootin, P., and Olsen, J., 1982, Prevalence and socioeconomic correlates of subfecundity and spontaneous abortion in Denmark, *Int. J. Epidemiol.* **11:**245.
12. Lindbohm, M.-L., Hemminki, K., and Kyyrönen, P., 1984, Parental occupational exposure and spontaneous abortions in Finland, *Am. J. Epidemiol.* **120:**370.
13. Kline, J., Stein, Z., Hatch, M., *et al.,* 1982, Surveillance of parental employment and spontaneous abortion, U.S. Department of Health and Human Services, National Institute of Occupational Safety and Health, Cincinnati, 10/82.
14. Figá-Talamanca, I., 1984, Spontaneous abortions among female industrial workers, *Int. Arch. Occup. Environ. Health* **54:**163.
15. Kavoussi, N., 1977, the effect of industrialization on spontaneous abortion in Iran, *J. Occup. Med.* **19:**419.
16. Heidam, L. Z., 1984, Spontaneous abortions among dental assistants, factory workers, painters, and gardening workers: a follow up study, *J. Epidemiol. Community Health* **38:**149.
17. Vaisman, A. J., 1967, Work in surgical theatres and its influence on the health of anaesthesiologists, *Eksp. Khir. Anest.* **12:**44 [in Russian].
18. Askrog, V., and Harvald, B., 1970, Teratogen effect of inhalationsanaestetika, *Nord. Med.* **83:**498.
19. Cohen, E. N., Bellville, J. W., and Brown, B. W., 1971, Anesthesia, pregnancy, and miscarriage: A study of operating room nurses and anesthetists, *Anesthesiology* **35:**343.

20. Knill-Jones, R. P., Moir, D. D., Rodrigues, L. V., *et al.*, 1972, Anesthetic practice and pregnancy, *Lancet* **1**:1326.
21. Rosenberg, P., and Kirves, A., 1973, Miscarriages among operating theatre staff, *Acta Anaesthesiol. Scand.* **53**:37.
22. Cohen, E. N., Brown, B. W., Bruce, D. L., *et al.*, 1974, Occupational disease among operating room personnel: A national study, *Anesthesiology* **41**:321.
23. Knill-Jones, R. P., Newman, B. J., and Spence, A. A., 1975, Anaesthetic practice and pregnancy: Controlled survey of male anaesthetists in the United Kingdom, *Lancet* **2**:807.
24. Göthe, C. J., Dahlgren, B.-E., Hallén, B., *et al.*, 1976, Narcotic gases as industrial hazard, *Lakartidningen* **73**:2553 [in Swedish].
25. Tomlin, P. J., 1979, Health problems of anesthetists and their families in the West Midlands, *Br. Med. J.* **1**:779.
26. Cohen, E. N., Brown, B. W., Wu, M. L., *et al.*, 1980, Occupational disease in dentistry and chronic exposure to trace anesthetic gases, *J. Am. Dent. Assoc.* **101**:21.
27. Pharoah, P. O. D., Alberman, E., Doyle, P., *et al.*, 1977, Outcome of pregnancy among women in anesthetic practice, *Lancet* **1**:34.
28. Rosenberg, P. H., and Vänttinen, H., 1978, Occupational hazards to reproduction and health in anesthetists and paediatricians, *Acta Anaesthesiol. Scand.* **22**:202.
29. Lauwerys, R., Siddons, M., Misson, C. B., *et al.*, 1981, Anesthetic health hazards among Belgian nurses and physicians. *Int. Arch. Occup. Environ. Health* **48**:195.
30. Spence, A. A., and Knill-Jones, R. P., 1978, Is there a health hazard in anaesthetic practice?, *Br. J. Anaesth.* **50**:713.
31. Vessey, M. P., Nunn, J. F., 1980, Occupational hazards of anaesthesia, *Br. Med. J.* **281**:696.
32. Edling, C., 1980, Anesthetic gases as an occupational hazard—A review, *Scand. J. Work Environ. Health* **6**:85.
33. Lane, G. A., Nahrwold, M. L., Tait, A. R., *et al.*, 1980, Nitrous oxide is fetotoxic, xenon is not, *Science* **210**:899.
34. Axelsson, G., and Rylander, R., 1982, Exposure to anaesthetic gases and spontaneous abortion: Response bias in a postal questionnaire study, *Int. J. Epidemiol.* **11**:250.
35. Hemminki, K., Kyyrönen, P., and Lindbohm, M.-L., 1985, Spontaneous abortions and malformations in the offspring of nurses exposed to anesthetic gases, cytostatic drugs and other potential health hazards in hospitals based on registered information of outcome, *J. Epidemiol. Community Health* **39**:141.
36. Hemminki, K., Mutanen, P., Saloniemi, I., *et al.*, 1982, Spontaneous abortions in hospital staff engaged in sterilising instruments with chemical agents, *Br. Med. J.* **285**:1461.
37. Hemminki, K., Mutanen, P., and Niemi, M.-L., 1983, Spontaneous abortions in hospital sterilising staff (Letter), *Br. Med. J.* **286**:1976.
38. Jakubova, Z. N., Shamova, N. A., Miftakhova, F. A., *et al.*, 1976, Gynecological disorders in workers engaged in ethylene oxide production, *Kaz. Med. Z.* **57**:558 [in Russian].
39. Shumlina, A. V., 1975, Menstrual and child-bearing functions of female workers occupationally exposed to the effects of formaldehyde, *Gig. Tr. Prof. Zabol.* **19**:18 [in Russian].
40. Sun, M., 1984, OSHA rule is curbed by budget office, *Science* **225**:603.
41. Pastorfide, G. B., and Goldstein, D. P., 1973, Pregnancy after hydatidiform mole, *Obstet. Gynecol.* **42**:67.
42. Walden, P. A. M., and Bagshawe, K. D., 1976, Reproductive performance of women successfully treated for gestational trophoblastic tumors, *Am. J. Obstet. Gynecol.* **125**:1108.

43. Selevan, S. G., Lindbohm, M.-L., Hornung, R. W., *et al.*, A case-referent study of occupational exposure to antineoplastic drugs and fetal loss in nurses (unpublished manuscript).
44. Kolmodin-Hedman, B., and Hedström, L., 1978, Enkätundersökning hos Kemika-lieexponerad laboratoriepersonal rörande spontanaborter, *Lakartidningen* **75**:3044.
45. Strandberg, M., Sandbäck, K., Axelsson, O., *et al.*, 1978, Spontaneous abortions among women in hospital laboratory, *Lancet* **1**:384.
46. Hansson, E., Jansa, S., Wande, H., *et al.*, 1980, Pregnancy outcome for women working in laboratories in some of the pharmaceutical industries in Sweden, *Scand. J. Work Environ. Health* **6**:131.
47. Axelsson, G., Jeansson, S., Rylander, R., *et al.*, 1980, Pregnancy abnormalities among personnel at a virological laboratory, *Am. J. Ind. Med.* **1**:129.
48. Axelsson, G., Lütz, C., and Rylander, R., 1984, Exposure to solvents and outcome of pregnancy in university laboratory employees, *Br. J. Indust. Med.* **41**:305.
49. Heidam, L. A., 1984, Spontaneous abortions among laboratory workers; a follow up study, *J. Epidemiol. Community Health* **38**:36.
50. Rom, W. N., 1980, Effects of lead on reproduction, in: *Proceedings of a Workshop on Methodology for Assessing Reproductive Hazards in the Workplace* (P. F. Infante and M. S. Legator, ed.), p. 33, NIOSH Publication No. 81-100, U.S. Department of Health and Human Services, Washington, D.C.
51. Nordström, S., Beckman, L., and Nordenson, I., 1979, Occupational and environmental risks in and around a smelter in northern Sweden: V. Spontaneous abortion among female employees and decreased birth weight in their offspring, *Hereditas* **90**:291.
52. Kolmodin-Hedman, B., Hedström, L., and Grönqvist, B., 1982, Menopausal age and spontaneous abortion in a group of women working in a Swedish steel works, *Scand. J. Soc. Med.* **10**:17.
53. Hemminki, K., Niemi, M.-L., Koskinen, K., *et al.*, 1980, Spontaneous abortions among women employed in the metal industry in Finland, *Int. Arch. Occup. Environ. Health* **47**:53.
54. Hemminki, K., Niemi, M.-L., Kyyrönen, P., *et al.*, 1984, Spontaneous abortion as risk indicator in metal exposure, in: *Reproductive and Development Toxicity of Metals* (T. W. Clarkson, G. F. Nordberg, and P. R. Sager, eds.), p. 369, Plenum Press, New York.
55. Goncaruk, G. A., 1977, Problems related to occupational hygiene of women in production of mercury, *Gig. Tr. Prof. Zabol.* **5**:17 [in Russian].
56. Marinova, G., Cakarova, O., and Kaneva, Y., 1973, A study of the reproductive function in women working with mercury, *Probl. Akus. Ginek.* **1**:75 [in Russian].
57. Pavlova, L. B., 1983, On rational employment of pregnant machine tool operators, *Gig. Tr. Prof. Zabol.* **2**:34 [in Russian].
58. Vaughan, T. L., Daling, J. R., and Starzyk, P. M., 1984, Fetal death and maternal occupation, *J. Occup. Med.* **26**:676.
59. Wilson, J. G., 1977, Environmental chemicals, in: *Handbook of Teratology*, Vol. 1 (J. G. Wilson and F. C. Fraser, eds.), p. 357, Plenum Press, New York.
60. Hemminki, K., 1980, Occupational chemicals tested for teratogenicity, *Int. Arch. Occup. Environ. Health* **47**:191.
61. Hemminki, K., Franssila, E., and Vainio, H., 1980, Spontaneous abortions among female chemical workers in Finland, *Int. Arch. Occup. Environ. Health* **45**:123.
62. Hemminki, K., Lindbohm, M.-L., Hemminki, T., *et al.*, 1984, Reproductive hazards and plastics industry, in: *Industrial Hazards of Plastics and Synthetic Elastomers* (J. Järvisalo, P. Pfäffli, and H. Vainio, ed.), p. 79, Alan R. Liss, New York.

63. Ehrhardt, W., 1967, Experiences with the employment of women exposed to carbon disulphide, in: *International Symposium on Toxicology of Carbon Disulphide, Prague, 1966,* p. 240, Excerpta Medica Foundation, Amsterdam.

64. Taskinen, H., Lindbohm, M.-L., and Hemminki, K., 1985, Spontaneous abortions among pharmaceutical workers, *Br. J. Indust. Med.* **46:**199.

65. Lindbohm, M.-L., Hemminki, K., and Kyyrönen, P., Spontaneous abortions among women employed in the plastics industry, *Am. J. Indust. Med.* **8:**579.

66. Aldyreva, M. V., Klimona, T. S., Izyumova, A. S., et al., 1975, The influence of phthalate plasticisers on the generative function, *Gig. Tr. Prof. Zabol.* **19:**25 [in Russian].

67. Härkönen, H., and Holmberg, P. C., 1982, Obstetric histories of women occupationally exposed to styrene, *Scand. J. Work Environ. Health* **8:**74.

68. Muhametova, I. M., and Vozovaja, M. A., 1972, Reproductive power and the incidence of gynaecological affections in female workers exposed to the combined effect of benzine and chlorinated hydrocarbons, *Gig. Tr. Prof. Zabol.* **11:**6 [in Russian].

69. Beskrovnaja, N. J., 1979, Gynaecological morbidity in women workers in the rubber industry, *Gig. Tr. Prof. Zabol.* **8:**36 [in Russian].

70. Kestrup, L., and Källen, B., 1982, Outcome of pilot study in pregnancy at Trelleborg Ab 1973–1980, in: *Scandinavian Rubber Conference, May 21–22, 1981, Symp. Proc.* 2; Kirjapaino Öhrling, Nokia, p. 66.

71. Axelson, O., Edling, C., and Andersson L., 1983, Pregnancy outcome among women in a Swedish rubber plant, *Scand. J. Work Environ. Health* Suppl. 2 **9:**79.

72. Hemminki, K., Niemi, M.-L., Kyyrönen, P., et al., 1983, Spontaneous abortions and reproductive selection mechanisms in the rubber and leather industry in Finland, *Br. J. Ind. Med.* **40:**81.

73. Lindbohm, M.-L., Hemminki, K., Kyyrönen, P., et al., 1983, Spontaneous abortions among rubber workers and congenital malformations in their offspring, *Scand. J. Work Environ. Health* Suppl. 2 **9:**85.

74. Neubert, D., Zens, P., Rothenwallner, A., et al., 1973, A survey of the embryotoxic effects of TCDD in mammalian species, *Environ. Health Perspect.* **5:**67.

75. Smith, F. A., Schwetz, B. A., and Nitschke, K. D., 1976, Teratogenicity of 2,3,7,8-tetrachlorodibenzo-p-dioxin in CF-I mice, *Toxicol. Appl. Pharmacol.* **38:**517.

76. Smith, J., 1979, EPA halts most use of herbicide 2,4,5-T, *Science* **203:**1090.

77. Longo, L. D., 1980, Environmental pollution and pregnancy: Risks and uncertainties for the fetus and infant. *Am. J. Obstet. Gynecol.* **137:**162.

78. Santi, L., Boeri, R., Remotti, G., et al., 1982, Five years after Seveso, *Lancet* **1:**343.

79. Nordström, S., Beckman, L., and Nordenson, I., 1978, Occupational and environmental risks in and around a smelter in norther Sweden. III. Frequencies of spontaneous abortion, *Hereditas* **88:**51.

80. Hemminki, K., and Niemi, M.-L., 1982, Community study of spontaneous abortions: Relation to occupation and air pollution by sulfur dioxide, hydrogen sulfide, and carbon disulfide, *Int. Arch. Occup. Environ. Health* **51:**55.

81. Bjerkedal, T., and Lund, T. E., 1978, Yrke Och fødsel, Hygienisk institut, Universitetet i Oslo [in Norwegian].

82. Leck, I., 1977, Correlations of malformation frequency with environmental and genetic attributes in man, in: *Handbook of Teratology,* Vol. 3 (J. G. Wilson and F. C. Fraser, eds.), p. 243, Plenum Press, New York.

83. Registrar General, 1978, Occupational mortality 1970–1972. The registrar general's decennial supplement for England and Wales, pp. 1. Her Majesty's Stationery Office, London.

84. Hemminki, K., Mutanen, P., Saloniemi, I., *et al.*, 1981, Congenital malformations and maternal occupation in Finland: Multivariate analysis, *J. Epidemiol. Comm. Health* **35**:5.

85. Ericson, A., and Källén, B., 1979, Survey of infants born in 1973 or 1975 to Swedish women working in operating rooms during their pregnancies, *Anesth. Anal.* **58**:302.

86. Corbett, T. H., Cornell, R. G., Endres, J. L., *et al.*, 1974, Birth defects among children of nurse-anesthetists, *Anesthesiology* **41**:341.

87. Goethe, C. J., and Hoffman, O., 1977, The consequences on pregnancies of smoking and occupational exposures to anesthetic gases, in: *Proceedings of the Fourth Swedish–Yugoslaw Days of Occupational Medicine*, p. 11.

88. Cohen, E. N., Brown, B. W., Bruce, D. L., *et al.*, 1975, A survey of anesthetic health hazards among dentists, *J. Am. Dent. Assoc.* **90**:1291.

89. Halling, H., 1979, Suspected link between exposure to hexachlorophene and malformed infants, *Ann. NY Acad. Sci.* **320**:426.

90. Baltzar, B., Ericson, A., and Källén, B., 1979, Delivery outcome in women employed in medical occupations in Sweden, *J. Occup. Med.* **21**:543.

91. Baltzar, B., Ericson, A., and Källén, B., 1979, Pregnancy outcome among women working in Swedish hospitals, *N. Engl. J. Med.* **300**:627.

92. Norppa, H., Sorsa, M., Vainio, H., *et al.*, 1980, Increased sister chromatid exchange frequencies in lymphocytes of nurses handling cytostatic drugs, *Scand. J. Work Environ. Health* **67**:229.

93. Sorsa, M., Norppa, H., and Vainio, H., 1982, Induction of sister chromatid exchanges among nurses handling cytostatic drugs, in: *Indicators of Genotoxic Exosure, Banbury Report 13*, p. 341, Cold Spring Harbor Laboratory, Cold Spring Harbor, N.Y.

94. Waksvik, H., Klepp, O., and Brogger, O., 1981, Chromosome analyses of nurses handling cytostatic agents, *Cancer Treatm. Rep.* **65**:607.

95. Anderson, R. W., Puckett, W. H., Dana, W. J., *et al.*, 1982, Risk of handling injectable antineoplastic agents, *Am. J. Hosp. Pharm.* **39**:1881.

96. Bos, R. P., Leenars, A. O., Theuws, J. L. G., *et al.*, 1982, Mutagenicity of urine from nurses handling cytostatic drugs, influence of smoking, *Int. Arch. Occup. Environ. Health* **50**:359.

97. Falck, K., Gröhn, P., Sorsa, M., *et al.*, 1979, Mutagenicity in urine of nurses handling cytostatic drugs, *Lancet* **1**:1250.

98. Nguyen, T. V., Theiss, J. C., and Matney, T. S., 1982, Exposure of pharmacy personnel to mutagenic antineoplastic drugs, *Cancer Res.* **42**:4792.

99. Vainio, H., Falck, K., and Sorsa, M., 1984, Mutagenicity in urine of workers occupationally exposed to mutagens and carcinogens, in: *Biological Monitoring and Surveillance of Workers Exposed to Chemicals* (A. Aitio, V. Riihimäki, H. Vainio, eds.), p. 323, Hemisphere Publishing Co., Washington, D. C.

100. Staiano, N., Gallelli, J. F., Adamson, R. H., *et al.*, 1981, Lack of mutagenic activity in urine from hospital pharmacists admixing antitumor drugs, *Lancet* **1**:615.

101. Szigeti, M., Fekete, G., and Szollar, J., 1982, The effect of regular cytostatic handling on the sister chromatid exchanges in hospital nurses, *Mutat. Res.* **97**:227 (abs.).

102. IARC Monographs on the Evaluation of Carcinogenic Risk of Chemicals to Humans, 1981, *Some Antineoplastic and Immunosuppressive Agents*, Vol. 26, p. 441, International Agency for Research on Cancer, Lyon.

103. Sorsa, M., Hemminki, K., and Vainio, H., 1985, Occupational exposure to anticancer drugs—Potential and real health hazards *Mutat. Res.* **154**:135.

104. Hirst, M., Mills, D. G., Tse, S., *et al.*, 1984, Occupational exposure to cyclophosphamide, *Lancet* **1**:186.

105. Erickson, J. D., Cochran, W. M., and Anderson, C. E., 1979, Parental occupation and birth defects. A preliminary report, *Contrib. Epidemiol. Biostatist. 1:*107.
106. Kucera, J., 1968, Exposure to fat solvents: A possible cause of sacral agenesis in man, *J. Pediatr.* **72:**857.
107. Meirik, O., Källén, B., Gauffin, U., *et al.*, 1979, Major malformations in infants born of women who worked in laboratories while pregnant, *Lancet* **2:**91.
108. Blomqvist, U., Ericson, A., Källén, B., *et al.*, 1981, Delivery outcome for women working in the pulp and paper industry, *Scand. J. Work Environ. Health* **7:**114.
109. Ericson, A., Källén, B., Meirik, O., *et al.*, 1982, Gastrointestinal atresia and maternal occupation during pregnancy, *J. Occup. Med.* **24:**515.
110. Ericson, M., Källén, B., Zetterström, R., *et al.*, 1984, Delivery outcome of women working in laboratories during pregnancy, *Arch. Environ. Health* **39:**5.
111. Holmberg, P. C., 1979, Central-nervous-system defects in children born to mothers exposed to organic solvents during pregnancy, *Lancet* **1:**177.
112. Holmberg, P. C., and Nurminen, M., 1980, Congential defects of the central nervous system and occupational factors during pregnancy. A case referent study, *Am. J. Ind. Med.* **1:**167.
113. Holmberg, P. C., Hernberg, S., Kurppa, K., *et al.*, 1982, Oral clefts and organic solvent exposure during pregnancy, *Int. Arch. Occup. Environ. Health* **50:**371.
114. Holmberg, P. C., 1977, Central nervous defects in two children of mothers exposed to chemicals in the reinforced plastics industry, *Scand. J. Work Environ. Health* **3:**212.
115. Hemminki, K., Saloniemi, I., Kyyrönen, P., *et al.*, 1982, Gastroschisis and omphalocele in Finland in the 1970s: Prevalence at birth and its correlates, *J. Epidemiol. Community Health* **35:**289.
116. Olsen, J., 1983, Risk of exposure to teratogens amongst labortory staff and painters, *Dan. Med. Bull.* **30:**24.
117. World Health Organization, 1983, Working group on women and occupational health risks, EURO reports and studies 76. *Report on a WHO Meeting, Budapest Feb. 16–18, 1982,* WHO Regional Office for Europe, Copenhagen.
118. Nordström, S., Beckman, L., and Nordenson, I., 1979, Occupational and environmental risks in and around a smelter in northern Sweden. VI. Congenital malformations, *Hereditas* **90:**297.
119. Koos, B. J., and Longo, L. D., 1976, Mercury toxicity in the pregnant woman, fetus and newborn infant, *Am. J. Obstet. Gynecol.* **126:**390.
120. Chang, L. W., Wade, P. R., Pounds, J. G., *et al.*, 1980, Prenatal and neonatal toxicology and pathology of heavy metals, *Adv. Pharmacol. Chem.* **17:**195.
121. Harada, M., 1978, Congenital minamata disease: Intrauterine methylmercury poisoning, *Teratology* **18:**285.
122. Amin-Zaki, L., Elhassani, S. B., Majeed, M. A., *et al.*, 1974, Intrauterine methylmercury poisoning in Iraq, *Pediatrics* **54:**587.
123. Amin-Zaki, L., Majeed, M. A., Elhassani, S. B., *et al.*, 1979, Prenatal methylmercury poisoning, clinical observations over five years, *Am. J. Dis. Child.* **133:**172.
124. Clarkson, T. W., Cox, C., Marsh, D. O., *et al.*, 1981, Dose-response relationship for adult and prenatal exposures to methylmercury, in: *Measurement of Risks* (G. G. Barg and H. D. Maillie, eds.), p. 111, Plenum Press, New York.
125. Snyder, R. D., 1971, Congenital mercury poisoning, *N. Engl. J. Med.* **284:**1014.
126. Reggiani, G., 1982, Toxicology of TCDD and related compounds: observations in man, in: *Chlorinated Dioxins and Related Compounds: Impact on the Environment* (O. Hutzinger, ed.), p. 463, Pergamon Press, Oxford.

127. Kuratsune, M., Yoshimura, T., Matsuzaka, J., *et al.,* 1972, Epidemiologic study on Yusho, a poisoning caused by ingestion of rice oil contaminated with a commercial brand of polychlorinated biphenyls, *Environ. Health Perspect.* **1:**119.
128. Miller, R. W., 1971, Cola-colored babies. Chlorobiphenyl poisoning in Japan, *Teratology* **4:**211.
129. Yamashita, F., 1977, Clinical features of chlorobiphenyls (PCBs)-induced fetopathy, *Paediatrician* **6:**20.
130. Shiota, K., 1976, Fetal accumulation of polychlorinated biphenyls (PCBs). A consideration on the problem of human prenatal exposure to environmental pollutants, *Congen. Anomal.* **16:**9.
131. Renwick, J. H., 1972, Hypothesis—Anencephaly and spina bifida are usually preventable by avoidance of specific but unidentified substance present in certain potato tubers, *Br. J. Prev. Soc. Med.* **26:**67.
132. Renwick, J. H., 1973, Anencephaly and potatoes, *Lancet* **1:**96.
133. Emanuel, I., 1972, Non-tuberous neural-tube defects, *Lancet* **2:**879.
134. Smith, C., Watt, M., Boyd, A. E. W., and Holmes, J. C., 1973, Anencephaly, spina bifida, and potato blight in the Edinburgh area, *Lancet* **1:**269.
135. MacMahon, B., Yen, S., and Rothman, K. J., 1973, Potato blight and neural-tube defects, *Lancet* **1:**589.
136. Elwood, J. H., and Nevin, N. C., 1973, Factors associated with anencephalus and spina bifida in Belfast, *Br. J. Prev. Soc. Med.* **27:**73.
137. Elwood, J. H., and MacKenzie, G., 1973, Associations between the incidence of neurological malformations and potato blight outbreaks over 50 years in Ireland, *Nature (Lond.)* **243:**476.
138. Elwood, J. M., 1973, Anencephaly and potato blight in Eastern Canada, *Lancet* **1:**769.
139. Field, B., and Kerr, C., 1973, Potato blight and neural-tube defects, *Lancet* **2:**507.
140. Kinlen, L., and Hewitt, A., 1973, Potato blight and anencephalus in Scotland, *Br. J. Prev. Soc. Med.* **27:**208.
141. Masterson, J. G., Frost, C., Bourke, G. J., *et al.,* 1974, Anencephaly and potato blight in the Republic of Ireland, *Br. J. Prev. Soc. Med.* **28:**81.
142. Roberts, C. J., Revington, C. J., and Loyd, S., 1973, Potato cultivation and storage in South Wales and its relation to neural tube malformation prevalence, *Br. J. Prev. Soc. Med.* **27:**214.
143. Clarke, C. A., McKendrick, O. M., and Sheppard, P. M., 1973, Spina bifida and potatoes, *Br. Med. J.* **3:**251.
144. Spiers, P. S., Pietrzyk, J., Piper, J. M., *et al.,* 1974, Human potato consumption and neural-tube malformation, *Teratology* **10:**125.
145. Nevin, N. C., and Merrett, J. D., 1975, Potato avoidance during pregnancy in women with a previous infant with either anencephaly and/or spina bifida, *Br. J. Prev. Soc. Med.* **29:**111.
146. Fedrick, J., 1970, Anencephalus and the local water supply, *Nature (Lond.)* **227:**176.
147. Fielding, D. W., and Smithells, R. W., 1971, Anencephalus and water hardness in South-West Lancashire, *Br. J. Prev. Soc. Med.* **25:**217.
148. Lowe, C. R., Roberts, C. J., and Lloyd, S., 1971, Malformations of central nervous system and softness of local water supplies, *Br. Med. J.* **2:**357.
149. Crawford, M. D., Gardner, M. J., and Sedgwick, P. A., 1972, Infant mortality and hardness of local water supplies, *Lancet* **1:**988.
150. Morton, M. S., Elwood, P. C., and Abernethy, M., 1976, Trace elements in water and congenital malformations of the central nervous system in South Wales, *Br. J. Prev. Soc. Med.* **30:**36.

151. St. Leger, A. S., Elwood, P. C., and Morton, M. S., 1980, Neural tube malformations and trace elements in water, *J. Epidemiol. Community Health* **34**:186.
152. Elwood, J. M., and Goldman, A. J., 1981, Water composition in the etiology of anencephalus, *Am. J. Epidemiol.* **113**:681.
153. Tung, T. T., Anh, T. K., Tuyen, B. Q., *et al.*, 1971, Clinical effects of massive and continuous utilization of defoliants on civilians, *Vietnamese Stud.* **29**;53.
154. Rose, H. A., and Rose, S. P. R., 1972, Chemical spraying as reported by refugees from South Vietnam, *Science* **177**:710.
155. Honoroff, I., 1973, *Down's Syndrome—It Can Happen Here. A Report to the Consumer.* III (50). 1–4, Sherman Oaks, California.
156. Advisory Committee on 2,4,5-T, 1971, *Report to the Administrator of the Environmental Protection Agency*, U.S. Environmental Protection Agency, Washington D. C.
157. Sare, W. H., and Forbes, P. I., 1972, Possible dismorfogenic effects of an agricultural chemical: 2,4,5-T, *NZ Med. J.* **75**:37.
158. Cutting, R. K., Phuoc, T. H., Ballo, J. M., *et al.*, 1970, *Congenital Malformations, Hydatidiform Moles and Stillbirths in the Republic of Vietnam 1960–1969*, Department of Defense, US Government Printing Office No. 903.233, Washington D. C. (abs.).
159. Young, A. L., Calcagni, J. A., Thalken, C. E., *et al.*, 1978, *The Toxicology, Environmental Fate, and Human Risk of Herbicide Orange and Its Associated Dioxin*, USAF OEHL Technical Report TR-78-92. USAF Occupational and Environmental Health Laboratory, Washington, D.C.
160. Roan, C. C., and Morgan, D. P., 1972, Alleged effects on human health of the use of herbicides in the area around Globe, Arizona, *Arizona Community Pesticide Study Project*, University of Arizona, Tucson.
161. McQueen, E. G., Veale, A. M. O., Alewander, W. S., *et al.*, 1977, *2,4,5-T and Human Birth Defects*, June, Department of Health, New Zealand.
162. Hanify, J. A., Metcalf, P., Nobbs, C. L., *et al.*, 1981, Aerial spraying of 2,4,5-T and human birth malformations: An epidemiological investigation, *Science* **212**:349.
163. Field, B., and Kerr, C., 1979, Herbicide use and incidence of neural-tube defects, *Lancet* **1**:1341.
164. Thomas, H. F., 1980, 2,4,5-T use and congenital malformation rates in Hungary, *Lancet* **2**:214.
165. Brogan, W. F., Brogan, C. E., and Dadd, J. T., 1980, Herbicides and cleft lip and palate (letter), *Lancet* **2**:597.
166. Bruzzi, P., Bisanti, L., Borgana-Pignatti, C., *et al.*, 1981, Birth defects in the TCDD polluted area of Seveso: Results of a 4-years follow-up, provisional draft, August.
167. Infante, P. F., 1976, Oncogenic and mutagenic risks in communities with polyvinyl chloride production facilities, *Ann. NY Acad. Sci.* **271**:49.
168. Edmonds, L. D., Falk, H., and Nissim, J. E., 1975, Congenital malformations and vinyl chloride, *Lancet* **2**:1098.
169. Edmonds, L. D., Anderson, C. E., Flynt, J. W., Jr., *et al.*, 1978, Congenital central nervous system malformations and vinyl chloride monomer exposure: A community study, *Teratology* **17**:137.
170. Rapaport, I., 1959, Nouvelles recherches sur le mongolisme, A propos du role pathogénique du fluor, *Bull. Acad. Natl. Med. (Paris)* **143**:367.
171. Berry, W. T. C., 1958, A study on the incidence of mongolism in relation to the fluoride content of water, *Am. J. Ment. Defic.* **62**:634.
172. Erickson, J. D., Oakley, G. P., Flynt, J. W., *et al.*, 1976, Water fluoridation and congenital malformations: No association, *J. Am. Dent. Assoc.* **93**:981.
173. Needleman, H. L., Pueschel, S. M., and Rothman, K. J., 1974, Fluoridation and the occurrence of Down's syndrome, *N. Engl. J. Med.* **291**:821.

174. Knox, E. G., Armstrong, E., and Lancashire, R., 1980, Fluoridation and the prevalence of congenital malformations, *Community Med.* **2**:190.
175. Erickson, J. D., 1980, Down syndrome, water fluoridation, and maternal age, *Teratology* **21**:177.
176. Hemminki, K., Saloniemi, I., Luoma, K., *et al.*, 1980, Transplacental carcinogens and mutagens. Childhood cancer, malformations and abortions as risk indicators, *Toxicol. Environ. Health* **6**:115.
177. Hemminki, K., Saloniemi, I., Salonen, T., *et al.*, 1981, Childhood cancer and parental occupation in Finland, *J. Epidemiol. Community Health* **35**:11.
178. van Steensel-Moll, H., Valkenburg, H. A., and van Zanen, G. E., 1985, Childhood leukemia and parental occupation. A register-based case-control study, *Am. J. Epidemiol.* **121**:216.
179. Hakulinen, T., Salonen, T., and Teppo, L., 1976, Cancer in the offspring of fathers in hydrocarbon-related occupations, *Br. J. Prev. Soc. Med.* **30**:138.
180. Kantor, A. F., McCrea Curnen, M. G., Meigs, J. W., *et al.*, 1979, Occupations of fathers of patients with Wilm's tumour, *J. Epidemiol. Community Health* **33**:253.
181. Kwa, S. L., and Fine, L. J., 1980, The association between parental occupation and childhood malignancy, *J. Occup. Med.* **22**:792.
182. Zack, M., Cannon, S., Loyd, D., *et al.*, 1980, Cancer in children of parents exposed to hydrocarbon-related industries and occupations, *Am. J. Epidemiol.* **111**:329.
183. Peters, J. M., Preston-Martin, S., and Yu, M. C., 1981, Brain tumors in children and occupational exposure of parents, *Science* **213**:235.
184. Sanders, B. M., White, G. C., and Draper, G. J., 1981, Occupations of fathers of children dying from neoplasms, *J. Epidemiol. Community Health* **35**:245.
185. Vianna, N., Kovasznay, B., Polan, A., *et al.*, 1984, Infant leukemia and paternal exposure to motor vehicle exhaust fumes, *J. Occup. Med.* **26**:679.
186. Coté, C. J., Meuwissen, J. J., and Pickerning, R. J., 1974, Effects on the neonate of predisone and azathioprine administered to the mother during pregnancy, *J. Pediatr.* **85**:324.
187. Holmes, G. E., and Holmes, F. F., 1978, Pregnancy outcome of patients treated for Hodgkin's disease. A controlled study, *Cancer* **41**:1317.
188. McKeen, E. A., Mulville, J. J., Rosner, F., *et al.*, 1979, Pregnancy outcome in Hodgkin's disease, *Lancet* **2**:590.
189. Hornung, S. J., Hoppe, R. T., Kaplan, H. S., *et al.*, 1981, Female reproductive potential after treatment for Hodgkin's disease, *N. Engl. J. Med.* **304**:1377.
190. Rustin, G. J. S., Booth, M., Dent, J., *et al.*, 1984, Pregnancy after cytotoxic chemotherapy for gestational trophoblastic tumours, *Br. Med. J.* **228**:103.

CHAPTER 3

Neonatal Polycythemia and Hyperviscosity

TED S. ROSENKRANTZ and WILLIAM OH

1. Introduction

The syndrome of polycythemia and hyperviscosity in the newborn continues to be a problem for which many questions concerning etiology, incidence, diagnosis, pathophysiology, outcome, and appropriate management remain. Recent research also suggests that this is a syndrome of multiple etiologies that may affect multiple organs to varying degrees of severity.[1-4] Studies involving both infants and animal models have provided greater insight into the pathophysiology of the problem, although certain areas are still ill defined.

2. Definition

The definition of polycythemia and hyperviscosity has varied in many different studies. The confounding variables have included source and time of blood sampling as well as level of hematocrit and viscosity to be considered diagnostic. Hematocrit values of ≥65% are generally considered polycythemic. Using cord blood obtained from 108 full-term appropriate-for-gestational-age (AGA) infants, Gross *et al.*[5] established normal values for blood viscosity. Using these normal values, hypervis-

TED S. ROSENKRANTZ • Division of Neonatology, Department of Pediatrics, University of Connecticut Health Center, Farmington, Connecticut 06032. **WILLIAM OH** • Brown University Program in Medicine, Department of Pediatrics, Women and Infants Hospital of Rhode Island, Providence, Rhode Island 02908.

cosity at the various shear rates was defined as a viscosity value greater
than 2 standard deviations (SD) from the mean (Fig. 1). Ramamurthy
et al.[6] obtained umbilical vein, peripheral vein and capillary blood samples from a group of normal infants. Hyperviscosity was defined as a
viscosity value of >3 SD from the mean. These workers found this value
to coincide with umbilical venous hematocrits of ≥63%. A consistently
higher hematocrit was found in capillary as compared with the corre-
sponding peripheral venous blood and in peripheral venous blood as
compared with simultaneously obtained umbilical venous blood. A study
done previously by Oh and Lind[7] also showed a consistently higher
capillary hematocrit (10%) as compared with a simultaneously obtained
peripheral venous hematocrit. The data have been replotted, as shown
in Figure 2.

At this time it would seem reasonable to define polycythemia as a
hematocrit value of ≥65% from a freely flowing peripheral vein. Cor-

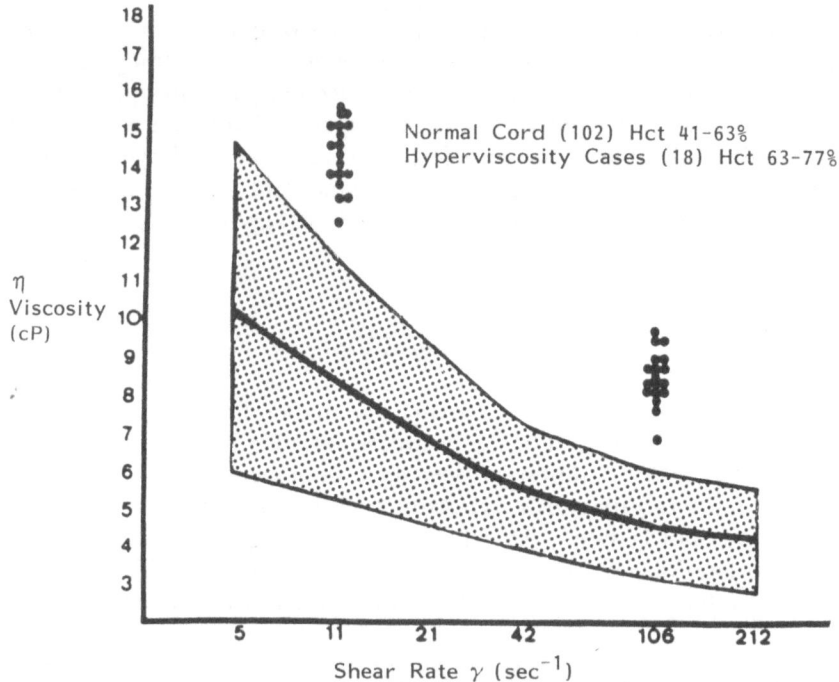

Figure 1. Shaded area represents viscosity of cord blood at shear rates from 2 to 212
sec^{-1} for 102 healthy full-term appropriate-for-gestational-age (AGA) infants (mean ±2
SD). Viscosity for 18 "symptomatic" infants is plotted at shear rates of 11 sec^{-1} and 106
sec.$^{-1}$ Hematocrit (Hct) values for each group are indicated. (From Gross *et al.*[5])

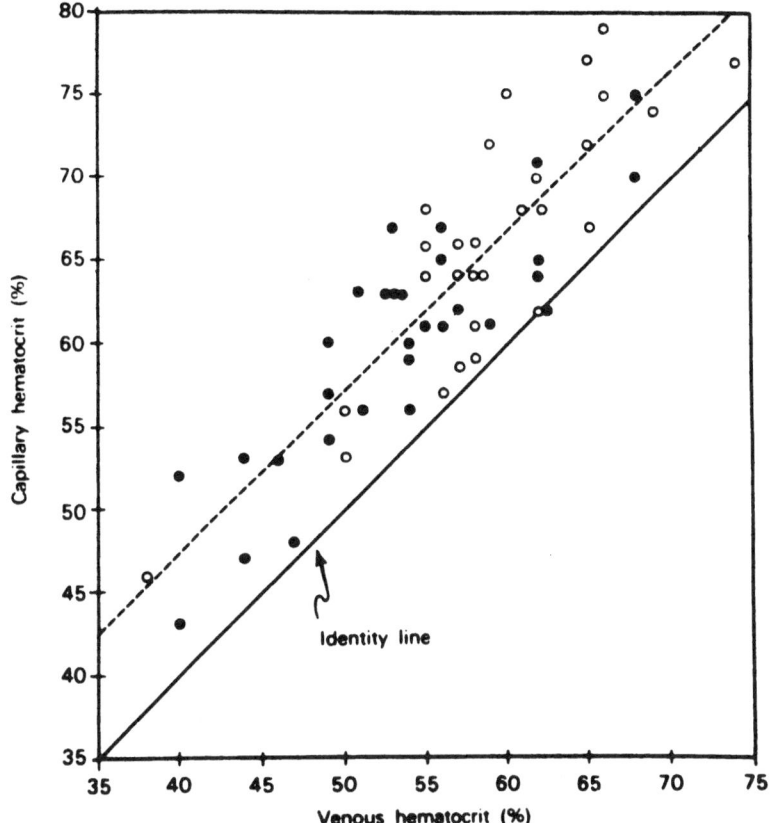

Figure 2. Correlation between capillary and venous blood hematocrit in newborn infants. (○) 2–6 hr; (●) 12–24 hr. (Modified from Oh and Lind.[7])

respondingly, hyperviscosity should be defined as a viscosity value of >2 SD greater than the norm (Fig. 1).

3. Incidence

It is commonly accepted that the incidence of polycythemia is 2–5%.[6,8–11] Factors known to influence this number include timing of cord clamping, population characteristics (high versus low risk), geographic area, sampling site, and postnatal age of sampling.[7–11] The incidence of hyperviscosity is slightly higher than that of polycythemia, as

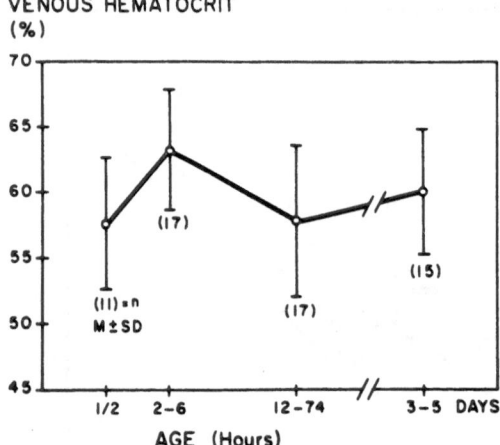

Figure 3. Changes in venous hematocrit during the first 5 days in infants who received placental transfusion at birth. (Modified from Oh and Lind.[7])

all infants with a hematocrit ≥65% will be hyperviscous, and a small portion of those with normal hematocrits may be hyperviscous on the basis of factors other than increased red blood cell (RBC) mass. The latter are infants whose blood viscosity is elevated because of increased plasma concentration of macroglobulin or decreased RBC deformability. Late cord clamping and "milking" of the cord appear to be associated with an increased hematocrit in the newborn infant.[12-15] At birth, the hematocrit values from the umbilical cord and peripheral vein are similar. Several hours after birth, however, those infants who receive placental transfusion by delayed cord clamping will have an elevation in blood hematocrit because of hemoconcentration. The hematocrit values will vary considerably during the first 24 hr of life according to the amount of blood transfused to the infant and subsequent hemoconcentration from this level (see Fig. 3).

As discussed in greater detail later, high-risk infants such as those with fetal distress, with intrauterine growth retardation (IUGR), or having a diabetic mother are at greater risk. Another important factor that determines the incidence of polycythemia and hyperviscosity is the altitude in which the population is located. Wirth and co-workers[8,9] performed large-scale screening studies in Denver, Colorado (1610 m above sea level) and in Norfolk, Virginia (sea level), two high-risk referral centers. The incidence at the Denver center was double that of Norfolk, suggesting that the lower atmospheric oxygen at high altitudes caused intrauterine fetal hypoxia with a resultant increase in RBC production and subsequent development of polycythemia.

4. Viscosity

Increased viscosity of the blood has traditionally been thought to cause the diminution of blood flow in the polycythemic infant that is ultimately responsible for the clinical pathology observed in these infants. It is appropriate to discuss thoroughly the physics of viscosity as well as how it affects blood flow in the vasculature of the newborn.

4.1. Definition

Viscosity was first defined by Poiseuille[16] as the ratio of shear stress to shear rate by the formula

$$\eta = \frac{(p - p') \, r^4 \, \pi}{8 \, l \, Q} = \frac{\text{shear stress}}{\text{shear rate}}$$

where η is the viscosity coefficient, $p - p'$ is the pressure gradient, r is the tube radius, l is tube length, and Q is flow.

More simply put, shear stress is the force per unit area applied in the direction of flow or, in the case of Poiseuille, the pressure gradient from one end of the capillary tube to the other times the radius to the fourth power.[17] Shear stress is expressed in dynes/cm^2. Shear rate refers to the velocity between two fluid planes, divided by the distance between them. Shear rate is expressed as sec^{-1}. Viscosity is expressed as dynes/sec per cm^{-2}, or poise. One centipoise is equal to the viscosity of water at 20°C.[18]

Poiseuille's work involved the flow of water through capillary tubes. He found that the ratio of shear stress to shear rate, and therefore viscosity, was constant. This relationship is true for homogeneous Newtonian fluids such as water. Blood, however, is a suspension of solid and fluid-filled particles in a solution and does not behave as a Newtonian fluid. As such, the shear stress/shear rate ratio is not constant.

To examine this relationship one must use an apparatus that will keep one of these variables constant while measuring the other. The most popular instrument for this procedure is a cone/plate microviscometer popularized by Wells et al.[19] Shear stress is measured at predetermined shear rates, allowing for calculation of viscosity.

Shear rates in the range of 100–300 sec^{-1} are thought to reflect conditions in large vessels such as the aorta, while shear rates of 11–25 sec^{-1} are more reflective of arterioles.[17] It should be kept in mind that measurements of viscosity in such apparatus reflect *in vitro* measurements and that other factors may alter the actual viscosity of body fluids such as blood in an *in vivo* environment.

4.2. Factors Affecting *in Vitro* Viscosity Measurements

Several factors may affect the determinants of *in vitro* blood viscosity values. These are described below.

4.2.1. Hematocrit

In the newborn infant, hematocrit, which represents RBC concentration, is the major determinant of whole blood viscosity. The relationship is logarithmic or curvilinear at all shear rates. The greatest changes

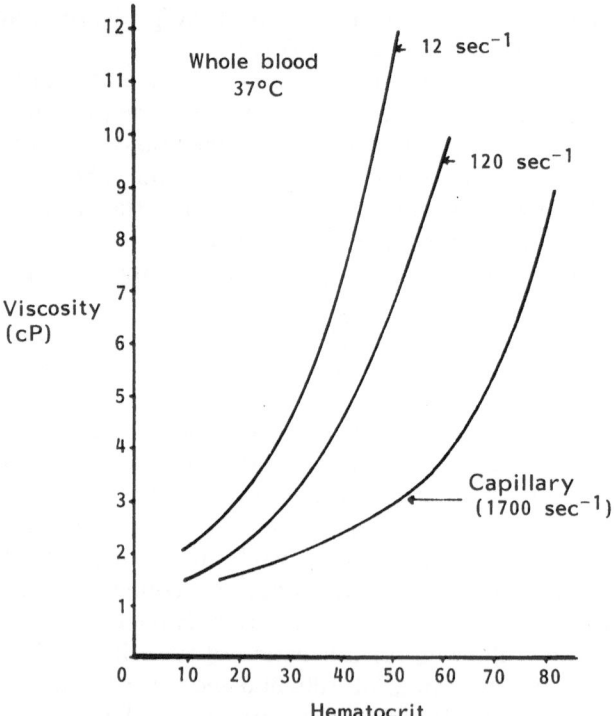

Figure 4. Comparison of viscosity–hematocrit diagrams of three shear rates. (From Wells *et al.*[20])

in the viscosity/hematocrit ratio occur at the lowest shear rates,[20,23] particularly when the hematocrit exceeds 65% (Fig. 4).

4.2.2. Plasma Proteins

In general, the plasma has a low viscosity of 1–1.5 centipoise (cP) and behaves like a Newtonian fluid.[18,21,24] That is, the viscosity is not affected by changes in the shear rate (Fig. 5). The protein and fibrinogen content of the plasma will directly affect its viscosity.[21] Preterm infants who have a low total protein will have a low plasma viscosity compared with full-term infants. Normal adult plasma is even higher. Adult syndromes of hyperviscosity can be attributed to abnormal or hyperproteinemia states such as diabetes and Waldenstrom's macroglobulinemia, but these conditions are not seen in the newborn.[22,26,27]

4.2.3. Red Blood Cell Deformability

The RBC contributes to the whole blood viscosity directly by being the most prominent particle suspended in the blood and due to its own intrinsic properties. The RBC is classically thought of as a static particle, a biconcave disc that will deform in order to fit through the capillary

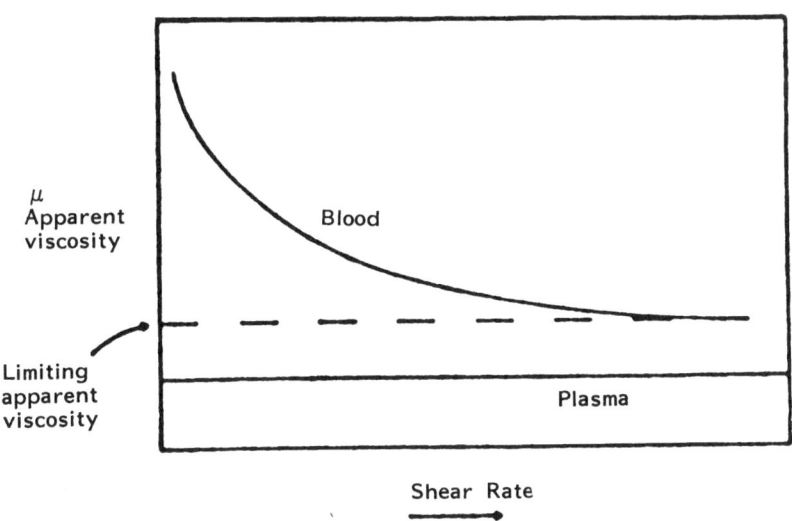

Figure 5. Change in apparent viscosity of blood with shear rate. Plasma has a constant viscosity. (From Charm and Kurland.[25])

beds of the body. Microscopic studies demonstrate that the RBC is a dynamic particle. The cell membrane moves around the internal fluid of the cell as the RBC makes its intravascular journey. Therefore, the physical characteristic of the RBC, which dictates its deformability, will also contribute to the whole blood viscosity.[24]

The membrane of the RBC is quite deformable. Older studies on RBC filterability suggested that the neonatal RBC was less deformable than the adult cell.[5] Recent, more sophisticated studies suggest the opposite.[27,29] The viscosity of the internal contents of the RBC is affected by cell age,[28] older cells having a higher viscosity due to increased hemoglobin concentration. At higher hematocrits, the internal viscosity of the cell plays a greater role in the whole blood viscosity. Indeed, it would appear that the internal viscosity increases with decreasing flow or shear rate.

4.2.4. White Blood Cells

The neonatal white blood cell (WBC) is larger and less deformable than the RBC. Few studies have been done to examine its role in the newborn except that an extremely high concentration of WBCs, as seen in congenital leukemia, can increase blood viscosity dramatically.[30–32]

4.2.5. Fibrinogen

Although the fibrin concentration of the plasma will have some effect on whole blood viscosity, it is minute.[21]

4.2.6. Platelets

Platelets, *per se*, do not seem to play a role in whole blood viscosity, although they are relatively inflexible particles compared with RBCs. Studies in adults suggest that platelet aggregates may contribute significantly to the viscosity of blood from adults with vaso-occlusive disease.[18] The existence of platelet aggregates in infants with polycythemia and hyperviscosity has not been documented although frequently theorized.

4.2.7. pH Value

Changes in pH value cause fluid shifts within the RBC and will change the blood viscosity.[18,33] Significant increases in blood viscosity are observed when the pH level is less than 7.0 and therefore may play a role in infants whose hyperviscosity is the result of an asphyxia-induced placental transfusion.

4.3. Factors Affecting Blood Viscosity *in Vivo*

4.3.1. Size of the Blood Vessels

Blood flow is high in large blood vessels and low in small blood vessels, hence the high shear rates (100–300 sec^{-1}) in the large blood vessels and low shear rates (11–25 sec^{-1}) in the small blood vessels. Because blood viscosity is higher at low shear rates, the viscosity of the blood will be higher in the small blood vessels. As seen in Figure 6, small changes in hematocrit result in large changes in viscosity at the lowest shear rates which occur in the smallest blood vessels.

4.3.2. Capillaries

The diameter of a capillary is in the range of 3–5 μm, whereas that of the neonatal RBC is approximately 8.5 μm, slightly larger than the adult erythrocyte. One would expect this size difference between the capillary and the RBC to increase viscosity further, but the opposite is true. In 1931, Fahraeus and Lindqvist described a phenomenon in which blood viscosity decreased as the radius of the capillary diminished[34] (see Fig. 7). This phenomenon has been confirmed and explained by modern-day techniques using capillaries as small as 3 μm. Blood takes on the characteristic of "bolus flow" when in a capillary.[24] Bolus flow demon-

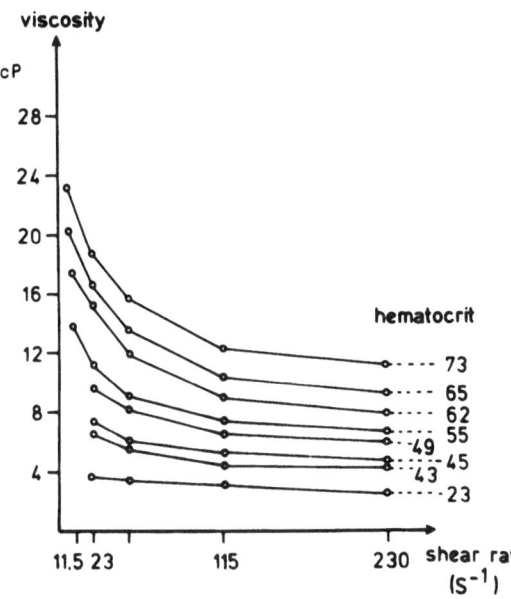

Figure 6. Variation of whole blood viscosity in eight newborn infants at different hematocrit values and shear rates. (From Bergqvist and Zetterman.[44])

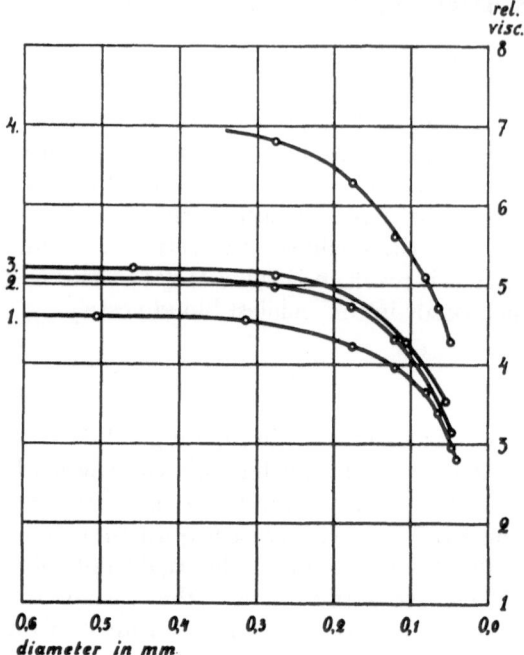

Figure 7.   Blood viscosity in small capillaries. (From Fahraeus and Lindqvist.[34])

strates high hemodynamic efficiency. Measurements of viscosity in the capillary are only 1.3 cP, approximately that of the plasma. This diminution in viscosity is independent of the hematocrit.[17] *In vitro* capillary pressure-flow studies have further confirmed this finding.[24] This implies that *in vitro* viscosity measurements may not reflect viscosity and organ blood flow at the capillary level. Dintenfass[18] suggested that blood viscosity may again increase in capillaries <4 μm in size.[18] Since the radius of capillaries in different organs varies, this may explain why changes in hematocrit and viscosity seems to have an effect on flow in some organs but none in other organs.

5. Hemodynamic Changes in Polycythemic and Hyperviscous States

Many problems experienced by the infant with polycythemia and hyperviscosity have been attributed to the diminished organ blood flow. It is therefore relevant to review the regulation of blood flow in the various organs of the body.

5.1. Cardiopulmonary Blood Flow

Most studies on cardiac performance during periods of polycythemia and hyperviscosity have used adult animals or newborn animals transfused with adult RBCs. Nonetheless, the results from most of these studies appear pertinent to the symptomatology observed in polycythemic and hyperviscous newborn infants.

Multiple studies have shown several changes to occur with increasing hematocrit and viscosity: (1) decreased cardiac output, (2) no change in oxygen transport or consumption in the myocardium and total body, and (3) increased pulmonary and systemic vascular resistance.

Using newborn piglets, Nowicki et al.[35] showed polycythemia to be associated with a decrease in cardiac output; however, due to an increase in oxygen content, the systemic oxygen delivery was unaffected by the reduced cardiac output. LeBlanc et al.[36] showed similar results in newborn puppies.

The decrease in cardiac output appears to be the result of a reduction in either stroke volume or heart rate, or both.[36–38] We performed a partial exchange transfusion with Plasmanate in 11 polycythemic and hyperviscous infants in order to reduce their hematocrit and blood viscosity. There was a significant rise in heart rate, reflecting an increase in cardiac output.[39] This is consistent with data that demonstrates the newborn infant's limited ability to increase stroke volume and thereby changes in cardiac output are reflected primarily by changes in heart rate.

In a series of experiments, Surjadhana and co-workers[37] demonstrated that myocardial blood flow and left ventricular flow were decreased with elevation of the hematocrit but that oxygen transport and consumption were normal. Subjecting the animals to hypoxia and thereby reducing oxygen content but not viscosity, these investigators demonstrated that both control and polycythemic animals appropriately increased myocardial blood flow to meet the tissue demand for oxygen. They concluded that the changes in myocardial blood flow observed were a result of autoregulation to changes in oxygen content and not viscosity.

The changes in systemic and pulmonary vascular resistance have been demonstrated by several authors.[38,40] Using newborn lambs, Fouron and Hebert[40] observed that increasing the hematocrit increases the pulmonary resistance proportionally greater than systemic resistance (see Fig. 8). At a hematocrit of 70%, pulmonary resistance equaled the systemic resistance (see Fig. 9). The left to right shunt through the ductus arteriosus reversed itself when the hematocrit exceeded 65–70%, resulting in a fall in the systemic arterial oxygen saturation. This may partly explain the cardiopulmonary symptoms observed in the neonates

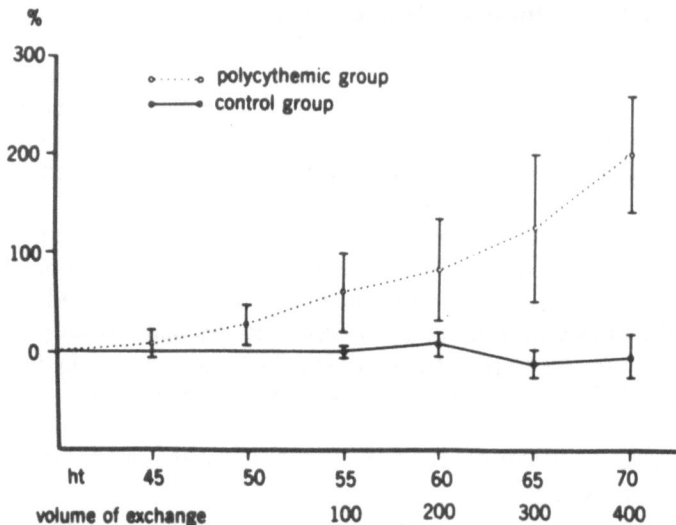

Figure 8. Percentage of changes of the pulmonary over the systemic vascular resistances. The starting point (0) corresponds to the value of the ratio before any exchange transfusion. In the polycythemic group (O · · · O), the percentage of changes in relationship to this point become significant at a hematocrit of 65% ($p < 0.05$). This difference is mainly due to the increase in pulmonary vascular resistance. In the control group (●——●), the changes are not significant. (From Fouron and Hebert.[40])

reported by Gatti *et al.*[41] and the cyanotic appearance observed by many clinicians.

5.2. Gastrointestinal Blood Flow

Studies in newborn puppies and piglets have shown that polycythemia and hyperviscosity results in a significant fall in blood flow to the unfed gastrointestinal (GI) tract.[35,42] Nowicki *et al.*[35] examined the effects of feeding on gut blood flow and oxygen utilization in polycythemic hyperviscous piglets. In the nonfed state, diminished gut blood flow was observed. The oxygen available to the GI tissue was unchanged, however, because of the increased arterial oxygen content. A decrease in oxygen extraction and uptake was observed as well. The reduction in oxygen uptake therefore is related to the tissue autoregulation of oxygen uptake rather than to availability. The reason for this pattern of oxygen transport in GI tissues during polycythemia and hyperviscosity is still unclear.

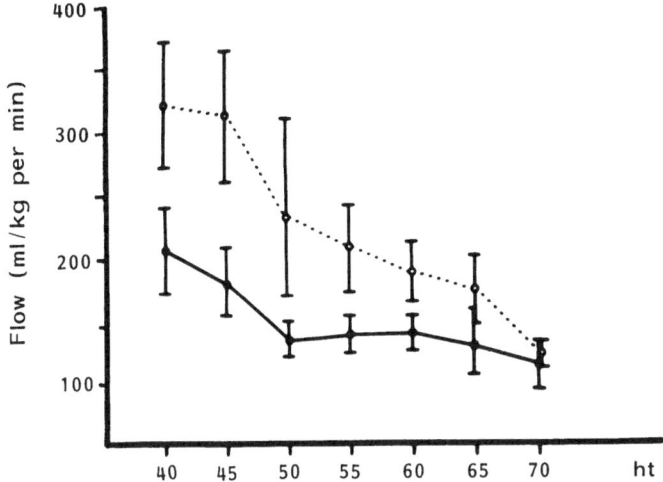

Figure 9. Pulmonary flows of the polycythemic group became significantly lower at a hematocrit of 65% ($p < 0.05$). The same is true for the systemic flows at a hematocrit of 70% ($p < 0.05$). (●———●) Systemic flow; (○···○) pulmonary flow. (From Fouron and Hebert.[40])

5.3. Renal Blood Flow

Kotagal and Kleinman[43] studied renal blood flow and function in the newborn puppy model of normovolemic polycythemia and hyperviscosity. Renal blood flow was unchanged by an elevation in hematocrit and viscosity. The decreased plasma volume led to diminished renal plasma flow (see Fig. 10). This resulted in a fall in glomerular filtration rate. An associated drop in urine output and Na^+ and K^+ excretion was found (see Figs. 11 and 12). The lack of change in systemic blood pressure and renal blood flow suggests that renal vascular resistance is not altered by increases in hematocrit and viscosity. It may be postulated that the Fahraeus-Lindqvist effect prevails in the kidney, accounting for the lack of change in blood flow. Oxygen delivery to the kidney is obviously increased due to the increase in arterial oxygen content.

In a study examining renal blood flow and function in a group of infants with early cord clamping (venous hematocrit: 50%) and late cord clamping (venous hematocrit: 62%[12]) soon after birth, the infants with late cord clamping had greater blood and RBC volumes, mean arterial blood pressure, and renal blood flow.[12] They also had a significantly higher glomerular filtration rate (GFR) and urine output. At 2–5 days of age, the blood pressures and renal blood flow became similar, as did

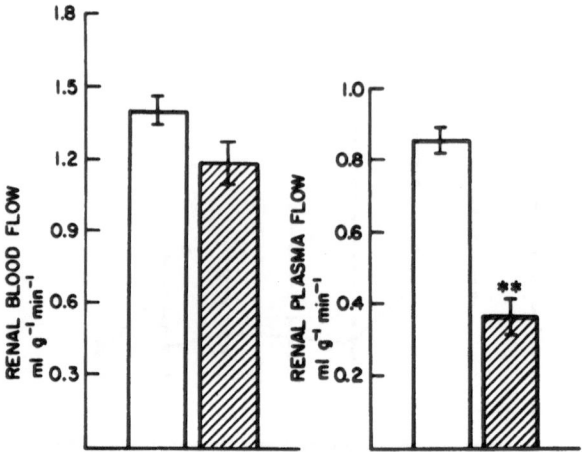

Figure 10. Renal blood flow and renal plasma flow before (unshaded) and after (shaded) polycythemia (mean ±SE). **$p < 0.01$. (From Kotagal and Kleinman.[43])

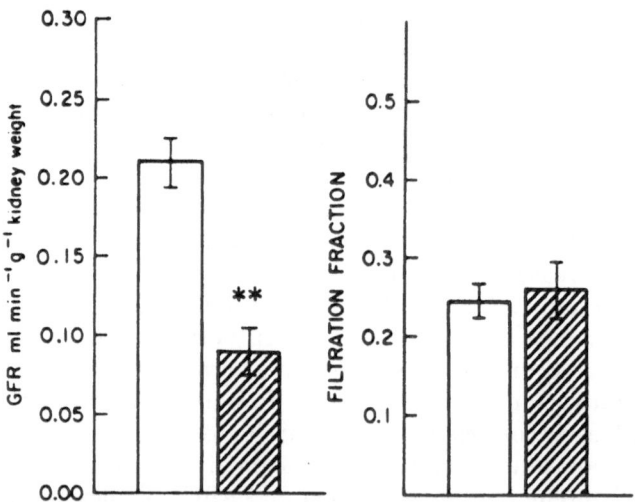

Figure 11. Glomerular filtration rate per gram kidney weight and filtration fraction before (unshaded) and after (shaded) polycythemia (mean ±SE). **$p < 0.01$. (From Kotagal and Kleinman.[43])

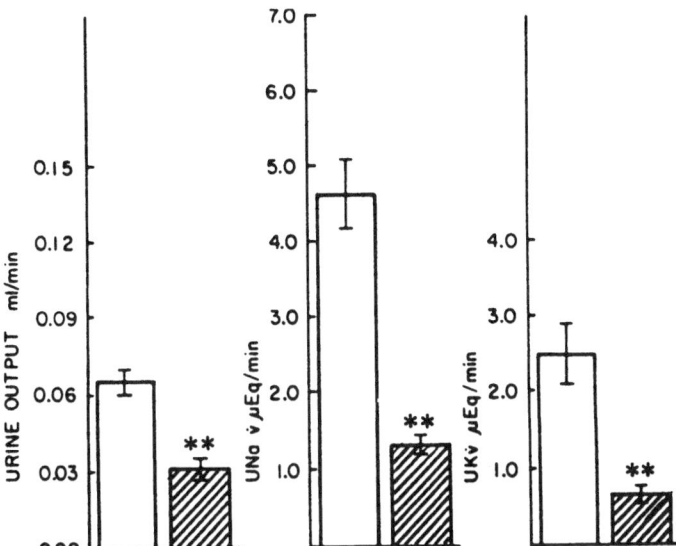

Figure 12.   Urine output, urine Na$^+$ and urine K$^+$ excretion before (unshaded) and after (shaded) polycythemia (mean ± SE). **$p < 0.01$. (From Kotagal and Kleinman.[43])

the various measures of renal function (see Fig. 13). The discrepancy between these two studies (Kotagal and Kleinman[43] and Oh *et al.*[12]) with reference to high hematocrit and renal function in the newborn is probably related to the blood volume difference in the two studies. In the puppy model, the elevation in hematocrit was produced by an isovolumetric exchange transfusion using packed RBCs.[12,43] Thus, the main effect on renal function was on the basis of high red cell mass and reduced plasma volume accounting for the lower renal plasma flow and glomerular filtration rates. In the human study, the high hematocrit was the result of hemoconcentration following an acute expansion of blood volume resulting from placental transfusion at birth. The high blood and plasma volume produced the expected results of higher renal blood flow, plasma flow, and GFR.

5.4.   Carcass Blood Flow

Initial studies of limb blood flow in newborn infants using venous occlusion plethysmography measured blood flow in skin and muscle. Thus, the measurements were influenced by the relatively large muscle

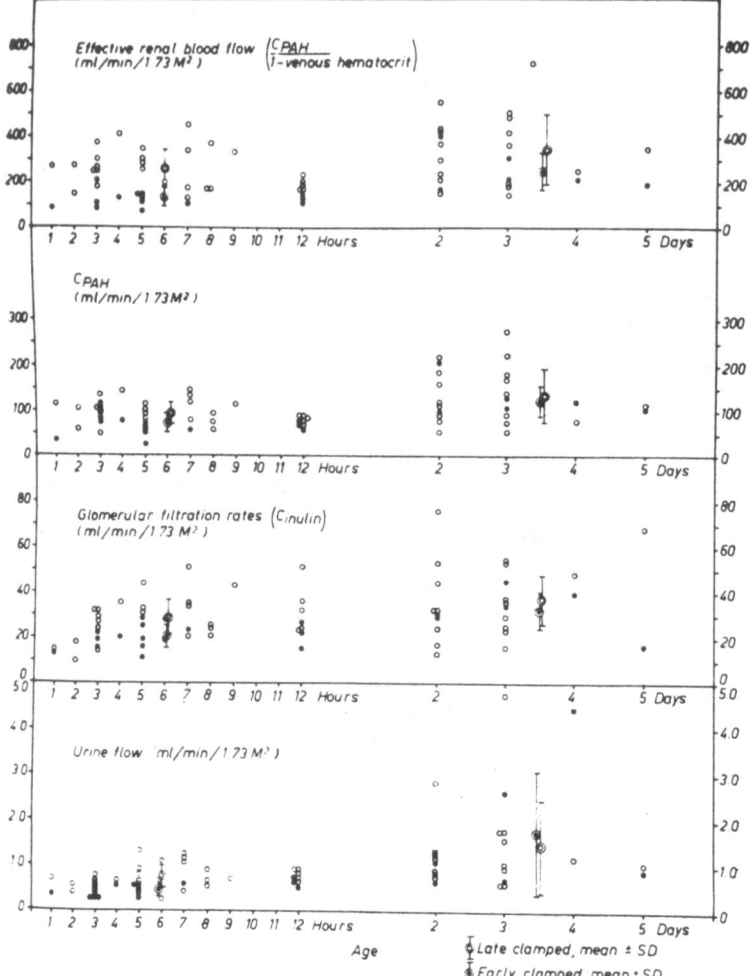

Figure 13. Urine flow, glomerular filtration rate, effective renal plasma, and blood flow in 69 infants with early and late cord clamping during the first 5 days of life. (From Oh et al.[12])

mass.[44,45] These studies were unable to show a relationship among hematocrit, viscosity, and peripheral blood flow. More sophisticated studies have now permitted separate measurements of muscle and skin.

Gustafsson et al.[46] examined blood flow in the isolated calf muscle of adult dogs. In the resting state, *in vivo* and *in vitro* viscosity measurements were higher and blood flow lower in the polycythemic state. While not directly measured in this experiment, oxygen delivery was approximately the same in both conditions. In working muscle, *in vivo* viscosity and blood flow were similar under both conditions. Owing to increased oxygen content, oxygen delivery to the muscle was higher during polycythemia. This experiment suggests that the Fahraeus-Lindqvist effect is operational and that muscle blood flow is regulated by metabolic activity.

Waffarn *et al.*[47] recently examined relative changes in cutaneous flow by measuring the changes in heat output of a transcutaneous P_{O_2}/P_{CO_2} monitor. Measurements were made prior to and after a partial exchange transfusion in a group of 10 polycythemic newborn infants, who were restrained under a radiant warmer. These workers found a 38% increase in cutaneous blood flow measurements after hematocrit reduction. No changes in P_{O_2}/T_{CO_2} or P_{CO_2}/T_{CCO_2} were found. They speculated that the lack of change in P_{O_2} and P_{CO_2} reflected adequate oxygen availability under polycythemic conditions and that oxygen delivery was probably similar before and after the exchange transfusion. Although the effect of viscosity was not isolated, it would appear that it does not have an adverse effect on cutaneous blood flow so as to prevent the metabolic needs of the skin from being met.

5.5. Brain Blood Flow

Recently, the changes in brain blood flow of infants with polycythemia were measured. Using Doppler techniques, we were able to demonstrate that infants with polycythemia and hyperviscosity have reduced cerebral blood flow velocity as compared with infants with normal hematocrit and viscosity (see Fig. 14). Partial exchange transfusion with plasmanate to reduce the hematocrit and viscosity resulted in an increase in cerebral blood flow velocity comparable to that of the control infants.[39]

Jones *et al.*[48] varied arterial oxygen content in newborn lambs by changing the hematocrit and P_{O_2} and examined the effects on brain blood flow. They concluded that there was a direct relationship between arterial oxygen content and blood flow. Viscosity, which was not measured, presumably varied with the changes in hematocrit and arterial oxygen content; thus, it might also play a role in the brain blood flow as observed by these investigators.

Using the newborn lamb model of polycythemia, we separated the factors of arterial oxygen content and viscosity in order to understand the role each might play in regulating cerebral blood flow.[49] We increased the hematocrit and viscosity to polycythemic and hyperviscous levels by performing isovolumetric exchange transfusions using newborn lamb packed RBCs (see Fig. 15). We observed an increase in arterial oxygen

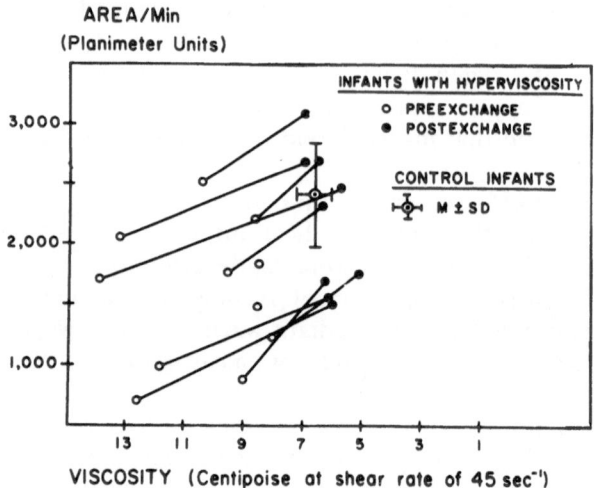

Figure 14. Individual values for area under the velocity curve per minute or cerebral blood flow velocity are plotted against viscosity. (From Rosenkrantz and Oh.[39])

content and decrease in cerebral blood flow. The animals were then infused with sodium nitrite, causing methemoglobin formation. This lowered the arterial oxygen content to control levels, while the hematocrit and viscosity remained elevated. Cerebral blood flow returned to control levels. Oxygen delivery remained constant throughout the study. We concluded that the reduced cerebral blood flow observed in polycythemic infants is a result of the elevated oxygen content and not of viscosity. Additional studies have demonstrated that oxygen uptake is also unaltered by polycythemia and hyperviscosity, thereby refuting the hypothesis that polycythemia and hyperviscosity is directly responsible for brain ischemia and hypoxia.[50]

Blood flow through the brain, like the heart, would appear to be subject to the Fahraeus-Lindqvist effect. That is, flow is unaffected by changes in viscosity but, rather, autoregulated to meet metabolic demands of the brain.

5.6. Fetal Blood Flow

Little information is available on the *in utero* effects of polycythemia and hyperviscosity on the fetus. Tenenbaum *et al.*[51] performed exchange transfusions in eight lamb fetuses using packed adult RBCs. This resulted in an increased hematocrit and viscosity but an unchanged um-

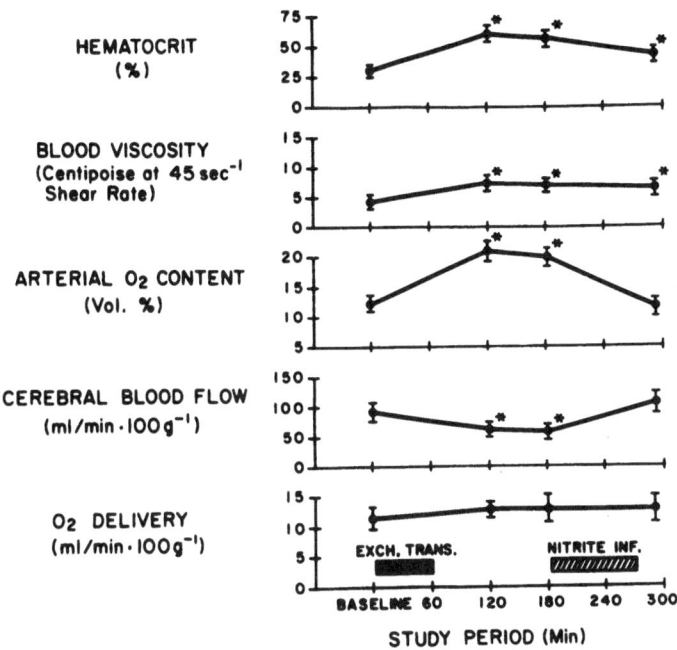

Figure 15. Hematocrit values, whole blood viscosity, arterial oxygen content, total brain blood flow, and oxygen delivery during study in seven newborn lambs. Data mean ± SD. *p < 0.01 versus baseline. (From Rosenkrantz et al.[49])

bilical venous oxygen content. Immediately after the exchange transfusion, they observed a significant decrease in umbilical blood flow and oxygen delivery. Because of increased extraction, fetal oxygen uptake was unchanged. This study suggests that viscosity may play a role in reduction of umbilical blood flow. It should be noted that this study examined the effect of isovolemic polycythemia, while the clinical situation probably represents a hypervolemic condition. Obviously there is a need for future research to determine the effect of long-standing polycythemia and hyperviscosity on fetal regional blood flow.

6. Etiology

The three major factors that may lead to polycythemia and hyperviscosity are chronic intrauterine hypoxia, perinatal asphyxia, and delayed cord clamping. Other causes and associations are maternal–fetal

**Table I. Factors Leading to Neonatal
Polycythemia and Hyperviscosity**

Chronic fetal hypoxia
   Infants of diabetic mother
   Intrauterine growth retardation
   Heavy maternal smoking
   Preeclampsia
Perinatal asphyxia
Placental transfusion at birth
Other factors
   Fetofetal transfusion
   Beckwith syndrome

hemorrhage, fetofetal transfusion, chromosomal abnormalities, including Trisomy 21, Beckwith Wiedemann syndrome, and neonatal hyperthyroidism[2,9,14,15,52] (see Table I).

The mechanism and time sequence for fetal transfusion *via* delayed cord clamping have been discussed.[15] To avoid excessive and acute expansion of blood volume, it is best to clamp the cord as soon as possible (within 10–15 sec after delivery of the buttocks) to avoid the problem of polycythemia.

Perinatal asphyxia remains a major cause of polycythemia. Philip *et al.*[53] examined placental residual volumes and fetal outcome. Those infants whose placental volumes were small had a significantly high rate of fetal distress and low Apgar scores. Similar studies by Flod and Ackerman[54] and Yao and Lind[55] yielded similar results.

Studies in the fetal lamb demonstrated that intrauterine hypoxia results in intrauterine placental transfusions.[56] Data from this study also suggested that fetal vasodilation may occur as part of the mechanism that results in the increased fetal blood volume.

Twin-to-twin transfusion is a well-documented cause of polycythemia.[57,58] This usually involves a monochorionic placenta with twin-to-twin vascular anastomoses in which flow from one twin to the other is not reciprocal. The result is a polycythemic large twin and a small anemic twin.

Fetuses with abnormal intrauterine growth—SGA or LGA—are at particularly high risk for polycythemia.[59] Widness *et al.*[60] showed that more of these infants who are polycythemic will have elevated erythropoietin levels as compared with AGA-polycythemic infants. These workers concluded that these high levels of erythropoietin were the result of chronic hypoxia related to placental insufficiency. Studies by Philipps *et al.*[61] demonstrated hypoxia in the hyperglycemic lamb fetus.

Thus hypoxia may explain the high incidence of polycythemia in the infant of the diabetic mother.

7. Clinical Symptoms

The clinical symptoms associated with polycythemia and hyperviscosity occur in multiple organ systems. The following discussion focuses on the physiologic basis of these symptoms.

A review of the literature reveals the following frequencies of clinical symptoms attributable at least in part to polycythemia (see Table II). The studies presented are those involving a large number of polycythemic infants in which early symptoms were investigated. In addition, Gatti et al.[41] reported on a prospective series of 629 infants. Twenty-five were polycythemic, but none had any symptoms.

Whereas a number of studies have noted an increased incidence of polycythemia in growth retarded infants, Hakanson and Oh[64] found a similar percentage of "polycythemic" symptoms in those infants with normal hematocrit and those who were polycythemic. This emphasizes the point that the symptoms observed in polycythemic infants may be

Table II. Frequency of Clinical Symptoms Attributed in Part to Polycythemia[a]

	Investigation			
Clinical symptoms	Gross et al.[5] (N = 18) (%)	Ramamurthy and Brans[6] (N = 54) (%)	Black et al.[62] (N = 111) (%)	Goldberg et al.[63] (N = 20) (%)
Cyanosis	89	17	7	nr
Plethora	83	63	nr	nr
Tremulous/jittery	67	13	nr	nr
Abnormal EEG	33	nr	nr	nr
Seizures	28	0	0	nr
Respiratory distress	44	4	10	15
Cardiomegaly	17	nr	nr	85
Lethargy/poor feeding	nr	50	+	55
Hyperbilirubinemia	50	6	nr	5
Abnormal blood smear	50	nr	nr	nr
Thrombocytopenia	39	nr	nr	25
Hypoglycemia	33	nr	27	40
Hypocalcemia	6	nr	nr	0

[a] nr, not reported or examined; +, greater incidence compared with the control group.

the result of other perinatal problems associated with polycythemia, such as asphyxia or poor intrauterine nutrition, and not directly due to the increased hematocrit and viscosity.

7.1. Blood Volume and Body Water

Polycythemic infants tend to have increased blood volumes when corrected for body weight.[12,65,66] This holds true for preterm and term infants, although there is a fair amount of variation from infant to infant. This is not surprising when one considers that the two most common etiologies of polycythemia are delayed cord clamping and perinatal asphyxia with placental-to-fetus transfusion. Saigal and Usher[52] showed a significant relationship between the degree of hypervolemia and cardiorespiratory problems. However, the causal relationship between blood volume and magnitude of respiratory symptoms remains obscure and needs further investigation.

A series of studies by Thorton and Brans and co-workers[66,67] demonstrated that polycythemic infants, when compared to their normocythemic counterparts, have similar total body water, mean extracellular water, mean intracellular water and mean interstitial water. Plasma volumes also seem to be normal in polycythemic infants.[12,66]

7.2. Cardiopulmonary Symptoms

The most frequently reported findings attributed to cardiopulmonary dysfunction are cyanosis, tachypnea, cardiomegaly, and "plethora" of the lung fields on the X-ray film of the chest.[4,5,41,52,68] Although the infants may have a red-blue color, the arterial PO_2 (PaO_2) usually reveals normal oxygenation. The respiratory distress may in part be due to elevated pulmonary blood pressure and ductal shunting, which may be secondary to hyperviscosity. The increased fluid content from transudation may also cause decreased lung compliance.[68] In general, most investigators report resolution of the cardiorespiratory symptoms with hemodilution.

7.3. Gastrointestinal Symptoms

Multiple series have reported on infants with poor feeding or vomiting.[60,69,70] In addition, there appears to be a significant risk for the development of necrotizing enterocolitis (NEC).[71,72] Many infants who are polycythemic and hyperviscous also have experienced either perinatal asphyxia or IUGR, or both, which in themselves are risk factors for the development of NEC. Thus, it is still unclear whether the direct association of polycythemic hyperviscosity and NEC is indeed real or is partly moderated by other risk factors such as fetal hypoxia.

LeBlanc et al.[73] recently examined the intestinal histology of dogs up to 24 hr after the induction of polycythemia. They found a 58% incidence of NEC. This is consistent with Nowicki's blood flow and oxygen uptake data in the piglet which suggest that the bowel may experience some hypoxia in the unfed state.[35]

Black et al.[74] recently reported on a group of 93 polycythemic infants who were randomized to either be observed or receive a partial exchange transfusion. Six percent of the observed infants had serious GI signs as compared with 51% of the infants receiving the exchange transfusion. One-third of the treated infants had X-ray evidence of pneumotosis intestinalis. This study suggests that exchange transfusion is the most important contributing factor in the development of NEC in these infants.

7.4. Renal Function

Acute renal failure has been reported in an infant with polycythemia[75]; however, the precise mechanism involved is unclear. In infants with polycythemia and normal blood volume, plasma volume will be reduced. The expected result would be low renal plasma flow, GFR, and urine flow. In infants who have high blood volume from a placental transfusion at birth, renal plasma flow, GFR, and urine flow rate are actually higher than in those with a lower blood volume. In addition, the perinatal asphyxia often associated with a placental transfusion at birth may have the direct effect of hypoxic/ischemic renal damage, resulting in reduced renal function. This discrepancy in physiologic measurement and clinical reports underscores the need for further study to clarify this issue of renal function in these infants.

7.5. Hypoglycemia

Hypoglycemia is frequently found in infants who are polycythemic even after such compounding issues as IUGR are considered.[5,58,62,63] Leake et al.[76] and Creswell et al.[77] examined the etiology in newborn polycythemic lambs. Both groups speculated about the roles of decreased glucose production and increased glucose uptake, but neither came to any finite conclusion. Thus, the etiology still seems unanswered. The following is presented as one explanation. Glucose is contained almost exclusively in the plasma fraction of blood that is reduced in polycythemia. Cardiac output and blood/plasma flow to most organs are reduced. This results in increased extraction of the available glucose and a decreased venous concentration. In addition, decreased liver blood/plasma flow may limit the exit of glucose produced through gluconeogenesis. This combination theoretically should lead to decreased glucose concentration of blood and plasma.

7.6. Hematologic Complications

Several centers have reported an association of polycythemic and hematologic abnormalities including thrombocytopenia and/or a decrease in the antithrombin III (AT-III) level. Disseminated intravascular coagulation (DIC) has been reported by one investigator, but others have not been able to confirm this finding.[78–80] Several explanations have been given for the thrombocytopenia. They include impaired production due to tissue hypoxia, predominance in the marrow of erythropoietic cells, slow spleen blood flow, and decreased plasma fraction with normal concentration.[79–83] Platelet counts seem to recover spontaneously in all series.

Low AT-III is found in asphyxiated infants.[84] It would seem reasonable that perinatal asphyxia may be responsible for the low AT-III levels observed in a portion of infants with polycythemia.[84,85]

7.7. Neurologic Manifestations

7.7.1. Neonatal Period

Numerous papers have reported infants with polycythemia and hyperviscosity to be lethargic, irritable, and tremulous and to have seizures during the neonatal period.[5,6,52,62,63] There are two case reports of cerebral infarcts.[88,87] In a controlled study, Goldberg et al.[63] showed abnormalities in the Prechtl and Brazelton examinations of these infants. These examinations slowly improved spontaneously. Hemodilution via partial plasma exchange transfusion did not significantly accelerate the process of recovery. van der Elst et al.[69] also performed the Brazelton examination on a group of neonates. Three groups were studied. Forty-nine infants with polycythemia were randomly assigned to either be observed or receive a partial exchange transfusion. A third group was composed of control infants. The Brazelton and Prechtl examination at 10 days of age showed the two polycythemic groups to be similar. The treated group was different from the control group in three of four categories, while the observed group only differed in one of four categories.

It would seem that polycythemic infants are different in their state behavior and neurologic function during the first week of life and that partial plasma exchange transfusion does not appear to facilitate improvement.

7.7.2. Long-Term Sequelae

Five series of patients have been followed from 8 months to 6 years in an effort to identify long-term disability that might be attributable to neonatal polycythemia and hyperviscosity. The first published series was by van der Elst et al.[69] The data involve the same three groups of infants previously discussed. At 8 months, a modification of the Griffith Developmental Score was administered. All infants in all three groups had normal neurologic examinations. Developmental scores were similar in all three groups.

Goldberg et al.[63] re-evaluated her previously described treated, observed, and control patients at 8 months. The Bayley Scales of Infant Development, Milani-Comparetti Postural Reflex Examination, medical history, and neurologic and physical examination were completed. There were no differences in the Bayley scores of the three groups. Neurologic examinations found abnormalities in 67% of the nontreated, 50% of the treated, and 17% of the control infants. Whereas there were no statistical differences among the three groups, there appeared to be a difference between the hyperviscous group and the control infants but no difference between treated and nontreated hyperviscous infants. Of concern was the high incidence of spastic diplegia found in the two groups of hyperviscous infants.

Black and colleagues[62] followed a group of 111 infants who had neonatal hyperviscosity and 110 control infants. Follow-up examinations were performed between 1 and 3 years of age and included the Bayley Scales, Denver Developmental Screening Test, physical and neurologic examinations, as well as medical history. Forty-two of the hyperviscous infants had received partial exchange transfusions during the newborn period. Patients were not randomized, but rather the sicker infants tended to receive this therapy. The follow-up data exhibited no difference in mental development in any of the groups, but a significant number (compared with the control group) of the hyperviscous infants had motor delays with no difference between the treated and observed hyperviscous groups. Twenty-five percent of the hyperviscous group had neurologic abnormalities, especially spastic diplegia. In all, 43% of the treated, 35% of the observed, and 11% of the control infants had handicaps ($p < 0.005$). Again, treatment did not seem to change in outcome.

More recently, Black et al.[88] completed another study to evaluate the effect of partial transfusions in infants with polycythemia and hyperviscosity. These workers evaluated 93 infants with polycythemia and hyperviscosity who were randomly assigned to treated and nontreated groups. No differentiation was made between symptomatic and asymptomatic infants. Only 80% of the infants were available for follow-up evaluation at 1 and/or 2 years (59% at 1 year and 61% at 2 years). No differences were observed at the 1 year evaluation. At 2 years of age, the treated group had fewer neurologic abnormalities. Black and coworkers also analyzed the neonatal morbidity of the partial transfusion and found a significantly higher incidence of necrotizing enterocolitis in the treated group.

Host et al.[79] reported a subset of polycythemic infants from data collected as part of a community health project. Follow-up at 2.5 years of age included a Denver Developmental Screening Test and health questionnaire. A second questionnaire was also evaluated at 6 years of age. A high percentage (80%) of the infants identified with a venous hematocrit of 65% completed the study. Basically all the infants were normal, except for one child with hypocalcemic seizures secondary to rickets.

In summary, it appears that polycythemic infants are neurologically "depressed" during the neonatal period. Studies to evaluate long-term neurologic and developmental outcome, particularly with reference to the benefits of partial exchange transfusions, are less definitive. Most studies indicate a less favorable outcome in the polycythemic and hyperviscous infant. In regard to the beneficial effect of treatment to lower the hematocrit and blood hyperviscosity, the only study that indicates a beneficial effect of such a procedure is that of Black et al.[88]

8. Management

The most common specific therapy for polycythemia and hyperviscosity is partial exchange transfusion, utilizing either saline, fresh frozen plasma, partial protein fraction, or dilute albumin as the exchange solution. All seem to be equally effective. The volume used for the exchange is as follows:

$$\frac{[\text{Hct (observed)} - \text{Hct (desired)}] \times \text{blood volume}^{89}}{\text{Hct (observed)}}$$

There are adequate data and understanding of the pathophysiology responsible for some of the symptoms observed in infants with polycythemia and hyperviscosity. These symptoms include cardiopulmonary embarrasment, renal failure, and hypoglycemia. Our present knowledge probably supports the efficacy of hemodilutional therapy to ameliorate these symptoms. The effectiveness of therapy for the prevention of neurologic and developmental sequelae is less conclusive. Only the randomized study by Black et al.[88] in polycythemic and hyperviscous infants appears to support the need for treating these infants. Infants who are polycythemic and hyperviscous but asymptomatic during the perinatal period are the population who present the most challenge and controversy with respect to the indication for treatment with partial exchange transfusions. This issue is complicated by the lack of good follow-up studies to evaluate the long-term outcome of asymptomatic polycythemic and hyperviscous infants. The issue of treatment will remain controversial until good data are obtained in the future.

References

1. Wood, J. L., 1952, Plethora in the newborn infant associated with cyanosis and convulsions, *J. Pediatr.* **54:**143.
2. Michael, A. F., and Mauer, A. M., 1961, Maternal–fetal transfusion as a cause of plethora in the neonatal period, *Pediatrics* **28:**458.
3. Minkowski, A., 1962, Acute cardiac failure in connection with neonatal polycythemia (in monovular twins and single newborn infants), *Biol. Neonate* **4:**61.
4. Danks, D. M., and Stevens, L. H., 1964, Neonatal respiratory distress with a high hematocrit, *Lancet* **2:**499.
5. Gross, G. P., Hathaway, W. E., and McGaughey, H. R., 1973, Hyperviscosity in the neonate, *J. Pediatr.* **82:**1004.
6. Ramamurthy, R. S., and Brans, Y. W., 1981, Neonatal polycythemia. I. Criteria for diagnosis and treatment, *Pediatrics* **68:**168.
7. Oh, W., and Lind, J., 1966, Venous and capillary hematocrit in newborn infants and placental transfusion, *Acta Paediatr. Scand.* **55:**38.
8. Wirth, F. H., Goldberg, K. E., and Lubchenco, L. O., 1979, Neonatal hyperviscosity. I. Incidence, *Pediatrics* **63:**833.
9. Stevens, K., and Wirth, F. H., 1980, Incidence of neonatal hyperviscosity at sea level, *J. Pediatr.* **97:**118.

10. Brooks, G. I., and Backes, C. R., 1981, Hyperviscosity secondary to polycythemia in the appropriate for gestational age neonate, *JAOA* **80:**415.
11. Reisner, S. H., Mor, N., Levy, Y., and Merlob, P., 1983, Incidence of neonatal polycythemia, *Isr. J. Med. Sci.* **19:**848.
12. Oh, W., Oh, M. A., and Lind, J., 1966, Renal function and blood volume in newborn infants related to placental transfusion, *Acta Paediatr. Scand.* **56:**197.
13. Oh, W., Blankenship, W., and Lind, J., 1966, Further study of neonatal blood volume in relation to placental transfusion, *Ann. Paediatr.* **207:**147.
14. Yao, A. C., Moinian, M., and Lind, J., 1969, Distribution of blood between infants and placenta after birth, *Lancet* **2:**871.
15. Linderkamp, O., 1981, Placental transfusion: Determinants and effects, *Clin. Perinatol.* **9:**559.
16. Poiseuille, J. L. M., 1840, Recherches expérimentales sur le mouvement des liquides dans les tubes de très petits diamètres, *C.R. Acad. Sci.* **11:**961, 1041.
17. van der Elst, C. W., Malan, A. F., and de v. Heese, H., 1977, Blood viscosity in modern medicine, *S. Afr. Med. J.* **52:**526.
18. Dintenfass, L., 1968, Blood viscosity, internal fluidity of the red cell, dynamic coagulation and the critical capillary radius as factors in the physiology and pathology of circulation and microcirculation, *Med. J. Aust.* **1:**688.
19. Wells, R. E., Penton, R., and Merrill, E. W., 1961, Measurements of viscosity of biologic fluids by core plate viscometer, *J. Lab. Clin. Med.* **57:**646.
20. Wells, R. E., and Merrill, E. W., 1961, Influence of flow properties of blood upon viscosity–hematocrit relationships, *J. Clin. Invest.* **41:**1591.
21. Linderkamp, O., Versmold, H. I. T., Riegel, K. P., and Betke, K., 1984, Contributions of red cells and plasma to blood viscosity in preterm and full-term infants and adults, *Pediatrics* **74:**45.
22. Bergqvist, G., 1974, Viscosity of the blood in the newborn infants, *Acta Paediatr. Scand.* **63:**858.
23. Shohat, M., Reisner, S. H., Mimoini, F., and Merlob, P., 1984, Neonatal polycythemia. II. Definition related to time of sampling, *Pediatrics* **73:**11.
24. Burton, A. C., 1966, Role of geometry, of size and shape, in the microcirculation, *Fed. Proc.* **25:**1753.
25. Charm, S. E., and Kurland, G. S., 1974, *Blood Flow and Microcirculation*, pg. 14, Wiley, New York.
26. Wells, R., 1970, Syndromes of hyperviscosity, *N. Engl. J. Med.* **283:**183.
27. Somer, T., and Ditzel, J., 1981, Clinical and rheological studies in a patient with hyperviscosity syndrome due to Waldenstrom's macroglobulinemia, *Bibl. Haematol.* **47:**242.
28. Linderkamp, O., Wu, P. Y. K., and Meiselman, H. J., 1982, Deformability of density separated red blood cells in normal newborn infants and adults, *Pediatr. Res.* **16:**964.
29. Smith, C. M., Prasler, W. J., Tukey, D. P., *et al.*, 1981, Fetal red cells are more deformable than adult red cells, *Blood* **58:**35a (abs.).
30. Lichtman, M. A., 1970, Cellular deformability during maturation of the myeloblast, *N. Engl. J. Med.* **283:**943.
31. Lichtman, M. A., 1973, Rheology of leukocytes, leukocyte suspensions, and blood in leukemia, *J. Clin. Invest.* **52:**350.
32. Miller, M. E., 1975, Developmental maturation of human neutrophil motility and its relationship to membrane deformability, in: *The Phagocytic Cell in Host Resistance* (J. A. Bellanti and D. H. Dayton, ed.), p. 295, Raven Press, New York.
33. Rand, P. W., Austin, W. H., Lacombe, E., and Barker, N., 1968, pH and blood viscosity, *J. Appl. Physiol.* **25:**550.

34. Fahraeus, R., and Lindqvist, T., 1931, The viscosity of the blood in narrow capillary tubes, *Am. J. Physiol.* **96:**562.

35. Nowicki, P., Oh, W., Yao, A., Hansen, N. B., and Stonestreet, B. S., 1984, Effect of polycythemia on gastrointestinal blood flow and oxygenation in piglets, *Am. J. Physiol.* **247** (Gastrointest. Liver Physiol. 10):G220.

36. LeBlanc, M. H., Kotagal, V. R., and Kleinman, L. I., 1982, Physiological effects of hypervolemic polycythemia in newborn dogs, *J. Appl. Physiol.* **53:**865.

37. Surjadhana, A., Rouleau, J., Boerboom, L., and Hoffman, J. I. E., 1978, Myocardial blood flow and its distribution in anesthetized polycythemic dogs, *Circ. Res.* **43:**619.

38. Brashear, R. E., 1980, Effects of acute plasma for blood exchange in experimental polycythemia, *Respiration* **40:**297.

39. Rosenkrantz, T. S., and Oh, W., 1982, Cerebral blood flow velocity in infants with polycythemia and hyperviscosity: Effects of partial exchange transfusion with Plamanate, *J. Pediatr.* **101:**94.

40. Fouron, J. C., and Hebert, F., 1973, The circulatory effects of hematocrit variations in normovolemic newborn lambs, *J. Pediatr.* **82:**995.

41. Gatti, R. A., Muster, A. J., Cole, R. B., and Paul, M. H., 1966, Neonatal polycythemia with transient cyanosis and cardiorespiratory abnormalities, *J. Pediatr.* **69:**1063.

42. Kotagal, V. R., Keenan, W. J., Reuter, J. H., et al., 1977, Regional blood flow in polycythemia and hypervolemia, *Pediatr. Res.* **11:**394.

43. Kotagal, V. R., and Kleinman, L. I., 1982, Effect of acute polycythemia on newborn renal hemodynamics and function, *Pediatr. Res.* **16:**148.

44. Bergqvist, G., and Zetterman, R., 1974, Blood viscosity and peripheral circulation in newborn infants, *Acta Paediatr. Scand.* **63:**865.

45. Linderkamp, O., Strohhacker, I., Versmold, H. T., et al., 1978, Peripheral circulation in the newborn: Interaction of peripheral blood flow, blood pressure, blood volume and blood viscosity, *Eur. J. Pediatr.* **129:**73.

46. Gustafsson, L., Applegren, L., and Myrvold, H. E., 1980, The effect of polycythemia on blood flow in working and non-working skeletal muscle, *Acta Physiol. Scand.* **109:**143.

47. Waffarn, F., Cole, C. D., and Huxtable, R. F., 1984, Effects of polycythemia and hyperviscosity on cutaneous blood flow and transcutaneous pO_2 and pCO_2 in the neonate, *Pediatrics* **74:**389.

48. Jones, M. D., Traystman, R. J., Simmons, M. A., and Molteni, R. A., 1981, Effects of changes in arterial O_2 content on cerebral blood flow in the lamb, *Am. J. Physiol.* **240** (Heart Circ. Physiol. 9):H209.

49. Rosenkrantz, T. S., Stonestreet, B. S., Hansen, N. B., et al., 1984, Cerebral blood flow in the newborn lamb with polycythemia and hyperviscosity, *J. Pediatr.* **104:**276.

50. Rosenkrantz, T. S., and Philipps, A. F., 1985, Cerebral carbohydrate metabolism in polythemic newborn lambs, *Pediatr. Res.* **19:**319A.

51. Tenenbaum, D. G., Piasecki, G. J., Oh, W., Rosenkrantz, T. S., and Jackson, B. T., 1983, Fetal polycythemia and hyperviscosity: Effect in umbilical blood flow and fetal oxygen consumption, *Am. J. Obstet. Gynecol.* **147:**48.

52. Saigal, S., and Usher, R. H., 1977, Symptomatic neonatal plethora, *Biol Neonate* **32:**62.

53. Philip, A. G. S., Yee, A. B., Rosy, M., et al., 1969, Placental transfusion as an intrauterine phenomenon in deliveries complicated by fetal distress, *Br. Med. J.* **2:**11.

54. Flod, N. E., and Ackerman, B. D., 1971, Perinatal asphyxia and residual placental blood volume, *Acta Paediatr. Scand.* **60:**433.

55. Yao, A. C., and Lind, J., 1969, Effect of gravity on placental transfusion, *Lancet* **2:**505.

56. Oh, W., Omori, K., Emmanouilides, G. C., and Phelps, D. I., 1975, Placenta to lamb fetus transfusion in utero during acute hypoxia, *Am. J. Obstet. Gynecol.* **122:**316.

57. Sacks, M. O., 1959, Occurrence of anemia and polycythemia in phenotypically dissimilar single ovum human twins, *Pediatrics* **24:**604.
58. Schwartz, J. L., Maniscalco, W. M., Lane, A. T., and Currao, W. J., 1984, Twin transfusion syndrome causing cutaneous erythropoiesis, *Pediatrics* **74:**527.
59. Humbert, J. R., Abelson, H., Hathaway, W. E., and Battaglia, F. C., 1969, Polycythemia in small for gestational age infants, *J. Pediatr.* **75:**812.
60. Widness, J. A., Garcia, J. A., Oh, W., and Schwartz, R., 1982, Cord serum erythropoietin values and disappearance rates after birth in polycythemic newborns, *Pediatr. Res.* **16:**218A.
61. Philipps, A. F., Dubin, J. W., Matty, P. J., and Raye, J. R., 1982, Arterial hypoxemia and hyperinsulinemia in the chronically hyperglycemic fetal lamb, *Pediatr. Res.* **16:**653.
62. Black, V. D., Lubchenco, L. D., Luckey, D. W., *et al.*, 1982, Developmental and neurologic sequelae of neonatal hyperviscosity syndrome, *Pediatrics* **69:**426.
63. Goldberg, K., Wirth, F. H., Hathaway, W. E., Guggenheim, M. A., Murphy, J. R., Braithwaite, W. R., and Lubchenco, L. O., 1982, Neonatal hyperviscosity. II. Effect of partial plasma exchange transfusion, *Pediatrics* **69:**419.
64. Hakanson, D. O., and Oh, W., 1980, Hyperviscosity in the small-for-gestational age infant, *Biol. Neonate* **37:**109.
65. Rawlings, J. S., Pettet, G., Wiswell, T. E., and Clapper, J., 1982, Estimated blood volumes in polycythemic neonates as a function of birth weight, *J. Pediatr.* **101:**594.
66. Brans, Y. W., Shannon, D. L., and Ramamurthy, R. S., 1981, Neonatal polycythemia. II. Plasma, blood and red cell volume estimates in relation to hematocrit levels and quality of intrauterine growth, *Pediatrics* **68:**175.
67. Thorton, C. J., Shannon, D. L., Hunter, M. A., Ramamurthy, R. S., and Brans, Y. W., 1983, Body water estimates in neonatal polycythemia, *J. Pediatr.* **102:**113.
68. Oh, W., Wallgren, G., Hanson, J. S., and Lind, J., 1967, The effects of placental transfusion on respiratory mechanics of normal term newborn infants, *Pediatrics* **40:**6.
69. van der Elst, C. W., Moteno, C. D., Malan, A. F., and de V Heese, H., 1980, The management of polycythemia in the newborn infant, *Early Hum. Dev.* **4:**393.
70. Host, A., and Ulrich, M., 1982, Late prognosis in untreated neonatal polycythemia with minor or no symptoms, *Acta Paediatr. Scand.* **71:**629.
71. Leake, R. D., Thanopoulos, B., and Nieberg, R., 1975, Hyperviscosity syndrome associated with necrotizing enterocolitis, *Am. J. Dis. Child.* **129:**1192.
72. Hakanson, D. O., and Oh, W., 1977, Necrotizing enterocolitis and hyperviscosity in the newborn infant, *J. Pediatr.* **90:**458.
73. LeBlanc, M. H., D'Cruz, C., and Pate, K., 1984, Necrotizing enterocolitis can be caused by polycythemic hyperviscosity in the newborn dog, *J. Pediatr.* **105:**804.
74. Black, V. D., Rumack, C. M., Lubchenco, L. O., and Koops, B. L., 1985, Gastrointestinal injury in polycythemic term infants, *Pediatrics* **76:**225.
75. Herson, V. C., Raye, J. R., Rowe, J. C., and Philipps, A. F., 1982, Acute renal failure associated with polycythemia in a neonate, *J. Pediatr.* **100:**137.
76. Leake, R. D., Chan, G. M., Zakauddin, S., *et al.*, Glucose perturbation in experimental hyperviscosity, *Pediatr. Res.* **14:**1320.
77. Creswell, J. S., Warburton, D., Susa, J. B., *et al.*, 1981, Hyperviscosity in the newborn lamb produces perturbation in glucose homeostasis, *Pediatrics* **15:**1348.
78. Rivers, R. P. A., 1975, Coagulation changes associated with a high haematocrit in the newborn infant, *Acta Paediatr. Scand.* **64:**449.
79. Katz, J., Rodriquez, E., Mandini, G., and Branson, H. E., 1982, Normal coagulation findings, thrombocytopenia, and peripheral hemoconcentration in neonatal polycythemia, *J. Pediatr.* **101:**99.

80. Henriksson, P., 1979, Hyperviscosity of the blood and haemostasis in the newborn infant, *Acta Paediatr. Scand.* **68:**701.

81. Shaikh, B. S., and Erslev, A. J., 1978, Thrombocytopenia in polycythemic mice, *J. Lab. Clin. Med.* **92:**765.

82. Jackson, C. W., Smith, P. J., Edwards, C. C., and Whidden, M. A., 1979, Relationship between packed cell volume, platelets and platelet survival in red blood cell-hypertransfused mice, *J. Lab. Clin. Med.* **94:**500.

83. Meberg, A., 1980, Transitory thrombocytopenia in newborn mice after intrauterine hypoxia, *Pediatr. Res.* **14:**1071.

84. Voorhies, T. M., Lipper, E. G., Lee, B. C. P., *et al.,* 1984, Occlusive vascular disease in asphyxiated newborn infants, *J. Pediatr.* **105:**92.

85. Peters, M., ten Cate, J. W., Koo, L. H., and Breederveld, C., 1984, Persistent antithrombin III deficiency: Risk factor for thromboembolic complication in neonates small for gestational age, *J. Pediatr.* **105:**310.

86. Merchant, R. H., Agarwal, M. B., Joshi, N. C., and Parekh, S. R., 1983, Neonatal polycythemia—A potentially serious disorder, *Indian J. Pediatr.* **50:**149.

87. Amit, M., and Camfield, P. R., 1980, Neonatal polycythemia causing multiple cerebral infarcts, *Arch. Neurol.* **37:**109.

88. Black, V. D., Lubchenco, L. O., Koops, B. L., Poland, R. L., and Powell, D. P., 1985, Neonatal hyperviscosity: Randomized study of effect of partial plasma exchange on long-term outcome, *Pediatrics* **75:**1048.

89. Glader, B., 1977, Erythrocyte disorders in infancy, in: *Diseases of the Newborn* (A. J. Schaffer and M. E. Avery, ed.), p. 625, W.B. Saunders, Philadelphia.

CHAPTER 4

Maternal Psychoactive Substance Use and Its Effect on the Neonate

BARRY S. ZUCKERMAN, STEVEN J. PARKER,
RALPH HINGSON, JOEL J. ALPERT,
and JANET MITCHELL

1. Introduction

This chapter reviews the impact of maternal psychoactive drug use during pregnancy on the newborn. Substances such as tobacco, coffee, alcohol, and marijuana are commonly used by women during pregnancy, whereas other substances such as heroin, methadone, diazepam, barbiturates, and amphetamines are used less frequently. Drugs such as cocaine and phencyclidine appear to be used more frequently now than in the past. Some of these drugs when used during pregnancy have well-documented teratogenic effects, while for others, particularly marijuana, little information is available. For cocaine and phencyclidine only a small number of case reports are available.

Teratogenicity refers to the ability of a drug consumed in pregnancy to cause a birth defect or other adverse fetal outcome. Thalidomide dramatically brought attention to the possibility that drug use during pregnancy can result in structural damage to the newborn. Whereas

BARRY S. ZUCKERMAN, STEVEN J. PARKER, and JOEL J. ALPERT • Department of Pediatrics, Boston City Hospital, Boston University School of Medicine, Boston, Massachusetts 02118. RALPH HINGSON • Section of Social and Behavioral Sciences, Boston University School of Public Health, Boston, Massachussetts 02118. JANET MITCHELL • Department of Obstetrics and Gynecology, Boston City Hospital, Boston University School of Medicine, Boston, Massachussetts 02118.

teratogenic effects have traditionally been associated with major structural defects, intrauterine growth retardation (IUGR), and neurobehavioral dysfunction may be more common and sensitive effects of drugs consumed during pregnancy. Alcohol,[1] aminopterin,[2] cigarette smoking,[3] coumadin,[4] dilantin,[5] heroin,[6] and methadone[7] have been conclusively associated with intrauterine growth deficiency in humans. Marijuana may also be associated with decreased birth weight,[8] although conflicting information exists. As Jones and Charnoff[9] point out, the small number of identified pharmacologic agents causing IUGR may be due either to few existing drugs that result in IUGR or to the difficulty in identifying drugs of low teratogenicity whose manifestations, such as smaller size at birth, are relatively common.

Neurobehavioral functioning of newborns may be the most sensitive indicator of subtle effects of psychoactive drugs consumed during pregnancy. Neurobehavioral differences of newborns exposed to psychoactive substances *in utero* may reflect either permanent CNS damage or a transient drug or withdrawal effect on CNS functioning. Even a transient behavioral dysfunction may have an indirect effect on later childhood functioning by its impact on parental caretaking, an effect consistent with the transactional model of development proposed by Sameroff and Chandler.[10] For example, an infant who is irritable may cry more. Excessive crying is reported as a reason for battering by 80% of abusing parents whose infants were less than 1 year old.[11] Another example might be lethargic infants who may not elicit sufficient caretaking from the mother, which may contribute to a cycle of failure to thrive. The cycle may be further compounded by a mother less sensitive to her infant's signals because of her own drug use.

This chapter discusses the pharmacology of the drug as well as animal data and human clinical and epidemiologic information. The methodologic limitations of the studies are discussed in an effort to explain the variability of results and limitations of research findings.

1.1. Methodologic Considerations

Information regarding the teratogenic effects of drugs on humans is generated by animal studies and human clinical and epidemiologic reports. By controlling for many confounding variables, animal models provide experimental information unlikely to be achieved in human studies. Their predictive value for human outcomes is limited, however. Despite their limitations, clinical reports serve as initial observations that generate hypotheses for subsequent research studies. Epidemiologic studies define the incidence of an event and factors associated with its occurrence. Retrospective epidemiologic studies are hindered by their general reliance on hospital records, which often are incomplete and reflect variable reporting of events. Prospective epidemiologic studies avoid some of these problems. The two major methodologic problems of human studies assessing the teratogenic potential of psychoactive drugs are the interrelationship of other factors (confounding variables) with the drug under study that may affect the newborn independently and the validity of self-reported drug use as a measure of drug use.

1.1.1. Validity of Self-Reported Drug Use

Because some drugs are illegal and considered socially undesirable, clinical studies may suffer from significant underreporting of their use during pregnancy. Underreporting of all drugs, or selective underreporting of some, may obscure their effects or cause misattribution of drug effects to another factor, such as nutrition, or to another drug.

Alcohol consumption, particularly among those who drink the most, appears to be underreported.[12] One study suggests that alcohol consumption in the United States National Survey data reflects only about one-half to two-thirds of the national per-capita consumption.[13]

A pilot study conducted at Boston City Hospital raises further questions about the validity of self-reported drug use during pregnancy.[14] Seventy-five pregnant women were interviewed about their consumption of marijuana and other drugs. In addition, a urine sample was analyzed for the presence of marijuana metabolites. This urine assay detects marijuana metabolites 5–7 days after smoking one marijuana cigarette. Eighteen women (24%) had urine samples positive for the presence of marijuana metabolites. Eight of these women (12.5%) reported not having smoked marijuana the previous week. While all eight women reported having used marijuana at some point, four of them reported using marijuana before but not during their pregnancy. The other four women acknowledged using marijuana during their pregnancy but not during the week before the interview. If the investigators had relied on self-reporting alone they would have missed 15% (4 of 27) of the women who used marijuana during pregnancy. A misclassification of 15% of women who consume marijuana during pregnancy might result in an underestimation of the association between marijuana use and neonatal growth.

If illicit substances such as marijuana or cocaine are more often unreported than legal substances such as alcohol or cigarettes, researchers may misattribute the effects of illicit psychoactive substances to alcohol or cigarettes. A recent study demonstrates that pregnant women who knew they would have their urine tested for drugs reported more marijuana use during pregnancy than women whose urine was not tested.[15] The self-reported incidence of cigarette smoking and alcohol intake were similar. This may help explain the reported consistent association between cigarette smoking and lower birth weight and the lack of consistency concerning the effects of illicit or socially undesirable substances on birth weight. Pregnant women may feel particular pressure to underreport certain health habits if they believe those habits will damage their unborn infants or the drug is illegal. Thus, prospective studies that quantify drug usage objectively are necessary before firm conclusions can be drawn regarding the potential risks of a drug on fetal development.

1.1.2. Confounding Variables

Efforts to identify and confirm the effects of a single substance such as alcohol, marijuana, or even more commonly used drugs, are complicated because it is unusual for humans to use or abuse only one drug. Those who smoke cigarettes are more likely to drink alcohol. Those who drink alcohol are more likely to use marijuana. Women addicted to heroin or methadone are more likely to use a variety of other drugs, including barbiturates, diazepam, cocaine, and alcohol. In addition, the type and extent of malformations may be due to genetic factors or the developmental stage at which the fetus is exposed. As a result, the same drug exposure may produce a variety of changes in newborn outcome, and a variety of drugs may produce similar outcomes.

Assessing the effect of any single drug or health variable is difficult and requires carefully designed studies with samples large enough to provide multivariate data analysis. A statistical approach is needed because experimental studies manipulating drug exposure in humans is unethical, and it is unlikely that a woman would use only one drug without other associated risk factors during pregnancy. Only through analytic statistical techniques that control for confounding variables can the independent impact of a single agent be assessed.

Low birth weight is an example of a common outcome. The following factors are known to be associated with low birth weight: nutrition (as measured by prepregnancy weight and pregnancy weight gain), cigarette smoking, sex and race of the infant, chronic medical conditions before or during pregnancy, previous history of miscarriages, age of the mother, and socioeconomic status. Many of these factors are highly intercorrelated. For example, a study[8] of the effect of alcohol consumed during pregnancy demonstrated the interrelationship between the level of alcohol consumption and some of these other factors (Table I). Women who drank alcohol had more risk factors than did women who did not drink, and the more a women drank, the more risk factors she had. Compared with infants whose mothers did not drink alcohol during pregnancy, infants whose mothers did weighed 228 g less ($p < 0.04$). However, when other confounding variables were analytically controlled, the birth-weight difference was only 51 g, which was statistically insignificant. This concrete example illustrates how false conclusions could be drawn by not fully considering the role of confounding variables.

1.2. Studies in Animals

Data from animal studies provide a model to study the effects of drugs while controlling for other factors that are difficult or impossible to control in human studies. The timing of drug intake during pregnancy, the dose of the drug, social and environmental factors, use of other drugs, and other health-related factors including nutrition can be

Table I. Characteristics of Mothers Whose Babies Were Examined at Boston City Hospital, February 1977 to October 1979, According to Alcoholic Drinks Consumed during Pregnancy[a,b]

	Average drinks/day (%)			
	0 (N = 1056)	0–0.99 (N = 452)	1.00–1.99 (N = 77)	2.00+ (N = 45)
Cigarette smoking, 1 or more packs daily	14	17	12	44
Drug use ever				
Marijuana	30	46	58	73
LSD	1	4	5	18
Amphetamines	4	10	15	22
Sedatives	3	5	12	15
Heroin	1	2	13	27
Drug use during pregnancy				
Marijuana	9	21	25	44
Either sedatives, LSD, tranquilizers, or heroin	0.4	2	3	7
Previous miscarriage or abortions	27	33	36	56
Age <21	38	30	39	22
3 or more previous pregnancies	13	14	28	42
Father drank 2+ drinks daily	3	8	12	17

[a] From ref. 8.
[b] Total of 1690 mothers, 60 not included here.

experimentally controlled in animal studies. However, there are methodologic problems in animal studies, including difficulty in controlling for nutritional utilization even when pair-fed controls are used, the lack in inhalation models for cigarettes and marijuana, choosing a dose for animals equivalent to the human dose, and species-specific differences among animal reactions to teratogens. Thus, there are important limitations in extrapolating from animal data to humans. For instance, thalidomide was found not to be teratogenic in most animals but is a major teratogen in humans.

2. Cigarette Smoking

2.1. Introduction

It was first noted during the 1940s that maternal exposure to tobacco smoke during pregnancy led to increased stillbirth and reduced birth weight in offspring of laboratory animals.[16,17] Not until 1957, however, was this relationship demonstrated in humans. Simpson[18] was the first to demonstrate that cigarette smoking during pregnancy was associated with lower birth weight and that the more cigarettes smoked, the greater the decrease in birth weight. In 1959, Lowe[19] not only confirmed the relationship between cigarette smoking and low birth weight but demonstrated that low birth weight was not due to confounding variables such as maternal age, parity, prepregnancy weight, or duration of gestation. Subsequent studies have confirmed this relationship and have linked cigarette smoking during pregnancy with other adverse fetal and neonatal outcomes. In spite of this information, smoking during pregnancy continues. A survey conducted in 1977 demonstrates that only 35% of women smokers stopped smoking during pregnancy, while another 32% decreased their amount of smoking.[20]

2.2. Pharmacology

Cigarette smoke contains more than 2000 pharmacologically active substances.[21] Most of these chemical agents are in the gas phase of cigarette smoke and include carbon monoxide, nitrous oxide, cyanide, and other compounds. Only a small number of these compounds are found in the particulate phase of cigarette smoke and include nicotine and hydrocarbon products. The pharmacologic effects of these compounds vary, and only a few of them have been studied specifically for their impact on the fetus.

Nicotine is the most studied substance and is considered the compound primarily responsible for the pharmacologic effects of smoking. Nicotine is readily absorbed by the lungs. Blood nicotine levels vary according to the duration and intensity of inhalation, number of inhalations per cigarette, brand of the cigarette, and the presence or absence of filters. Nicotine is water and lipid soluble and is rapidly distributed throughout the body. It is metabolized by the liver, kidneys, and lungs, into two main metabolites: cotinine and nicotine-1-N-oxide. Nicotine and its metabolites are primarily eliminated by the kidney. Fifty percent is eliminated during the first 2 hr after smoking a cigarette, and 25% more of the drug is eliminated over the subsequent 22 hr.

Nicotine is known to cross the placenta. However, levels of nicotine in the placenta and fetus appear to be species specific and may vary depending on the stage of pregnancy.[22] The pharmacologic effect of nicotine includes stimulation of the release of catecholamines from peripheral nerve cells and the adrenal glands. In a study of eight chronic smokers at 34 weeks gestation, Quigley et al.[23] demonstrated increased levels of norepinephrine and epinephrine within $2\frac{1}{2}$ min of smoking a cigarette. These neurochemical changes were associated with an increase in maternal pulse and blood pressure followed by an increase in fetal heart rate (FHR). Since these catecholamines do not cross the placenta, the fetal response might be due to direct effect of nicotine on the fetal adrenergic system or an indirect effect of uterine vasoconstriction.

2.3. Studies in Animals

Animal studies generally agree with the human epidemiologic findings associating cigarette smoking with low birth weight, spontaneous abortion, and behavioral dysfunction.[22] Malformations are seldom seen except at high doses of nicotine, which is usually injected intraperitonally or subcutaneously. Inhalation models for animals are not well developed at this time.

2.4. Studies in Humans

2.4.1. Spontaneous Abortion

The relationship between cigarette smoking and spontaneous abortion has been documented in numerous studies. When other risk factors are controlled, women who smoke cigarettes during pregnancy are 1.2–1.8 times more likely to have a spontaneous abortion as those who did not smoke.[24,25] The mechanism for this epidemiologic association has not been identified but might include abnormalities in placental development or dysfunction in hormones that sustain pregnancy, such as progesterone or prolactin.

2.4.2. Sudden Infant Death Syndrome

A case-control study demonstrated that mothers of victims of sudden infant death syndrome (SIDS) were more likely to smoke cigarettes either during pregnancy or after their baby was born.[26] Two studies in which data were prospectively collected also demonstrate that maternal cigarette smoking significantly increases the likelihood of SIDS.[27,28]

2.4.3. Apgar Scores

Three studies have indicated that maternal cigarette smoking during pregnancy is associated with low Apgar scores.[29–31] These studies do not assess whether cigarette smoking or other factors during pregnancy contribute to lower Apgar scores when obstetric, labor, and delivery risks are controlled analytically. When these potentially confounding factors were controlled in a study of 1709 mother–child pairs at Boston City Hospital, no significant independent association was demonstrated between cigarette smoking and Apgar scores.[32] Nor did this study demonstrate any difference between cigarette smoking and Apgar score on the univariate analysis.

2.4.4. Teratogenic Potential

The results of studies assessing the association between cigarette smoking during pregnancy and congenital malformations are conflicting. The British Perinatal Mortality Survey ($N = 17,418$) demonstrated that maternal smoking was associated with congenital heart defects, even when age, parity, and social class were controlled.[33] However, the United States Collaborative Perinatal Project ($N = 50,282$) did not demonstrate this association.[34] In the U.S. study, the total number of malformed babies was unrelated to maternal smoking. However, several categories of malformations did demonstrate a somewhat increased relative risk for children of women who smoke during pregnancy, including malformations of the CNS, hypospadias, inguinal hernia, and eye and ear malformations. A third large study ($N = 18,631$) demonstrated increased risk of cleft palate and/or cleft lip in infants of mothers who smoked during pregnancy.[35] Other studies report no association between congenital malformations and maternal smoking.[36–38] These studies have smaller sample sizes than the previous studies, which could account for the lack of a positive relationship. However, the lack of reported consistent malformations or of a pattern of malformations suggests that cigarette smoking may not by itself cause malformations.

2.4.5. Birth Weight

Studies assessing the association between cigarette smoking during pregnancy and birth weight consistently demonstrate a decrease in birth weight as well as an increased percentage of low-birth-weight infants (2500 g or less). In addition, a dose-related response between the number of cigarettes smoked and decrease in birth weight as well as the percentage of low-birth-weight infants is demonstrated. Abel[22] summarizes the effect of cigarette smoking on birth weight. The babies of smokers have reductions in birth weight from 40 to 430 g, with an average weight reduction of about 200 g as compared with the birth weights of nonsmokers. These findings remain consistent when numerous variables are controlled. For white mothers, the incidence of low-birth-weight babies ranges from 4.8% for women who do not smoke, to 8% for women who smoke 1–10 cigarettes per day, to 13.4% for women who smoke more than 20 cigarettes per day. For black women, the incidence of low-birth-weight babies ranges from 8.3% for women who do not smoke, to 13.6% for women who smoke 1–10 cigarettes per day, to 22.7% for women who smoke more than 20 cigarettes per day. Studies comparing infant birth weights show that mothers who quit smoking during pregnancy have babies with higher birth weights than do mothers who continue to smoke during pregnancy.

While smoking during pregnancy decreases growth, the nature of the growth deficit in terms of newborn body composition has only been recently assessed.[39] Anthropometric indices of subcutaneous fat deposition and lean body mass were assessed in infants of 109 smokers and 176 nonsmokers. Whereas birth weight, length, and head circumference were smaller for infants of smoking mothers, there was no difference between the two groups of infants in any of the skinfold measurements or in the calculated cross-sectional fat area of the upper arm. These new data suggest that the reduction in birthweight of infants whose mothers smoke is due primarily to a decrease in the lean body mass of the newborn, while deposition of subcutaneous fat is relatively unaffected. In addition to decreased birth weight, babies of mothers who smoke have been shown in some studies to have decreased birth length[40] and decreased head circumference.[41]

Numerous mechanisms have been proposed to explain the relationship between cigarette smoking and low birth weight. Some studies demonstrate that cigarette smokers gain less weight, so that undernutrition is the mediating variable.[42] Another hypothesis is that women who smoke are constitutionally different from nonsmokers; it is this difference that accounts for birth-weight differences in children.[43] Studies reviewed by Abel[22] do not support these hypotheses.

The most commonly accepted hypothesis is that smoking results in fetal hypoxia. Smoking increases the level of carbon monoxide in the blood. Carboxyhemoglobin is formed, which reduces the oxygen-carrying capacity of the blood resulting in fetal hypoxia. Both pregnant smokers and the infants of pregnant smokers have higher levels of carboxyhemoglobin than do nonsmokers or infants of nonsmokers.[44,45] Carbon monoxide also increases the affinity of oxygen for hemoglobin, thereby impairing the ability of the hemoglobin to release oxygen to the fetus. In addition to producing carbon monoxide, animal studies seem to indicate that nicotine indirectly decreases uterine blood flow, which also would produce hypoxia in the fetus.[46,47] Fetal hypoxia is thus caused by the multiple actions of agents associated with cigarette smoke; each mechanism associated with fetal hypoxia is probably additive in decreasing the birth weight of the fetus.

2.4.6. Neurobehavioral Effects

The impact of cigarette smoking during pregnancy on newborn behavior and on later child development has been assessed. On the Brazelton Neonatal Behavioral Assessment Scale (BNBAS) newborns of mothers who smoked during pregnancy performed less well on items covering an auditory component, such as habituating to sound or orienting to a voice as compared with newborns whose mothers did not smoke.[48] No other differences were noted. These two differences might be due to multiple comparisons alone. In this study, mothers were matched for age, social class, and parity. Infants did not differ on birth weight, sex, obstetric factors, or duration of labor. This study did not control for other factors, such as alcohol use.

Another study found that newborns exposed *in utero* to greater amounts of alcohol and nicotine performed less well on two operant conditioning tasks: head turning and sucking.[49] Landesman-Dwyer *et al.*[50] observed that newborns of heavier smoking and drinking women coughed and sneezed more and were less visually alert. Other studies have demonstrated more crying[51] and poorer autonomic regulation.[52]

These studies do not demonstrate a clinically significant impact on neonatal behavior that can be independently attributed to cigarette smoking. Because of the difficulty in identifying newborns who are only exposed to cigarette smoking and not to other factors that would affect their behavior, it is unlikely that clinically important differences will be demonstrated. If there are differences, however, current research indicates that they will be small.

Long-term follow-up evaluation of children's cognitive and developmental functioning seems to indicate that, when sociodemographic factors are controlled, children exposed to cigarette smoking *in utero* do less well on tests of cognitive, psychomotor, language, and general academic achievement, including reading and mathematics. Whereas differences are statistically significant between children exposed to cigarette smoking *in utero* versus children who are not, differences are small compared with other factors that affect children's performance.[53,54]

2.5. Summary

Cigarette smoking during pregnancy is associated with lower birth weights presumably due to fetal hypoxia. A higher incidence of spontaneous abortions and SIDS is also documented. There is no strong evidence linking cigarettes with congenital malformations, lower Apgar scores, or neurobehavioral dysfunction.

3. Caffeine

3.1. Introduction

Caffeine is the most widely used drug in North America.[55] More than 1 billion kg of coffee is consumed annually in the United States alone. All known agricultural civilizations have discovered indigenous sources of caffeine-containing beverages.[56] In one study, 5% of pregnant women drank more than four coups of coffee per day, whereas only 60% drank no coffee at all.[57] In addition, coffee drinkers are three to four times more likely to smoke cigarettes during pregnancy. Despite its ubiquitous usage, few studies have explored the effect of caffeine on pregnancy and neonatal outcome.

3.2. Pharmacology

Caffeine is a methylxanthine alkaloid with powerful CNS stimulant effects on the cerebral cortex, medulla, and spinal cord. Caffeine also

**Table II. Amount of Caffeine in Commonly Used
Beverages**

Beverage	mg caffeine/cup
Coffee (brewed)	112
Coffee (instant)	66
Tea	27
Tea (in United Kingdom)	70
Cola	30–45

directly stimulates the myocardium, dilates coronary blood vessels, constricts cerebral blood vessels, relaxes bronchiolar muscles, causes a mild diuresis, and augments gastric secretion. The average caffeine content is listed in Table II.

Following absorption, caffeine is distributed into all body compartments. Less than one-half is bound to plasma proteins, allowing for a higher concentration in the cerebral spinal fluid than other xanthines. It is eliminated primarily by metabolism in the liver.

During pregnancy, the half-life of caffeine slowly increases from 6 hr during the first trimester to 18 hr during the third trimester.[58] Studies suggest that caffeine is transported through the placenta into the fetus, where concentrations may be even higher than in the maternal plasma.[59] The half-life of caffeine in the term neonate is approximately 80 hr.[60]

3.3. Studies in Animals

Caffeine has been shown to penetrate the preimplantation blastocyst of the rabbit.[61] Despite its early uptake into fetal tissues and its potent mutagenic effect on bacteria, evidence points to a lack of teratogenic potential in mammalian tissue cultures.[56] To achieve mutagenesis in mammalian cells, doses of 250–800 mg/kg per day are required. No study using less than 50 mg/kg per day has been associated with chromosomal abnormalities or gross congenital anomalies in the rat.

Pups born to mothers ingesting 120 mg/kg per day of caffeine were shown to be more active in the perinatal period.[56] Elevated norepinephrine levels have been found in newborn guinea pigs born to caffeine-ingesting mothers and may be responsible for the hyperactivity.[62] Rats ingesting 70 mg/kg per day of caffeine delivered pups with decreased fetal cerebral weights as well as diminished DNA and RNA protein in the brain.[63] Caffeine also diminishes lipid synthesis on cultured glial and neuronal cells, which could have detrimental effects *in vivo* on brain structure and function.[64]

3.4. Studies in Humans

3.4.1. Teratogenic Potential

Initial reports[65–67] implicated caffeine intake with a wide variety of anomalies. However, these studies had few subjects, used anecdotal case report methodology, lacked controls, and did not quantify the daily caffeine consumption or other drug usage. More recent studies[57,68,69] have shown no significant increases in congenital anomalies associated with coffee drinking during pregnancy. For example, a study from Finland,[68] which boasts the highest per-capita coffee consumption in the world (including a 96% incidence in coffee consumption in women and a 70% consumption during pregnancy), did not find more frequent malformations among infants born to coffee drinkers.

3.4.2. Perinatal Morbidity

In a large retrospective study, coffee drinkers had a significant increase in premature rupture of membranes, even when covariables were controlled, as well as a higher incidence of breech presentation. Although these mothers delivered children with lower birth weight, the relationship disappeared when maternal smoking was factored out. No other pregnancy complications were noted in coffee drinkers.[57]

3.4.3. Neurobehavioral Outcomes

Two studies demonstrate an association between maternal caffeine use and newborn behavior. One study demonstrates an inverse relationship between coffee consumption during pregnancy and activity level and motor coordination on the BNBAS when alcohol and cigarette smoking were held constant.[70] Another study associated caffeine use during pregnancy with a higher incidence of abnormal reflexes, whereas coffee use before pregnancy is associated with poorer orientation and greater arousal and irritability even when other variables and coffee consumption during pregnancy are controlled.[71]

3.5. Summary

Coffee is a commonly ingested drug during pregnancy. It appears to have little teratogenic potential in humans. Pregnancy outcomes are generally benign, with reported problems usually due to concomitant cigarette smoking. Subtle neurobehavioral sequelae in the neonate await further study.

4. Alcohol

4.1. Introduction

The association between alcohol consumption during pregnancy and adverse neonatal outcome was brought to scientific and public awareness by two reports during the early 1970s.[1,72] The report by Jones, which described a "characteristic pattern of malformation" of eight children of chronic alcoholics, served as a major stimulus for research on the teratogenicity of alcohol.

Alcoholic beverages vary in alcoholic content. The concentration of alcohol in beer is approximately 4%, in table wine 12%, and in most hard liquor drinks 50%. Based on the percentage of alcohol, a 12-ounce can of beer is approximately equivalent to a 4-ounce glass of wine or one mixed drink containing an ounce of 100-proof hard liquor. This type of calculation allows comparability among drinks in calculating the amount of alcohol ingested.

4.2. Pharmacology

Alcohol is quickly absorbed from the gastrointestinal tract by passive diffusion and is rapidly distributed throughout the body. Because it is water soluble, alcohol distributes throughout all body water compartments. Absorption is positively affected by factors such as the concentration of alcohol in the drink and an empty stomach. Alcohol is primarily metabolized to acetaldehyde in the liver. Both alcohol and acetaldehyde cross the placenta[73] and have been show *in vitro* to reduce protein synthesis.[74]

4.3. Studies in Animals

Animal studies consistently demonstrate adverse affects on fetal viability, newborn growth, and morphology.[22] However, there are methodologic concerns regarding animal studies on alcohol. First, the method of administration varies. Injection and intubation of ethanol are stressful to the mother, and maternal stress is known to be independently associated with adverse outcomes in the offspring. The most accepted method of administration is adding alcohol to a liquid diet, in which animals consume greater amounts of water than on a regular diet. The increased fluid intake may have adverse metabolic or renal effects.

Second, even if adequate nutrition is ingested by the animal, alcohol is known to impair the absorption, utilization, and metabolism of nutrients.[75] Thus, even with appropriate pair-fed control groups, adverse effects of alcohol in the fetus may actually be nutritionally related.[76] Although the mechanism is not clear, alcohol is known to impair protein synthesis in many adult and fetal tissues, including the brain.[77]

4.4. Studies in Humans

4.4.1. Fetal Alcohol Syndrome

The specific pattern of malformations described by Jones et al.[78] was called the fetal alcohol syndrome (FAS). More recently the Fetal Alcohol Study Group of the Research Society of Alcoholism has established formal minimal criteria needed for the diagnosis of FAS. The child must have signs in each of these three categories to conform to the diagnosis of FAS:

1. Prenatal and/or postnatal growth retardation (weight, length, and/or head circumference below the tenth percentile when corrected for gestational age)
2. Central nervous system involvement (signs of neurologic abnormality or developmental delay)
3. Characteristic facial dysmorphology with at least two of three signs: microcephaly (head circumference below the third percentile), short palpebral fissures, poorly developed philtrum, thin upper lip, and/or flatting of the maxillary area.

These criteria were developed from 250 reported cases of FAS.

These cases represented very careful descriptions of the physical characteristics of the children but varied widely in the extent to which health habits and other characteristics of the mothers were detailed. Thus, other facts known to influence fetal development may have been missed. In addition, it is unusual for a syndrome to be named by its etiologic agent, as was FAS. This may have led to neglecting important research questions. Since one of the key components of the syndrome is believed to be alcohol, clinicians may pay more attention to a mother's alcohol consumption than to her other habits. It is also unlikely that babies with features compatible with FAS are reported in the absence of alcohol use during pregnancy.

In two studies comparing infants born to alcoholic and to nonalcoholic women, conflicting results have been noted. Both studies had significant methodologic problems. In one, alcoholism was not systematically recorded, and in the other, infant data were taken from birth certificates. In the first study, the Collaborative Perinatal Project, infants of the alcoholic mothers who were identified were significantly more likely to have lower weight, shorter length, smaller palpebral fissures, and more cardiac murmurs at birth. Significant differences in head circumference were not found.[78]

In the other study, Russell[79] compared 223 children born to 145 diagnosed alcoholics and 276 children born to 185 women seen in the alcoholism department with other psychiatric disorders. An additional control group was drawn from birth certificates matched for sex, maternal age, race, and education. No congenital malformations were recorded on the birth certificates of children born to alcoholics, and only one was recorded in either of the control groups. The low rate of congenital malformations probably reflects either inadequate examination or recording, or both. Infants born to alcoholics had lower birth weights than did those infants born to women in the control groups. By contrast, mothers who did not start drinking until after the birth of their baby also had infants who were smaller at birth than did control infants. This raises questions about whether index and control groups were really comparable on other characteristics that might influence birth weight.

The reported incidence of FAS appears to be low. Five cases were identified by nonblinded examinees in an unselected population of 12,000. Other studies have identified one case in a study population of 1690,[9] one case out of 322 patients,[81] and two out of 1529 cases.[82] The variability in reported incidence could be due to numerous factors, including the differences in health behaviors, drug use, medical histories of alcoholic women, or genetic susceptability. Possible genetic vulnerability to alcohol exposure *in utero* was observed in a pair of fraternal twins born to an alcoholic mother, one of whom had greater reduction in all growth parameters than the other twin.[83]

4.4.2. Specificity of Fetal Alcohol Syndromes or Features Compatible with Fetal Alcohol Syndrome

Because the reported incidence of the FAS is rare, Hanson *et al.*[82] developed criteria to be used to classify infants as having features compatible with FAS (CFAS). This classification is an attempt to identify an association between lower levels of drinking and less extensive fetal dysmorphology. Each infant is rated according to several criteria: (1) small size for gestational age (weight, length, or both less than the third percentile); (2) microcephaly (head circumference less than the third percentile); (3) short palpebral fissures (less than 1.8 cm wide in infants greater than or equal to 36 weeks gestational age); and (4) multiple dysmorphic features (two or more significant dysmorphic features judged by clinical observation, including broad low nasal bridge, epicanthal folds, thin upper lip, hypoplastic philtrum, small nails, limitation of joint movement, large hemangiomas, abnormal palmar crease patterns, cardiac murmurs, and ear anomalies. Infants are classified as having CFAS features if rated abnormal on at least two of the four criteria. One of the two must be either short palpebral fissures or multiple dysmorphic features.

CFAS feature may not be specific to alcohol. Of 1384 infants examined in a study of the effect of alcohol on fetal development conducted at Boston City Hospital, 31 (2.3%) had CFAS features.[8] Women who smoked marijuana during pregnancy were five times more likely than nonusers to deliver a child with CFAS features ($p < 0.001$). Women who gained less than 5 lb during pregnancy were 2.6 times more likely to deliver a CFAS child than were those who had average weight gain ($p < 0.001$). The relative risk for women exposed to x-rays was 2.8, compared with women who were not exposed ($p < 0.02$). By contrast, the relative risk for women who averaged two or more drinks daily compared wth nondrinkers was only 0.6 and not significant. This is the only study that attempts to identify a possible association between factors other than alcohol and CFAS.

CFAS features may reflect a final common pathway of numerous agents or combination of agents, rather than a specific teratogenic effect of alcohol. This may be more true of fetal alcohol effects, which are identified when two of three areas (growth, dysmorphology, and CNS-related development) demonstrate abnormality. While some investigators consider the facial dysmorphology the most unique aspect of FAS, a recent report demonstrates a similarity between the facial appearance in FAS and the face of children born to mothers who have phenylketonuria.[84] A similar-appearing syndrome was also seen in the offspring of epileptic women who take Dilantin during pregnancy.[85] In reviewing her work and other studies regarding cranial facial dysmorphogenesis,[86] Sulik concludes that the FAS phenotype may not be unique to alcohol. Animal studies suggest that teratogen exposure, such as might be seen with high levels of alcohol during the primitive streak stage of development, interferes with formation of the prechordal mesoderm. At this stage of development, teratogens must get to the embryo by diffusion, as the placenta is not yet formed. A teratogenic process at this stage of development will result in craniofacial brain and eye defects noted in severe forms of FAS. This is on the mild end of the spectrum of malformations which extends to holoprosencephaly. Other agents or a combination of agents (such as other drugs or radiation) may also interfere with embryogenesis at this stage. The combination of alcohol and marijuana in mice and rats is more toxic to the fetus than either drug alone.[87] The association of alcohol and the constellation of dysmorphic features known as FAS may exist because alcohol is a frequently used teratogen but not necessarily a unique one.

4.4.3. Birth Weight

In addition to FAS, numerous studies have examined the impact on the newborn of various levels of alcohol consumption before and during pregnancy. The association between low birth weight and high levels of alcohol consumption is the most common finding in these studies.[88–91]

The best-controlled study, conducted by Little,[92] demonstrated a relationship between moderate levels of alcohol consumption and a decrease in birth weight. Of 902 consecutive patients in a health-maintenance organization (HMO), 801 agreed to participate in the study. Sixty-six of 73 subjects who reported consuming one or more ounces of absolute alcohol per day before pregnancy were studied. The effects of maternal age, weight, parity, number of cigarettes smoked, gestational age, and sex of the child were held constant through regression analysis. Drinking an average of one or more ounces of absolute alcohol per day before pregnancy was associated with an average decrease of 90 g in birth weight. Drinking that amount during late pregnancy (months 5–8) was associated with an average 160-g drop in birth weight.

The study made a considerable effort to control for several confounding variables. Some potentially important variables were not examined, however, including maternal illness during pregnancy and maternal weight gain. Since this study is frequently cited as demonstrating an impact of moderate drinking (one ounce of alcohol per day or two drinks), it is important to acknowledge that these unexplored variables may have explained the small differences in birth weight.

A number of other studies do not demonstrate an association between alcohol consumption and lower birth weight.[8,93–95] The advantage of many of these studies is their attempt to control for numerous relevant confounding variables. Hingson *et al.*[8] studied 1690 mother/infant pairs at Boston City Hospital and controlled for more than 40 variables. In this study, alcohol consumption was analyzed in numerous ways, including frequency of drinking, usual quantity of consumption on days the subjects drank, and average daily volume of alcohol consumption. Regardless of which measure was used, the pattern of results was the same. This study demonstrated no association between any of these separate variables of alcohol consumption and neonatal birth weight, length, head circumference, or congenital abnormality. However, maternal drinking before pregnancy was significantly related to shortened gestation. While this study and others controlled for numerous confounding variables, the number of heavy drinkers was small and the results are only suggestive that moderate drinking is not associated with low birthweight. No inference about the impact of heavy drinking on the neonate can be drawn.

An assessment of the infants of heavy drinkers results in different findings. An analysis conducted by members of the same research team reported on a subgroup of women who were interviewed prenatally regarding their alcohol use.[90] In this group of mothers, heavy drinking, defined by consumption of more than five drinks on some occasions and at least 45 drinks per month, was reported by 43 women (9%). All but six of these heavy-drinking mothers were matched to lesser-drinking and nondrinking mothers on the following variables: parity, ethnicity, cigarettes, marijuana use, prepregnancy weight, mother's age, baby's sex, and gestational age. The heavy-drinking women had significantly more babies whose length, weight, and head circumference were below the tenth percentile for gestational age. In addition, more of the babies from this group had congenital abnormalities.

This comparison between the findings of two analytic methods of the same study population is instructive. The findings of studies comparing heavy drinkers to nondrinkers suggest that there may be a threshhold after which drinking has an adverse effect rather than a linear relationship between drinking and birth weight. Another explanation is that unknown confounding variables explain the differences between the two groups.

In conclusion, alcohol consumption during pregnancy may have an adverse effect on birth weight, at least when consumption is high. Whether this impact is attributable only to alcohol or to a combination of factors, including alcohol, remains unclear at this time. Findings from a recent study suggest that the impact of drinking alcohol may have a greater effect on smokers than on nonsmokers.[96] Thus, isolating a single cause of abnormal growth in newborns is very difficult due to the interrelationship of numerous factors associated with a poor neonatal outcome.

4.4.4. Behavioral Teratogenicity

A withdrawal syndrome in newborns of alcoholic mothers has been described in three papers involving eight infants.[97-99] The mothers of these babies are all described as alcoholics who were intoxicated at the time of delivery. There is no mention of other drugs taken during pregnancy. Therefore, it is unclear whether these babies' behavioral symptoms were due entirely to alcohol or a combination of alcohol and other drugs. Behavioral assessment of newborns demonstrate that alcohol consumption during pregnancy is associated with a poorer ability to habituate and a lower level of arousal.[100] One study elegantly demonstrated dysfunction in the regulation of states of consciousness in newborns exposed to alcohol *in utero*. Using a special pressurized mattress, neonates of mothers who were heavy alcohol users during pregnancy demonstrate poor state regulation, as manifested by a decrease in total amount of sleep and an increase in the fragmentation of sleep periods.[101] Because alcohol use is frequently interrelated with other drug use during pregnancy, these drugs also need to be assessed for effects on newborn behavior. In a study assessing the effects of prenatal exposure to smoking, caffeine, and small amounts of alcohol, an independent effect on behavior is seen for alcohol and caffeine but not for cigarette smoking.[71]

In a follow-up study of their initial sample, Streissguth *et al.*[102] demonstrated an effect of maternal alcohol use during pregnancy on 4-year-old children's attentional abilities, which was measured by a computer operator vigilance system. This effect was independent of cigarette smoking, birth order, maternal education, nutrition, and caffeine.

4.5. Prenatal Intervention

Providing care for the pregnant alcohol abuser requires a comprehensive approach, including a strong psychosocial component that utilizes counseling, education, and/or psychotherapy. Because the alcohol abuser may be more difficult to identify, Rosett and Weiner[104] developed a simple 10-question drinking history (TQDH) that is easily incorporated into a prenatal record. These questions address the frequency and the amount of beer, wine, or liquor consumed and whether a change has occurred over the past year. Test–retest reliability is reported between 89 and 100%. When women do not have a drinking problem, the 10 questions require less than 5 min to administer. For women who are abusing alcohol, their questionnaire provides a focus for discussing the possible adverse effects of their drinking on their unborn baby.

Rosett et al.[90] described a positive effect of an intervention program for heavy-drinking women during pregnancy. Among 469 women, 9% ($N = 43$) were categorized as heavy drinkers—women who consumed at least five drinks on some occasions and no fewer than 45 drinks per month. Twenty-three of these women participated in at least three counseling sessions at the prenatal clinic. Of the 23 women, 16 abstained or reduced their alcohol consumption significantly below heavy levels before the third trimester. Infants born to mothers who reduced heavy drinking did not differ in birth weight, length, or head circumference from offspring of rare or moderate drinkers. However, the infants of the reduced drinkers did demonstrate a higher frequency of congenital abnormalities than did the infants of rare or moderate drinkers. This analysis does not indicate whether other health habits, such as cigarette smoking and nutrition, also changed in response to their interventions. It may be that changes in other habits or a combination of habits accounts for the improvement in intrauterine growth.

The improvement in intrauterine growth suggests that the identification and therapy of heavy-drinking women are essential components of prenatal care. Rosett and Weiner[104] maintain that while traditional treatment of alcoholism is pessimistic, pregnancy is a time when women are very motivated around issues of their own bodies and the well-being of their unborn child. The use of chlordiazepoxide and other benzodiazepines and anticonvulsants for the heaviest drinkers were limited because of their potential risk to the fetus. Disulfiram (Antabuse), also suspected as a possible teratogen, was not used.

4.6. Summary

Consumption of large amounts of alcohol during pregnancy appears to be associated with lower birth weight. Fetal alcohol syndrome appears to be rare, and features compatible with this diagnosis may not be uniquely attributable to alcohol.

5. Marijuana Use

5.1. Introduction

Marijuana use is most common among individuals in their late teens and early 20s. The number of people using marijuana, especially women, has increased during the past 10–15 years. In a review, Abel[22] points out that the percentage of adults 18 years and over who have ever used marijuana increased from 39% to 60%, while adults aged 18–25 who used marijuana during the past month rose from 17% to 28%. Table III indicates percentages of women using marijuana during pregnancy. The range of use during pregnancy reported in these studies varies and may be due to different populations, assessment techniques, or variability due to self-reporting. Only recently have studies assessed the relationship of marijuana use to neonatal outcome.

5.2. Pharmacology

Marijuana is the name given to flowering tops from the plant *Cannabis sativa*. More than 400 chemicals have been identified in the cannabis plant.[102] The principal psychoactive ingredient in marijuana is 1-Δ^9-tetrahydrocannabinol (Δ^9-THC).

The principal route of administration of marijuana in humans is by inhalation. More than one-half the Δ^9-THC present in a marijuana cigarette is absorbed.[105] Δ^9-THC has a high affinity for lipids and therefore accumulates in fatty tissues throughout the body.[106] A single dose of cannabis in humans takes as much as 30 days to be excreted with a half-life in tissues of about 7 days.[107] Most of the Δ^9-THC is metabolized in the liver and eliminated in the feces.[108]

Marijuana affects numerous factors relating to reproductive functioning. Inhibition of luteinizing hormone (LH) by 50–90% following marijuana ingestion lasts for 6–24 hr, depending on the dose.[109] In five

Table III. Percentage of Women Using Marijuana during Pregnancy

Study site	Sample size	Users	Ref.
Boston	1659	14%	8
Ottawa	217	13%	119
Boston	12,424	10%	120
Australia	7,301	5.4%	94

women who were either postmenopausal or ovariectomized and who received cannabis in the form of one marijuana cigarette of known purity, Kolodny[110] found an 80% decrease in the follicle-stimulating hormone (FSH) and LH levels within 60–90 min. Δ^9-THC appears to be the primary component of marijuana that decreases gonadotropin release.[111] Because these gonadotropins are already depressed during pregnancy, it is unclear whether marijuana further supresses them.

Although the placenta does screen the fetus from some constituents of marijuana, radiolabeled Δ^9-THC is known to cross the placenta.[112] Placenta transfer is higher in early pregnancy than in late pregnancy. Since Δ^9-THC crosses the placenta, it can potentially have a direct effect on the fetus. Marijuana, similar to cigarettes, produces increased carbon monoxide levels in the blood and decreases uterine blood flow. Both mechanisms can result in fetal hypoxia.[52]

On the basis of the high use of marijuana by women of childbearing age, its impact on known reproductive factors and the knowledge that marijuana crosses the placenta, it is important to assess whether marijuana during pregnancy has an adverse impact on the neonate.

5.3. Studies in Animals

The animal literature on the effects of maternal marijuana exposure during pregnancy has recently been summarized by Abel.[22] Malformations are not consistently observed and usually occur only at high marijuana levels obtained by intraperitoneal administration. An appropriate inhalation model has not yet been developed. Although IUGR is observed in many animal studies, marijuana administration also results in decreased food and water consumption during pregnancy.[13] To control for decreased intake, pair-fed controls are used. These animals are only given the amount of food and water consumed during the previous day by the drug group. Recently, Abel[114] published results of a study comparing offspring of pregnant rats orally administered Δ^9-THC with pair-fed and watered controls. The drug-treated rats exhibited a significant dose-related decrease in pregnancies carried to term, weight gain during pregnancy, and birth weight. A particular protective role of good nutrition is suggested by a study demonstrating that marijuana plus an enriched protein diet prevented marijuana induced developmental problems, such as delayed onset of the righting reflex, eye opening, and visual placing.[115]

A possible synergistic effect of marijuana and alcohol has recently been demonstrated.[87] In two different species, marijuana plus alcohol caused a significant increase in fetal mortality, whereas the fetal mortality for either drug alone did not differ from pair-fed controls. Thus, the combination of two commonly used drugs has a greater negative impact than that associated with either drug alone.

In studies assessing chromosome damage in cells of animals, no effects are demonstrated when cells are incubated with Δ^9-THC.[116] This finding is consistent with studies in human subjects.[117]

5.4. Studies in Humans

5.4.1. Epidemiologic Research in Humans

Epidemiologic data concerning the effects on fetal development of human marijuana use during pregnancy are limited and inconsistent. Only a handful of studies have been reported. Greenland *et al.*[118] compared 35 regular marijuana users with 35 nonusers matched by age, ethnicity, parity, and center of care. Women more than 30 weeks pregnant were excluded, as were those with medical problems and those who reported the use of other illicit psychoactive drugs during the 3 weeks prior to pregnancy. Each subject's drug use history was supplemented by laboratory determinations of urine canabinoids. Marijuana users had lower income and less education, and a higher proportion of users were black or Hispanic. They also exhibited higher consumption of tobacco and alcohol than did nonusers. Antepartum, intrapartum, postpartum, and neonatal clinic data were collected from medical records.

Significantly, more marijuana users exhibited precipitous labor and their infants were significantly more likely to exhibit meconium staining (5% vs. 25%). Statistical adjustment for other risk factors, e.g., income, smoking, alcohol use, and time of first prenatal visit, did not alter results. The percentage of subjects with precipitous labor and meconium staining increased proportionally to the reported frequency of marijuana use. Although not significant, marijuana users exhibited higher levels of anemia, poor weight gain, suspected IUGR, and prolonged or arrested labor.

Whereas this study used biochemical markers to assess marijuana use, so many prenatal outcomes were examined that chance alone might yield statistically significant differences. Furthermore, the sample size was so small that meaningful differences may not have been considered statistically significant. Thus, although suggestive, the results need to be interpreted cautiously.

Tennes and Blackard[95] examined 278 offspring of mothers interviewed before and after delivery at two public hospital outpatient obstetric clinics. Use of caffeine, nicotine, over-the-counter drugs, illnesses, fevers, exposure to irradiation, and use of alcohol, marijuana and illicit drugs was ascertained. Infant outcomes were obtained from the infants' medical records. Multiple regression analyses revealed no significant independent relationship between marijuana use and shorter duration of gestation or low infant birth weight or length. Nor was an association observed between marijuana use and minor or major congenital abnormalities. As with the previously mentioned studies, however, the small sample size was a severely limiting factor, and it is possible that clinically meaningful relationships did not produce statistical significance.

Only four studies of humans have examined samples of sufficient size to adequately control for potential confounding effects of other maternal habits, such as smoking, drinking, or other illicit drug use.

In a study of 583 women who were interviewed during the prenatal period and after delivery, Fried et al.[119] observed a statistically significant reduction of 0.8 weeks gestation among offspring of mothers who smoked six or more marijuana joints per week during pregnancy even when effects of cigarette smoking, alcohol use, parity, mother's prepregnancy weight, and sex of the infant were controlled analytically.

An independent association with maternal marijuana use and lower birth weight was not observed. The small sample size in this study relative to the others cited may have precluded identification of meaningful differences in birthweight between offspring of users and nonusers. Even after potential confounders were controlled analytically, the birth weight of infants of these heavy marijuana users was 78 g smaller, but this was not statically significant.

Linn et al.,[120] at the Boston Hospital for Women, interviewed the largest number of women to date. Of 17,136 women who delivered at the hospital between August 1977 and March 1980, 12,718 women were interviewed shortly after delivery. Infant outcomes were obtained from the infant medical records. Women were asked whether they used marijuana during pregnancy and, if so, whether they used it on an occasional, weekly, or daily basis. Other maternal characteristics, such as previous stillbirths, maternal ponderal index, education, race, cigarette smoking, alcohol use, age, welfare status, previous miscarriages, and induced labor, were controlled. No independent association was observed between marijuana use and duration of gestation of less than 37 weeks or birth weight below 2500 g. A suggestive odds ratio of 1.36 was observed between the use of marijuana and infants having major malformations based on the coding schemes developed for the Congenital Malformations Surveillance Program at the Centers for Disease Control in Atlanta.

The 95% confidence interval was 0.97–1.91, indicating that the relationship approached, but did not quite reach, statistical significance at $p < 0.05$. However, of the 10 independent variables in the analysis, marijuana use was the most highly predictive of a malformation. Univariate analyses revealed that infants born to women who smoked marijuana during pregnancy had lower Apgar scores ($p < 0.05$). A multivariate analysis of this outcome variable was not provided.

A study of 1690 mother–child pairs at Boston City Hospital by Hingson *et al.*[8] compared infants of 234 mothers who reported marijuana use during pregnancy to the infants of nonusers. Other maternal characteristics that might influence fetal growth and development, such as cigarette smoking, maternal drinking, weight gain during pregnancy, maternal height, prepregnancy weight, and medical history, were controlled analytically. Marijuana use was found to be independently associated with lower infant birth weight and length. Women who used marijuana less than three times per week during pregnancy delivered infants 95 g smaller than infants of nonusers, and women who used marijuana three or more times per week delivered babies 139 g smaller than infants of nonusers. In comparison, women who smoked one pack or more of cigarettes daily delivered infants 83 g smaller than did nonusers.

The same study did not identify significant independent associations between maternal marijuana use and shorter duration of gestation, presence of congenital malformation, or lower 1- or 5-min Apgar scores. The study found, however, that among a variety of maternal habits and characteristics, maternal marijuana use was the strongest independent predictor of whether a mother delivered an infant with a combination of anomalies considered compatible with fetal alcohol syndrome. This finding underlines the possibility that marijuana use may contribute independently to the development of abnormalities heretofore thought to be exclusively caused by excessive alcohol use during pregnancy. It is also possible that interactions may occur that are detrimental to fetal growth when more than one of these substances is used simultaneously, similar to the synergistic effect of alcohol and marijuana for animals reported by Abel.

Most recently, another large sample of 7310 births was studied by Gibson *et al.*[94] Mothers of the infants were interviewed extensively during both the prenatal and postnatal periods about their health and health habits. Marijuana use was classified as nonuser, up to once a week, and more than once per week. Five percent of women smoked marijuana during pregnancy; of these only 5% used it habitually. Marijuana users were significantly more likely to deliver premature infants even when parity, maternal age, alcohol, and tobacco use were controlled analytically. Among women who used marijuana once a week, 25% reported premature births. Marijuana use was also associated independently with low birth weight ($p < 0.05$) but this relationship was not found when only full-term infants were examined. No significant independent relationships were observed between marijuana use and low Apgar scores, congenital malformations, or perinatal death.

On balance, the literature based on human studies of the possible effects of marijuana on fetal development is limited and inconsistent. Only three studies have reported the possible independent relationship between marijuana use and adverse fetal development in samples of more than 1000 mother–child pairs.[9,94,120] Of those, only Gibson *et al.*[94] used a truly prospective design where mothers were interviewed before delivery.

That these studies each found an association between marijuana use and some adverse pregnancy outcome clearly points to a need for more research on the topic. But the lack of consistency in specific effects suggests considerable caution before ascribing pregnancy risk to maternal marijuana use.

5.4.2. Neurobehavioral Functioning

Only one study has assessed the impact of maternal marijuana consumption and neonatal neurobehavioral functioning.[121] Using the BNBAS, more newborns of heavy marijuana smokers either did not respond to a light stimulus or did not habituate to it. In addition, the newborns of the marijuana smokers demonstrated more tremors and startles in addition to being less successful at self-quieting. By 30 days postdelivery, there did not appear to be any differences between the infants of marijuana users and those of nonusers. This preliminary study should be interpreted cautiously because of the small sample size of heavy users and possible impact of confounding variables.

5.5. Summary

Studies have suggested associations between marijuana use in pregnancy and various adverse neonatal outcomes. Clearly, more research must be done before any firm conclusions can be reached. In addition, recent data[14] indicating the underreporting of its use during pregnancy necessitate laboratory verification of self-report in these studies.

6. Opiate Use

6.1. Introduction

In 1680 Sydenham wrote "among the remedies which has pleased Almighty God to give man to relieve his sufferings, none is so universal and efficacious as opium." Opiate alkaloids include heroin, morphine, methadone, and codeine. Currently more than 200,000 people in this country are addicted to opiates. In New York City alone, an estimated 3000 passively addicted babies are born each year.[122] As New York City contains one-third to one-half of all addicts in the country, it has been extrapolated that 6000–9000 babies are born every year to addicted mothers in the United States, an incidence of 1–2 in 1000 births. There are currently 200,000–300,000 children in the United States who were exposed to opiates *in utero*.[123]

Perhaps no drugs of abuse have been more thoroughly studied during pregnancy than the opiates. However, significant methodologic problems are inherent in these studies, including (1) polydrug use, (2) nutritional factors, (3) poor documentation, (4) maternal health habits, and (5) limited outcome measures.

Heroin and/or methadone addicts commonly use many drugs of different classes, including alcohol, cigarettes, diazepam, barbiturates, amphetamines, and phencyclidine. The possibility of drug synergism in the adverse outcomes by the numerous drugs must always be considered in these studies and outcomes may be due to polydrug effects rather than to opiates *per se*.

Drug addicts often are malnourished. Decreased caloric intake and various nutritional deficiencies may compound adverse outcomes in the babies. Addicts are notoriously poor reporters of both the quantity and type of drug intake during pregnancy. In addition, street drugs are often impure mixtures of various drugs, making it difficult to ascertain exactly what has been ingested. An accurate quantification of drug usage during pregnancy is often impossible.

Addicts may have hazardous and unhealthy life-styles and often do not seek prenatal care. They are subject to numerous medical illnesses, such as hepatitis, subacute bacterial endocarditis, urinary tract infection, tuberculosis, venereal disease, anemia, and phlebitis. It is estimated that 40–50% of addicted women will manifest medical complications known to affect perinatal outcome unfavorably during pregnancy.[124]

Many studies do not include control groups in their analyses. In addition, it is almost impossible to find comparable matching controls.

The life-style of a drug abuser differs from that of other groups, no matter how well matched for socioeconomic status, race, or age.

Most studies analyze short-term outcomes, and these tend to be explicit, e.g., birth weight, malformations, or I.Q. scores in the first year. However, subtle changes in the morphology or neurobehavioral functioning in the infant are often not assessed, and important effects of drug taking during pregnancy may then be missed. In addition, the dropout rate in follow-up studies is very high. Assurances that no significant drug effects during pregnancy have been found in the newborn must be cautiously interpreted.

6.2. Pharmacology

Opium is obtained by drying the milky exudate of unripe poppy seeds, which are indigenous to Asia Minor. Opium powder contains more than 20 alkaloids, including morphine and codeine. Only simple modifications of the morphine compound are necessary to synthesize a host of semisynthetic alkaloids, including heroin, oxycodeine (Percodan), and hydromorphone (Dilaudid). Whereas the chemical structure of methadone is completely different from that of opiates, the pharmacologic properties are qualitatively similar.

The main effects of this group of drugs are on the CNS, where they produce analgesia, drowsiness, changes in mood, and mental clouding. Other effects include miosis, respiratory depression, peripheral vasodilation, and decreased intestinal peristalsis. Despite its major effects on the CNS, only small amounts pass the blood–brain barrier. The greatest concentration occurs in the kidneys, lungs, liver, and spleen. The major mode of excretion is in the urine after conjugation with glucoronic acid in the liver. Opiates are secreted in breast milk in small concentrations.[125]

6.3. Studies in Animals

Numerous animal studies show a deleterious effect of opiates on the fetus.[126–128] In general, a dose-dependent relationship between opiate usage during pregnancy and various adverse outcomes has been found. Lowered birth weights and increased neonatal mortality rates have been found in rat pups born to mothers given either heroin or methadone, or both, during pregnancy. This is due to a direct effect of the drug on the fetus and indirectly to the anorexia and decreased caloric intake following opiate exposure.[127] These outcomes are reduced but not eliminated when secondary effects such as malnutrition and polydrug use are controlled.[128]

Malformations due to opiates (particularly anomalies of the brain) have been observed when very large doses have been administered. Smaller doses, more closely approximating human usage, generally have not been shown to increase malformations in various species.[129]

Offspring of rats given methadone during pregnancy demonstrate postnatal hyperactivity, tremors, delayed motor development, and other behavioral changes.[130] Diminished levels of dopamine and norepinephrine in the forebrain areas of the rat have been found in pups born to addicted mothers.[131] Others have shown postnatal reductions in opioid receptor functioning.[132] Many suggest that the behavioral changes seen postnatally are caused by an altered neurochemistry in the neonate.[133]

6.4. Studies in Humans

6.4.1. Somatic Growth

There is ample evidence to relate adverse outcomes of pregnancy and newborn functioning to opiate use during pregnancy. The most consistent finding is a lowered mean birth weight in this population of infants (Table IV). It is clear from these studies that women who are involved in methadone maintenance programs deliver children with significantly higher birth weights than do multidrug users, although both groups have lower birth weights than those of control groups. Most have interpreted this finding to reflect the superior health care and life-style of women who are involved in such programs, rather than a lower toxicity of methadone on intrauterine growth.

Table IV. Birth Weights Associated with Drug Intake

Study	Methadone alone	Polydrug[a]	Control
Stimmel and Adamson[134]	2933	2763	3309
Zelson et al.[135]	2625	2464	—
Ostrea et al.[136]	2949	2765	—
Kandall et al.[137]	2961	2490	3176

[a] Polydrug is defined as usually taking either heroin or methadone, or both, and other psychoactive drugs.

There is evidence that both heroin and methadone have a direct adverse effect on somatic growth. Postmortum examinations of infants born to addicted mothers show a marked diminution in the cell number but not the cell size of various organs.[138] This pattern of somatic growth is different from that occurring secondary to maternal malnutrition, which yields a decreased cell number and cell size. Thus, the deleterious effect on somatic growth may be due to both a direct adverse effect of the opiates on organ cell number and to secondary effects of poor nutrition and maternal illness.

6.4.2. Perinatal Morbidity

The incidence of intrauterine growth retardation is 13% in street addicts, 7.5% for women in methadone treatment centers, and 2.7% of control groups.[124] Opiate abusers are far more likely to deliver preterm babies than are nonabusers.[134] It is estimated that 50% of street addicts and 20% of methadone-treated mothers will deliver low-birth-weight infants.[139] The combination of increased prematurity and IUGR is the cause for most of the perinatal morbidity and mortality in these children. One study documents a 70–80% incidence of neonatal morbidity in infants of addicted mothers versus 25% in nonaddicted neonates from a similar socioeconomic group.[124] The overall mortality rate for these infants is 5.7% compared with 1.6% of the control group.

The importance of good prenatal care on mortality is underscored by a study that demonstrates an 8% mortality rate for babies born of mothers who took methadone but did not have adequate prenatal care versus a 3% mortality rate when mothers involved in methadone programs also received consistent prenatal care.[139] Additional morbidity results from increased perinatal asphyxia and meconium staining in addicted infants[140] and an increased frequency of chromosomal damage in both mothers and infants.[141] An increase in obstetric complications such as spontaneous abortion, abruptio placenta, amnionitis, breech delivery, eclampsia, postpartum hemorrhage, and premature rupture of membranes are described in drug-dependent women.[139]

Two salutary effects of addiction during pregnancy have been reported. Opiates may accelerate the maturity of the lecithin/sphingomyelin ratio in fetal lungs, thereby improving respiratory function in the preterm infant.[142] A lowered incidence of hyperbilirubinemia is also seen in addicted infants, perhaps because of intrauterine induction of hepatic microsomal enzyme systems.[140]

6.4.3. Withdrawal during Prenancy

The fetus of an addicted mother is exposed to numerous deleterious agents and factors capable of seriously impairing neonatal functioning. However, there is some evidence that withdrawing from opiate use during pregnancy may present an even greater hazard to the fetus. A precipitous reduction of the methadone dose will precipitate a four- to fivefold increase in fetal epinephrine and norepinephrine excretion in the amniotic fluid.[143] At least five intrauterine deaths occurring during detoxification in the last trimester have been reported.[143] Furthermore, the monitoring of fetal distress during maternal narcotic withdrawal is made difficult due to a paradoxical increase in estriol levels despite increasing fetal distress. In addition, the drug withdrawing fetus has increased oxygen needs, which may be inadequately met in the intrauterine environment.[144] Further study in this area is needed to elucidate the relative benefits and risks of continuing versus discontinuing opiate use during pregnancy.

6.4.4. Neurobehavioral Studies

Passively addicted infants demonstrate neurobehavioral dysfunction from birth. An identifiable withdrawal syndrome occurs in 70–90% of infants born to addicted mothers.[124,135,140] Withdrawal symptoms include fist sucking, irritability, tremors, sneezing, high-pitched cry, hypertonicity, exaggerated primitive reflexes, stuffy nose, diaphoresis, diarrhea, and vomiting.[136] While some studies describe a higher rate of seizure activity during withdrawal,[145] other studies have not confirmed this finding. A significant thrombocytosis appearing after the first week of life has also been observed.[146]

Compared with heroin, methadone seems to cause more severe withdrawal symptoms, especially when administered at doses greater than 20 mg/day.[135,136] The symptoms of methadone withdrawal start later, usually beginning 18–36 hr (occasionally days and even weeks) after delivery, compared with the usual 4–24 hr onset of symptoms in heroin-exposed infants.[139] Withdrawal symptoms last longer for the methadone-addicted infants. The delayed and more intense withdrawal pattern for methadone-addicted infants may be due to prolonged fetal storage and delayed excretion of the drug.[147]

Up to 80% of infants who withdraw in the nursery will continue to have symptoms such as increased restlessness, agitation, tremors, decreased sleep, hyperphagia, colic, vomiting, and hyperacusis when discharged home. These "subacute" withdrawal symptoms usually resolve within 3–6 months.

The behavior of passively addicted neonates also has been studied by more refined techniques. The Brazelton Neonatal Assessment Scale has shown these babies to have a decreased capacity for alertness, self-quieting, and a poor ability to regulate their state of consciousness and orient to the environment.[148,149] Their sleep pattern is characterized by a more active rapid eye movement (REM) phase, less quiet sleep, and more time spent in indeterminant sleep, which implies a less organized CNS.[150] Analysis of feeding behavior in these infants has shown them to have lower rate and pressure to their sucking and a nutrient intake only one-half that of controls.[151]

There is no general agreement as to how or when to treat the abstinence syndrome. For mild symptoms, environmental maneuvers such as swaddling, pacifier, and a dark, quiet room are the usual approach to management. For moderate or severe withdrawal, a wide variety of pharmacologic agents have been employed, such as paregoric, phenobarbital, diazepam, and thorazine. There are currently no conclusive data to support the relative advantage of any of these agents over the others. However, most centers use one of the opiates.

6.5. Follow-up Studies

Follow-up studies of babies born to drug-dependent mothers are difficult to interpret, and there is no general agreement as to their significance. The confounding variables listed in the introduction contribute to the confusion. These include a lack of valid control groups, short-term follow-up only, high dropout rate of the subjects, relatively gross measures of behavioral and developmental functioning, concomitant medical illness, and malnutrition. In addition, the parent–child relationship and drug culture environment exert a profound influence on the development of the child, and it is difficult to separate these factors from possible organic risk due to prenatal drug exposure.

6.5.1. Health Outcomes

Infants born to addicted mothers have approximately a five times greater risk of developing SIDS during the first year of life.[152,153] In a 24-month follow-up, a second study has reported an increased incidence in these children of otitis media, abnormal neurologic findings including nystagmus, strabismus, and tone or coordination abnormalities.[154] Another study[155] found no increased incidence of medical illness but an increased rate of accidents in the first 12 months of life.

6.5.2. Somatic Growth

While opiates inhibit somatic growth prenatally, the persistence of this effect over time is minimal. Follow-up studies have shown no difference in weight and height compared to control groups at 18 months,[156] 24 months,[154,155] and 36 months.[157] Whereas the mean head circumference is also within normal limits in these groups, a higher percentage of microcephaly is present in children exposed to opiates prenatally.[154,156]

6.5.3. Developmental Outcome

Although interpretation is made difficult by confounding variables and limited outcome measures, studies generally fail to implicate opiate abuse during pregnancy as a direct cause of adverse developmental outcome. For example, scores on the Bailey infant test are usually within the normal range for these children on follow-up at 1 to 2 years.[155] Many studies show these developmental indices to be somewhat lower than controls but still within normal limits.[154,156] Others have suggested that more subtle measures of behavior such as a decreased attention span, perceptual motor difficulties, and hyperactivity may result from prenatal opiate exposure.[155] In many studies, the best predictor of long-term I.Q. score was maternal health during pregnancy and the postnatal home environment, but not the degree of maternal narcotic use during pregnancy. The attrition rate of the study population of opiate-addicted mothers may result in a self-selected population for these follow-up studies, causing inaccurate conclusions.

6.6. Prenatal Intervention

The availability of methadone to treat narcotic addiction during the 1960s generated the establishment of programs to care for and treat the addicted pregnant patient and her offspring. Since addiction is a psychological disorder as well as a physical dependence, these programs developed an interdisciplinary approach that included not only obstetric care but methadone maintenance and psychosocial supports.

Such programs have been shown to reduce maternal and infant

morbidity significantly, especially the incidence of low-birth-weight and neonatal withdrawal syndrome.[124]

In the interdisciplinary program to treat pregnant addicted women at Boston City Hospital, street addicts are given methadone in a dose high enough to eliminate other drug intake. The dose is subsequently reduced by 2–5 mg every 1–2 weeks, with the goal of a 20-mg/day maintenance dose. In a select group, inpatient total detoxification is attempted with frequent monitoring of fetal well-being through bio-physical profiles and nonstress tests. Other women are encouraged to increase their dose of methadone rather than take other drugs.

6.7. Summary

Opiate use during pregnancy is associated with significant morbidity during pregnancy. Well-established sequelae in the neonatal period include increased neonatal mortality and morbidity, suppressed birth weight, increased microcephaly, increased prematurity, and neonatal withdrawal syndrome. A direct effect of the drugs as well as numerous adverse health habits in the mother accounts for these outcomes.

7. Amphetamines

7.1. Introduction

During the early 1960s amphetamines were widely prescribed during pregnancy as a treatment of obesity.[158] During this period, studies reported an incidence of amphetamine use during pregnancy ranging from 0.5%[159] to 16%.[158] Amphetamines are rarely prescribed now, and use occurs mainly in drug-abusing mothers. The current incidence of use during pregnancy is unknown.

7.2. Pharmacology

Amphetamines are powerful CNS stimulants and sympathomimetic drugs. These drugs increase systolic and diastolic blood pressure, relax bronchial smooth muscle, stimulate the respiratory center, depress the appetite, and ameliorate fatigue. Unlike epinephrine, they easily cross the blood–brain barrier and cause a euphoric elevation of mood and a sense of increased energy and alertness. Amphetamines are ingested, snorted, and injected. Tolerance often develops to the central effects, requiring increasingly higher doses. This may result in a toxic psychotic syndrome weeks to months after continued use. Discontinuation of the drug after chronic use causes hypersomnia, fatigue, lassitude, and depression. The metabolism of these amines is complicated. They are excreted in the urine with approximately one-half of the drug unchanged and the rest metabolized by various pathways. These drugs are secreted in breast milk in concentrations three to seven times greater than in maternal plasma.[160]

7.3. Studies in Animals

D-Amphetamine is metabolized more slowly in the pregnant than in the nonpregnant mouse.[161] Transplacental transfer of this drug occurs, but it appears in the fetus in much lower concentrations than in the mother. It is speculated that a vasoconstrictive effect on the placental vessels may prevent the buildup of amphetamine in the fetus.

High doses of amphetamines cause malformations in mice and rabbits, although the data are not consistent.[162] Prenatal exposure to amphetamines results in increased malformations of the heart and great vessels of chicks.[163] A decrease in brain norepinephrine levels at birth is seen in rats exposed to D-amphetamine prenatally.[164] In addition, high-dose exposure has also been shown to effect the postnatal behavior of rats.[165,166]

7.4. Studies in Humans

7.4.1. Teratogenic Potential

Initial reports concerning amphetamines in pregnancy consisted of small samples. In one study, 5 of 11 patients with biliary atresia were thought to have been exposed to amphetamines during early pregnancy.[167] A case-control study of 184 infants with congenital heart disease found significant exposure to amphetamines during pregnancy, especially during the first trimester.[168]

The largest study of amphetamine use during pregnancy occurred in a retrospective study of 12,205 deliveries.[158] In this sample, 16% (or 1,992 women) were prescribed amphetamines during pregnancy for weight control, fatigue, and/or depression. This study found no increase in the incidence of severe congenital anomalies, including cardiac defects or biliary atresia, over the control group.

7.4.2. Perinatal Morbidity

Another retrospective study assessed the infants of 237 pregnancies in which amphetamines had been prescribed.[159] This study found no differences in length and head circumference of the neonates over the control groups but did find a modestly lower birth weight if the drug was taken after 28 weeks gestation. In both studies the doses of the drug were relatively low and well controlled and not confounded by polydrug usage.

In a study of 69 women who abused primarily amphetamines during pregnancy,[169] the infants' weight and lengths (corrected for gestational age) did not differ from those of the control group. However, these women experienced a higher incidence of preterm deliveries as well as increased pregnancy complications, including hypertension, poor weight gain, and more hospital admissions.

There are no systematic descriptions of the behavior of infants born to amphetamine-abusing mothers. Two reports[170,171] describe infants with symptoms of extreme lassitude as well as occasional restlessness, miotic pupils, and irritability. These symptoms of lethargy closely approximate those seen in adults withdrawing from amphetamine abuse.

7.5. Summary

There is no good evidence that amphetamines are a teratogen in humans, nor does this drug exhibit a significant effect on birth weight. An increased incidence of intrapartum complications and preterm delivery has been noted, as well as an ill-defined behavioral constellation in the newborn marked by lethargy.

8. Cocaine

8.1. Introduction

Cocaine is an extract of the leaves of coca plant. Cocaine abuse is the fastest-growing drug problem in the United States. For example, its use in college-age young adults has risen from seven million in 1972 to

33 million in 1982.[172] Despite its widespread use, its effect on pregnancy has not been well studied.

8.2. Pharmacology

Cocaine is easily absorbed from mucous membranes or gastric mucosa. Following absorption, it is degraded by plasma esterases and hepatic enzymes with a plasma half-life of 1 hr. Its main actions are to block nerve conduction locally, but its illicit abuse is due to its ability to stimulate the central nervous system. In addition, cocaine in low doses may slow the heart through central vagal stimulation but in high doses causes a sympathetic tachycardia. Cocaine potentiates the excitatory and inhibitory responses of sympathetically innervated organs.

8.3. Studies in Animals

Studies of possible teratogenicity of cocaine in rats have yielded conflicting results. When high doses (60 mg/kg) were given at days 7–9 of pregnancy, one study found markedly increased congenital anomalies in the offspring, including skeletal abnormalities, exencephaly, hydronephrosis, and cryptorchidism.[173] A similar study giving cocaine on days 8–12 of pregnancy yielded growth retardation in the offspring, thought to be secondary to a combination of maternal anorexia and placenta vasoconstriction, but no increase in congenital malformations.[174] Further research is needed to elucidate the possible teratogenic potential of cocaine.

8.4. Studies in Humans

To date there are few systematic studies of the effects of cocaine on pregnancy and neonatal outcome. Sporadic case reports have appeared in the literature. For example, two cases of maternal abruptio placenta were described in mothers who used cocaine during pregnancy.[175] Cocaine is possibly associated with transient hypertension and placental vasoconstriction, which may account for this effect. More recently, a controlled study examined the effects of cocaine use during pregnancy on newborn outcomes.[176] This study suggested a higher rate of spontaneous abortion in cocaine users, described four cases where the onset of labor with abruptio placenta occurred immediately following self-injection of cocaine, but could find no evidence of intrauterine growth retardation in the babies of cocaine users. This study also reported a deleterious effect of cocaine use during pregnancy on newborn neurobehavioral function. Specifically, on the Brazelton Neonatal Behavioral Assessment Scale, they found a depression of the babies' interactive abilities and impaired organization of states of consciousness compared to control groups. Methodologic issues such as small sample size, confounding variables, and designation of control groups do not allow firm conclusions at this time. We await further studies to precisely delineate cocaine's effects on pregnancy and on newborn outcomes.

9. Barbiturates

9.1. Introduction

During the late 1950s and early 1960s, prescription use of phenobarbital during pregnancy was at its peak. For example, 12% of the 9006 women in the Danish Perinatal Cohort from 1959–1961 were treated with barbiturates during pregnancy, usually for hypertension and/or sedation.[177] In a Collaborative Perinatal Project in the United States conducted in 1959–1961, 25% of the women received barbiturates in pregnancy.[177] Currently they are rarely prescribed during pregnancy except for seizure control. However, barbiturates now represent one of the most abused prescription drugs alone or in combination with other drugs.

9.2. Pharmacology

Barbiturates are sedative-hypnotic agents used to promote drowsiness and sleep. They have the capacity to depress a wide range of physiologic activity, including that of nerve, skeletal muscle, smooth muscle, and the myocardium. Tolerance develops after prolonged intake, probably from enhanced deactivation by the liver. These drugs are distributed to all body tissues and fluids and readily cross the placenta. Most are eventually transformed by the liver into inactive metabolites and excreted in the urine. Barbiturates are excreted in breast milk in small amounts.

9.3. Studies in Animals

In rats, phenobarbital exposure has been linked with a decreased brain growth, especially in the hippocampus and cerebellum.[177] It has also been linked with other teratogenic effects in mice (such as curly tail and phocomelia) in large doses.[178] Inhibition of pulmonary maturation in the fetal rabbit has been shown, presumably secondary to induction of liver enzymes that hasten steroid degradation.[179] Prenatal phenobarbital exposure in the rat blocks neonatal testosterone synthesis and interferes with normal masculinization in the postnatal period.[177,180]

9.4. Studies in Humans

Phenobarbital rapidly passes through the placenta into fetal tissues. In a study of 35 human fetuses aborted at 4–7 months, mothers were given phenobarbital anywhere from $\frac{1}{2}$ to 50 hr before the abortion. Traces were found in the fetus as early as 30 min, and peak levels were attained after 2 hr. The largest concentration of the drug was found in the fetal liver and fourth ventricle of the brain.[181]

Most studies evaluating the teratologic potential of phenobarbital have been conducted on women being treated with phenobarbital for epilepsy during pregnancy. Interpreting these studies is made difficult by a number of factors. First, most women were taking other medications in addition to the phenobarbital, such as diphenylhydantoin, which has a clearly established teratogenic potential. Thus, when present, malformations may be due to other drugs or to a teratogenic synergism between phenobarbital and the other drugs. Second, frequent seizures with their attendant hypoxia and acidosis may predispose to malformations. Third, phenobarbital lowers serum folic acid levels.[182] Since folic acid antagonists have been shown to be associated with a variety of malformations, a teratogenic result may be an indirect action of barbiturates.

Table V. Percentage of Malformations Associated with Phenobarbital

Study	Phenobarbital taken alone (%)	Phenobarbital and diphenylhydantoin (%)	Control (%)
Fedrick *et al.*[182]	4.9	22	5.6
Speidel and Meadow[183]	1.6	4.2	—
Lowe[184]	1.9	10	2.7
Annegers *et al.*[185]	12	—	—

Table V lists the percent of malformations in studies that examined women taking phenobarbital alone or in combination for seizure control during pregnancy. Because of the retrospective nature of these studies, the lack of control groups, and the variability of the malformations found, the issue is still not totally resolved. However, it appears that phenobarbital alone has little teratogenic potential. In addition, a larger retrospective study of 2784 cases of CNS, skeletal, or cranial facial defects in the Finnish report of congenital malformations showed no association between phenobarbital and birth defects.[186]

9.4.1. Neurobehavioral Functioning

The existence of withdrawal syndrome in infants exposed *in utero* to barbiturates is well established.[187–189] The onset of this syndrome occurs 3–14 days after delivery. The duration of symptoms typically ranges from 2 to 6 months. Symptoms described in this syndrome include tremors, hyperphagia, hyperreflexia, jitteriness, hypertonia, vomiting, sneezing, vasomotor instability, hyperacusis, and poor weight gain. These studies have reported decreased incidence of jaundice in these infants. Follow-up data on long-term functioning are lacking.

9.5. Summary

Barbiturates are rarely taken, licitly or illicitly, as a single drug. Present evidence does not appear to demonstrate a strong teratogenic effect in humans. Whether barbiturates might act synergistically with other drugs such as alcohol or marijuana remains unknown. A neonatal withdrawal syndrome is marked by later onset and prolonged symptomatology.

10. Phencyclidine

10.1 Introduction

Phencyclidine (PCP) was developed during the 1950s as a human anesthetic but was not approved because of adverse side effects, such as delirium, agitation, and hallucinations after anesthesia. Recently it has become a popular drug among teenagers and young adults. During 1976–1977, its use among 18–25-year-olds increased from 9.6 to 13.9%.[190] In young adults who abuse more than one drug, 32% take PCP also, making it the third most frequently abused drug after alcohol and marijuana. PCP is unusual in that it can act as a depressant, stimulant, or hallucinogen, depending on the dose, type of administration, and circumstance of usage. It appears in powdered, liquid, or tablet form and may be mixed with, or counterfeited as, other drugs. It can be swallowed, smoked, snorted, or ingested.

The incidence of PCP usage during pregnancy appears to be increasing. A study of 200 women randomly selected from a low-socioeconomic-status Hispanic population showed a startling 12% incidence of PCP in cord blood.[191] Another study of 2327 pregnant women showed 6.8% admitting to having used PCP but only 0.8% admitting to usage during pregnancy.[192] However, one-third of users during pregnancy were detected by urine tests only and had previously denied usage. Thus, usage during pregnancy may be higher than evidenced by self-report. These studies showed that women who took PCP during pregnancy also tended to smoke, drink alcohol, and take other drugs.

10.2. Pharmacology

Phencyclidine is a dissociative anesthetic agent related to ketamine. It is well absorbed following any route of administration and is subsequently metabolized by the liver. The plasma half-life is about 3 days, but this can be shortened by acidification of the urine and gastric suctioning.

10.3. Studies in Animals

In rats, large doses of PCP in pregnancy cause numerous malformations, including abnormalities of extremities, cleft palate, micrognathia, and cranial dysplasia.[193] PCP was found to cross the placenta in rabbits[194] and pigs.[195] It concentrates at a level 10 times greater in the fetal piglet plasma than that of the maternal sow.[195] Mice exposed to PCP were also found to be less advanced in the development of certain reflexes, including crawling and walking postnatally.[194]

10.4. Studies in Humans

10.4.1. Teratogenic Potential

The teratogenic potential of PCP during human pregnancy has not been addressed to date. A single case report[196] described an infant with multiple dysmorphic features born to a mother who admitted abusing mainly PCP during pregnancy. However, this mother also took other drugs during pregnancy. Further studies are necessary in this area.

10.4.2. Perinatal Morbidity

Studies on the relationship of PCP to other neonatal outcome are equally limited. In three studies[197,198] that looked at a total of 18 infants whose mothers took primarily PCP during pregnancy, birth weight, length, and head circumference was slightly smaller, but not significantly different from that of control groups. However, these babies were considered behaviorally distinctive and were characterized by an inability to regulate states of consciousness as well as poor consolability. They had sudden attacks of agitation and grimaces as well as an exaggerated reaction to sound. However, these children did not seem to manifest classic signs of withdrawal. No conclusions concerning the role of PCP in pregnancy and neonatal outcome can be drawn at this time.

11. Diazepam

11.1. Introduction

Diazepam (Valium) is used as an antianxiety agent and as a muscle relaxant. Its ability to depress the CNS seems to be due to an inhibitory effect on the reticular activating and limbic systems. The incidence of diazepam and related compound use during pregnancy is unknown. However, in a study of opiate abusers, Valium was the most widely used second drug in the sample. There is very little information to date on the effect of diazepam on the newborn.

11.2. Pharmacology

Diazepam is a benzodiazepine derivative, as are chlordiazepoxide (Librium) and oxazepam (Dalmane). Following oral absorption, a portion of the drug is excreted rapidly in the urine with a half-life of 7–10 hr, while the remainder is excreted slowly over 2–8 days. Mild tolerance to the drug and physical dependence are seen after prolonged use.

Diazepam found brief favor during the 1960s and 1970s as an intrapartum agent to control anxiety and blood pressure. Studies conducted during that time showed diazepam to rapidly cross the placenta.[199,200] In one infant it was detected in the fetal blood 10 min after intravenous administration to the mother.[201] Compared with adults, the fetus more slowly metabolizes and excretes diazapem, and levels are often higher than in maternal tissues.[201,202] A postmortem examination of a fetus whose mother took diazepam during pregnancy showed accumulation of the drug in lungs, heart, and brain.[200]

11.3. Studies in Animals

Large doses of diazepam in pregnant rats are related to a significant increase in cleft palates in the offspring.[203] Rats exposed to diazepam during pregnancy also show poor weight gain.[204] Prenatal exposure to diazepam during late gestation causes a decrease in norepinephrine levels and an increase in norepinephrine utilization in hypothalamus of the pup.[205] Another study has shown fewer opioid-binding sites in the rat cortex and striatum following *in utero* exposure.[206] These studies suggest that exposure of the evolving brain to diazepam may lead to specific and long-lasting alterations in the nervous system. Other studies[204,207] have shown altered postnatal behaviors in rats exposed to diazepam prenatally.

11.4. Studies in Humans

11.4.1. Teratogenic Potential

On the basis of animal studies, possible teratogenicity of diazepam in humans has focused on cleft lip and cleft palate. Using a case-control method, mothers of children with cleft lip or palate had a four- to five-fold increase in taking benzodiazepines during the first trimester over a group of controls.[208] However, the most recent review of the Birth Defects Study of the National Institute of Child Health could find no significant increase in the use of diazepam in the first trimester and oral clefts.[209] Another review of 445 children with oral clefts likewise found no association with the use of diazepam.[210] We can say that there is little evidence to associate diazepam and oral clefts.

11.4.2. Perinatal Morbidity

Intravenous diazepam during labor is related to a decrease in beat-to-beat variability of the fetal heart without changing the heart rate. The use of less than 30 mg diazepam 15 hr before delivery has few adverse behavioral effects on the newborn.[200] However, doses greater than 30 mg are associated with neonatal depression, as evidenced by apnea, a poor suck, hypotonia, and hyporeflexia.[211,212] Maternal administration of diazepam in the late states of delivery is associated with inadequate neonatal thermogenesis and an exaggerated fall in infants' temperature following delivery.[213,214]

There are only anecdotal case reports relating diazepam use during pregnancy and withdrawal symptoms in the neonate. One study[215] describes three infants born to mothers prescribed Valium during their pregnancy. These infants were indistinguishable from infants withdrawing from narcotics and manifested irritability, hypertonicity, hyperexcitability, tachypnea, and hyperphagia. Initial symptoms were noted 2–6 hr after delivery. At that time, urine screens were negative for narcotics, but positive for diazepam. Mild tremors persisting for 5–6 weeks after delivery were also reported.

11.5. Summary

Diazepam use during pregnancy has been associated with an increased incidence of oral clefts although recent studies refute this. The use of diazepam during delivery may lead to neonatal central nervous system depression and impaired thermogenesis. Withdrawal symptoms of the neonate may occur in mothers who have taken diazapem during pregnancy.

12. Summary

Psychoactive drugs consumed during pregnancy can be teratogenic to the fetus (Table VI). The most common form of teratogenicity is low birth weight and neurobehavioral dysfunction. Conclusive evidence is lacking to implicate any of the drugs discussed in this chapter with a specific malformation. Many unanswered questions remain, including the possible synergistic effect of psychoactive substances and whether drugs being used with increasing frequency, such as marijuana, cocaine, and phencyclidine, are teratogenic.

Deciding which substances taken during pregnancy are hazardous to the fetus is an issue of enormous importance for pregnant women. The results of this review emphasize the difficulty in isolating single factors as the cause of abnormal newborn development. Whereas there is a need to warn people about specific agents that may adversely influ-

Table VI. Teratogenicity of Psychoactive Drugs Based on Studies in Humans

	Controlled studies	Growth failure	Malformations	Neurobehavioral dysfunction
Cigarettes	+	+ +	−	+
Caffeine	+	−	−	+
Alcohol	+	+ +	+/−	+
Marijuana	+	+/−	+/−	+
Opiates	−	+ + + +	−	+ + + +
Amphetamines	−	−	−	+
Cocaine	+	N/A	N/A	+ +
Barbiturates	−	−	−	+ + +
Phencyclidine	−	N/A	N/A	+ +
Diazepam	−	N/A	−	+ +

ence fetal development, human studies that attempt to identify specific agents should be viewed cautiously. This update of substance abuse by the pregnant woman suggests that a life-style that combines smoking, drinking, and marijuana use is more marked a risk than the use of any single substance.

Acknowledgment

We thank Susan Simon for her help in preparing the manuscript. This work was supported by grant RO1 DAO3508-01 from the National Institute on Drug Abuse.

References

1. Jones, K. L., Smith, D. W., Ulleland, C. N., *et al.*, 1973, Pattern of malformation in offspring of chronic alcoholic women, *Lancet* 1:1267.
2. Milunsky, A., Graef, J. W., and Gaynor, M. F., 1968, Methotrexate induced congenital malformations with a review of the literature, *J. Pediatr.* 72:790.
3. Younoszai, N. K., Kacic, A., and Haworth, J. C., 1968, Cigarette smoking during pregnancy: The effect upon hematocrit and acid–base balance of the newborn, *Can. Med. Assoc. J.* 99:197.
4. Shaul, W. L., and, Hall, J. G., 1977, Multiple congenital anomalies associated with oral anticoagulants, *Am. J. Obstet. Gynecol.* 127:191.
5. Hanson, J. W., and Smith, D. W., 1975, The fetal hydantoin syndrome, *J. Pediatr.* 87:285.
6. Stone, M. L., Salerno, L. J., Green, M., *et al.*, 1971, Narcotic addiction in pregnancy, *Am. J. Obstet. Gynecol.* 109:716.
7. Zelson, C., Lee, S. J., and Casalino, M., 1973, Neonatal narcotic addiction, *N. Engl. J. Med.* 289:1216.

8. Hingson, R., Alpert, J., Day, N., *et al.*, 1982, Effects of maternal drinking and marijuana use on fetal growth and development, *Pediatrics* **70**:539.
9. Jones, K. L., and Charnoff, G. F., 1978, Drugs and chemicals associated with intrauterine growth deficiency, *Reprod. Med.* **21**:365.
10. Sameroff, A. J., and Chandler, M. T., 1975, Reproductive risk and the continuum of caretaking casuality, in: *Review of Child Development Research* (F. D. Horowitz, ed.), Vol. 4, pp. 187–243, University of Chicago Press, Chicago.
11. Weston, J., 1968, The pathology of child abuse, in: *The Battered Child* (R. Helfer and C. Kempe, eds.), pp. 80, University of Chicago Press, Chicago.
12. Fitzgerald, J., and Mulford, H., 1978, Distribution of alcohol consumption and problem drinking: Comparison of sales records and survey data, *J. Stud. Alcohol* **35**:879.
13. Amour, D., Pollich, J., and Stambul, H., 1976, *Alcoholism and Treatment*, Rand Corporation, Santa Monica, Calif.
14. Zuckerman, B. S., Hingson, R., Morelock, *et al.*, 1985, A pilot study assessing maternal marijuana use by urine assay during pregnancy, *Current Challenges to Methods of Drug Abuse Estimation* No. 57, pp. 84–93, NIDA Research Monograph Series.
15. Hingson, R., Zuckerman, R., Amaro, H., *et al.*, 1986 Maternal marijuana use and neonatal outcome: Uncertainty posed by self-reports, *Am. J. Public Health*, **76**:667.
16. Essenberg, J. M., Schwind, J. V., and Patras, A. B., 1940, The effects of nicotine on cigarette smoke on pregnant female albino rats and their offspring, *J. Lab. Clin. Med.*, **25**:708.
17. Schoeneck, F. J., 1941, Cigarette smoking in pregnancy, *N.Y. State. J. Med.* **41**:1945.
18. Simpson, W. J., 1975, A preliminary report of cigarette smoking and the incidence of prematurity, *Am. J. Obstet. Gynecol.* **73**:808.
19. Lowe, C. R., 1959, Effect of mothers' smoking habits on birth weight of their children, *Br. Med. J.* **2**:673.
20. Fielding, J. E., 1978, Smoking and pregnancy, *N. Engl. J. Med.* **298**:337.
21. U.S. Public Health Service, 1979, Smoking and Health, A Report of the Surgeon General, U.S. Department of Health, Education, and Welfare Publ. No. (PHS) 79-50066, Public Health Service, Office on Smoking and Health, Washington, D. C.
22. Abel, E. L., 1983, *Marihuana, Tobacco, Alcohol and Reproduction*, CRC Press, Boca Raton, Florida.
23. Quiglye, M. E., Sheehan, K. L., Wilkes, M. M., *et al.*, 1979, Effects of maternal smoking on circulatory catecholamine levels and fetal heart rates, *Am. J. Obstet. Gynecol.* **133**:685.
24. Kline, J., Stein, Z. A., and Susser, M., 1977, Smoking as a risk factor for spontaneous abortion, *N. Engl. J. Med.* **297**:793.
25. Himmelberger, D. U., Brown, B. W., and Cohen, E. N., 1978, Cigarette smoking during pregnancy and the occurrence of spontaneous abortion and congenital abnormality, *Am. J. Epidemiol.* **108**:470.
26. Bergman, A. B., and Wiesner, L. A., 1976, Relationship of passive cigarette smoking to sudden infant death syndrome, *Pediatrics* **58**:665.
27. Lewak, N., Va-den-Berg, B. J., and Beckwith, J. B., 1979, Sudden infant death syndrome risk factors: Prospective data review, *Clin. Pediatr.* **18**:404.
28. Naeye, R. L., Ladis, B., and Drage, J. S., 1976, Sudden infant death syndrome, *Am. J. Dis. Child.* **130**:1207.
29. O'Lane, J. M., 1963, Some fetal effects of maternal cigarette smoking, *Obstet. Gynecol.* **22**:181.
30. Garn, S. M., Johnson, M., Ridella, S. A., *et al.*, 1981, Effects of maternal cigarette smoking on Apgar scores, *Am. J. Dis. Child.* **135**:503.
31. Schramm, W., 1980, Smoking and pregnancy outcome, *Mo. Med.* **77**:619.

32. Hingson, R., Gould, J. R., Morelock, S., *et al.*, 1982, Maternal cigarette smoking, psychoactive substance use and infant Apgar scores, *Am. J. Obstet. Gynecol.* **144:**959.
33. Fedrick, J., Alberman, E., and Goldstein, H., 1971, Possible teratogenic effect of cigarette smoking, *Nature (London)* **231:**530.
34. Heinonen, O. P., 1976, Risk factors for congenital heart disease: A prospective study, in: *Birth Defects Risks and Consequences* (S. Kelly, E. B. Hook, D. T. Janerich, *et al.*, eds.), pp. 221–264, Academic Press, New York.
35. Andrews, J., and McGarry, J. M., 1972, A community study of smoking in pregnancy, *J. Obstet. Gynaecol. Br. Commonw.***79:**1057.
36. Peterson, W. F., Morese, K. N., and Kaltreider, D. F., 1965, Smoking and prematurity: A preliminary report based on study of 7740 caucasians, *Obstet. Gynecol.* **26:**775.
37. Kullander, S., and, Kallen, B., 1971, A prospective study of smoking and pregnancy, *Acta Obstet. Gynaecol. Scand.* **50:**83.
38. Richards, I. D., 1969, Congenital malformations and environmental influences in pregnancy, *Br. J. Prev. Soc. Med.* **23:**218.
39. Harrison, G. G., Branson, R. S., and Vaugher, Y. E., 1983, Association of maternal smoking with body composition of the newborn, *Am. J. Clin. Nutr.* **38:**757.
40. Miller, H. C., Hassanein, K., and Hensleigh, P., 1976, Fetal growth retardation in relation to maternal smoking and weight gain in pregnancy, *Am. J. Obstet. Gynecol.* **1:**55.
41. Davies, D. P., Gray, O. P., Ellwood, P. C., *et al.*, 1976, Cigarette smoking in pregnancy: Associations with maternal weight gain and fetal growth, *Lancet* **1:**385.
42. Rush, D., 1976, Cigarette smoking during pregnancy: The relationship with depressed weight gain and birth weight, in: *Birth Defects Risks and Consequences* (S. Kelly, E. B. Hook, D. T. Janerich, *et al.*, eds.), pp. 161–172, Academic Press, New York.
43. Yerushalmy, J., 1971, The relationship of parents' cigarette smoking to outcome of pregnancy—Implications as to the problem of inferring causation from observed association, *Am. J. Epidemiol.* **93:**443.
44. Heron, H. J., 1962, The effects of smoking during pregnancy: A review with a preview, *N. Z. Med. J.* **61:**543.
45. Cole, P., Hawkins, L. H., and Roberts, D., 1972, Smoking during pregnancy and its effect on the fetus, *J. Obstet. Gynaecol. Br. Commonw.* **79:**782.
46. Resnick, R., Brink, G. W., and Wiles, M., 1979, Catecholamine-mediated reduction in uterine blood flow after nicotine infusion in the pregnant ewe, *J. Clin. Invest.* **63:**1133.
47. Suzuki, K. T., Minel, L. J., and Johnson, E. E., 1980, Effect of nicotine upon uterine blood flow in the pregnant rhesus monkey, *Am. J. Obstet. Gynecol.* **136:**1009.
48. Saxton, D. W., 1978, The behaviour of infants whose mothers smoke in pregnancy, *Early. Hum. Dev.* **2:**363.
49. Martin, J. C., Martin, D. C., Lund, C., *et al.*, 1973, Maternal alcohol ingestion and cigarette smoking and their effect upon newborn conditioning, *Alcoholism Clin. Exp. Res.* **1:**243.
50. Landesman-Dwyer, S., Keller, L. S., and Streissguth, A. P., 1978, Naturalistic observations of newborns: effects of maternal alcohol intake, *Alcoholism Clin. Exp. Res.* **2:**171.
51. Woodson, E. M., DaCosta, P., Woodson, R. H., *et al.*, 1980, Maternal smoking and newborn behavior, presented at the International Conference on Infant Studies, New Haven, Conn.
52. Picone, T. A., Allen, L. H., Olsen, P. N., *et al.*, 1980, The effect of maternal weight gain and smoking during pregnancy on human neonatal behavior, presented at the Biennial meeting on the International Conference on Infant Studies, New Haven, Conn.

53. Butler, N. R., and Goldstein, H., 1973, Smoking in pregnancy and subsequent child development, *Br. Med. J.*, 4:573.
54. Dunn, H. G., McBurney, A. K., Ingram, S., *et al.*, 1977, Maternal cigarette smoking during pregnancy and the child's subsequent development. II. Neurological and intellectual maturation to the age of 6½ years, *Can. J. Publ. Health* 68:43.
55. Soyka, L., 1981, Caffeine ingestion during pregnancy: In utero exposure and possible effect, *Semin. Perinatol.* 4:305.
56. Timson, J., 1977, Caffeine, *Mutat. Res.* 47:1.
57. Linn, S., Schoenbaum, S., Monson, R., *et al.*, 1982, No association between coffee consumption and adverse outcomes of pregnancy, *N. Engl. J. Med.* 306:141.
58. Aldridge, A., Bailey, J., and Neims, A., 1981, The disposition of caffeine during and after pregnancy, *Semin. Perinatol.* 5:310.
59. Kirkinen, P., Jouppila, P., Koivula, A., *et al.*, 1983, The effect of caffeine on placental and fetal blood flow in human pregnancy, *Am. J. Obstet. Gynecol.* 147:939.
60. Parsons, W., Aranda, J., and Neims, A., 1976, Elimination of transplacentally acquired caffeine in fullterm neonates, *Pediatr. Res.* 10:333.
61. Fabro, S., and Sieber, S., 1969, Caffeine and nicotine penetrate the pre-implantation blastocyst, *Nature (London)* 233:410.
62. White, B., Simpson, C., Adams, J. and Harkins, D., 1978, Monoamine synthesis and caffeine induced locomotor activity, *Neuropharmacology* 17:511.
63. Tanaka, H., Nakazama, K., and Arima, M., 1983, Adverse effect of maternal caffeine ingestion on fetal cerebrum in the rat, *Brain Dev.* 5:397.
64. Volpe, J., 1981, Effects of methylxanthines on lipid synthesis in developing neural systems, *Semin. Perinatol.* 5:395.
65. Borlee, L., 1978, Le café, facteur de risque pendant la grossesse?, *Louvain Med.* 97:279.
66. Jacobson, M., Goldman, A., and Syme, R., 1981, Coffee and birth defects, *Lancet* 1:1415.
67. Weathersbee, P., Olsen, L., and Lodge, J., 1977, Caffeine and pregnancy, *Postgrad. Med. J.* 62:64.
68. Kurppa, K., Holmberg, P., Kuosma, E., and Saxen, L., 1983, Coffee consumption during pregnancy and selected congenital malformations: A nationwide case-control study, *Am. J. Publ. Health* 73:1397.
69. Rosenberg, L., Mitchell, A., Shapiro, S., and Slone, D., 1982, Selected birth defects in relation to caffeine-containing beverages, *J.A.M.A.* 247:1429.
70. Streissguth, A. P., Martin, D. C., and Bair, H. M., 1978, Neonatal Brazelton assessment and relationship to maternal alcohol use, Unpublished manuscript, University of Washington, Seattle.
71. Jacobson, S. W., Fein, G. G., Jacobson, J. L., *et al.*, 1984, Neonatal correlates of prenatal exposure to smoking, caffeine, and alcohol, *Infant Behavior and Development* 7:253–265.
72. Ulleland, C., Wennberg, R., Igo, R., *et al.*, 1970, The offspring of alcoholic mothers, *Pediatr. Res.* 4:474.
73. Ho, B. T., Fritchie, G. E., Idanpaan-Heikkila, J. E., *et al.*, 1972, Placental transfer of 14-C ethanol, *Am. J. Obstet. Gynecol.* 110:426.
74. Henderson, G. L., Hoyumpa, A. M., and Schenker, S., 1982, Effect of chronic and acute maternal alcohol consumption on fetal growth parameters and protein synthesis in fetal tissues, in: *Fetal Alcohol Syndrome: Animal Studies* (E. L. Abel, ed.), Vol. 3, pp. 151–158, CRC Press, Boca Raton, Florida.
75. Tabakoff, B., Nobel, E. P., and Warren, K. R., 1979, Alcohol, nutrition and the brain, in: *Nutrition and the Brain* (R. J. Wurtman and J. J. Wurtman, eds.), Vol. 4, pp. 159–213, Raven Press, New York.

76. Weinberg, J., 1984, Nutritional issues in perinatal alcohol exposure, *Neurobehav. Toxicol. Teratol.* **6:**261.
77. Wunderlich, S. M., Baliga, S., and Munro, H. N., 1979, Rat placental protein synthesis and peptide secretion in relation to malnutrition from protein deficiency in alcohol administration, *J. Nutr.* **109:**1534–1541.
78. Jones, K., Smith, D., Streissguth, A., *et al.*, 1974, Outcome of offspring in chronic alcoholic women, *Lancet* **1:**1076.
79. Russell, M., 1977, Intra-uterine growth in infants born to women with alcohol-related psychiatric diagnoses, *Alcohol. Clin. Exp. Res.* **1:**225.
80. Sokol, R. J., Miller, S. L., and Reed, G., 1980, Alcohol abuse during pregnancy: An epidemiologic study, *Alcohol. Clin. Exp. Res.* **4:**135.
81. Ouellette, E. M., Rosett, H. L., Rosman, N. P., *et al.*, 1977, Adverse effects on offspring of maternal alcohol abuse during pregnancy, *N. Engl. J. Med.* **297:**528.
82. Hanson, J. W., Streissguth, A. P., and Smith, D. W., 1978, The effects of moderate alcohol consumption during pregnancy on fetal growth and morphogenesis, *J. Pediatr.* **92:**457.
83. Christoffel, K. K., and Salabsky, T., 1975, Fetal alcohol syndrome in dyzygotic twins, *J. Pediatr.* **87:**963.
84. Lipson, A. H., Yu, J. S., O'Halloran, M. T., *et al.*, 1981, Alcohol and phenylketonuria, *Lancet* **1:**717.
85. Hill, R. M., 1976, Fetal malformations and antiepileptic drugs, *Am. J. Dis. Child.* **130:**923.
86. Sulik, K. K., 1984, Critical periods for alcohol teratogenesis in mice with special reference to the gastulation stage of embryogenesis, in: *Mechanisms of Alcohol Damage in Utero*, CIBA Foundation Symposium 105, pp. 124–141, Pitman Press, London.
87. Abel, E. L., 1985, Alcohol enhancement of marijuana-induced fetotoxicity, *Teratology* **31:**35–40.
88. Sokol, R. J., Miller, S. I., and Reed, G., 1980, Alcohol abuse during pregnancy: An epidemiologic model, *Alcohol. Clin. Exp. Res.* **4:**135.
89. Silva, V. A., Laronjeira, R. R., Dolnikoff, M., *et al.*, 1981, Alcohol consumption during pregnancy and newborn outcome: A study in Brazil, *Neurobehav. Toxicol. Teratol.* **3:**169.
90. Rosett, H. L., Weiner, L., Lee, A., *et al.*, 1983, Patterns of alcohol consumption and fetal development, *Obstet. Gynecol.* **61:**539.
91. Kaminsky, M., Franc, M., Lebouvier, M., *et al.*, 1981, Moderate alcohol use and pregnancy outcome, *Neurobehav. Toxicol. Teratol.* **3:**173.
92. Little, R., 1977, Moderate alcohol use during pregnancy and decreased infant birthweight, *Am. J. Publ. Health* **67:**1154.
93. Marbury, M. C., Linn, S., Monson, R. R., *et al.*, 1983, The association of alcohol consumption with outcome of pregnancy, *Am. J. Publ. Health* **73:**1165.
94. Gibson, G. T., Bayhurst, P. A., and Colley, D. P., 1983, Maternal alcohol, tobacco and cannabis consumption and the outcome of pregnancy, *Aust. N.Z. Obstet. Gynecol.* **23:**16.
95. Tennes, M. A., and Blackard, C., 1980, Maternal alcohol consumption, birth weight and minor physical anomalies, *Am. J. Obstet. Gynecol.* **138:**774.
96. Wright, J. T., Barrison, I. G., Lewis, I. G., *et al.*, 1983, Alcohol consumption, pregnancy and low birthweight, *Lancet* **1:**663.
97. Schaefer, O., 1962, Alcohol withdrawal syndrome in a newborn infant of a Yukon Indian mother, *Can. Med. Assoc. J.* **87:**1333.
98. Nichols, M. M., 1967, Acute alcohol withdrawal in a newborn, *Am. J. Dis. Child.* **113:**714.

99. Pierog, S., Chandauasu, C., and Wexler, L., 1977, Withdrawal symptoms in infants with the fetal alcohol syndrome, *J. Pediatr.* **90**:630.

100. Streissguth, A. P., Barr, H. M., and Martin, D. C., 1983, Maternal alcohol use and neonatal habituation assessed with the Brazelton scale, *Child. Dev.* **54**:1109.

101. Rosett, H. L., Snyder, J. A., and Santer, L. W., 1979, Effects of maternal drinking on neonatal stafe regulation, *Dev. Med. Child Neurol.* **21**:464.

102. Streissguth, A. P., Martin, D. C., Barr, H. M., *et al.*, 1984, Intrauterine alcohol and nicotine exposure: Affection and reaction time on 4 year old children, *Dev. Psychol.* **20**:533.

103. Turner, C. E., 1980, Marijuana research and problems: an overview, *Pharm. Int.* **1**:93.

104. Rosett, H. L., and Weiner, L., 1984, *Alcohol and the Fetus. A Clinical Perspective*, Oxford University Press, New York.

105. Renault, P. F., Schuster, C. R., Heinrich, R., *et al.*, 1971, Marihuana: Standardized smoke administration and dose effect curves on heart rate in humans, *Science* **174**:589.

106. Kreuz, D. S., and Axelrod, J., 1973, Delta-9-tetrahydrocannabinol: Localization in body fat, *Science* **179**:391.

107. Nahar, G. G., 1976, *Marijuana: Chemistry, Biochemistry, and Cellular Effects*, Springer-Verlag, New York.

108. Klausner, H. A., and Dingell, J. V., 1971, The metabolism and excretion of delta-9-tetrahydrocannabinol in the rat, *Lif. Sci.* **10**:49.

109. Smith, C. G., Besch, N. F., Smith, R. G., *et al.*, 1979, Effects of tetrahydrocannabinol on the hypothalamic-pituitary axis in the ovariectomized rhesus monkey, *Fertil. Steril.* **31**:335.

110. Kolodny, R., Masters, W., Kolodner, A., and Toro, G., 1974, Depression of plasma testosterone levels after chronic intensive marihuana use, *N. Engl. J. Med.* **290**:872.

111. Smith, C. G., 1979, Comparison of the effects of marijuana extract and delta-9-tetrahydrocannabinol on gonadotropin levels in the rhesus monkey, *Pharmacologist* **21**:204.

112. Indanpaan-Haikkila, J., 1969, Placental transfer of titrated 1 tetrahydrocannabinol, *N. Engl. J. Med.* **281**:330.

113. Abel, E. L., 1975, Cannabis: Effects on hunger and thirst, *Behav. Biol.* **15**:235.

114. Abel, E. L., 1984, Effects of delta 9-THC on pregnancy and offspring in rats, *Neurobehav. Toxicol. Teratol.* **6**:29–32.

115. Charlebois, A. J., and Fried, P. A., 1980, Interactive effects of nutrition and cannabis upon rat perinatal development, *Dev. Psychobiol.* **13**:591.

116. Glatt, H., Ohlsson, A., Argurell, S., *et al.*, 1979, delta-1-tetrahydrocannabinol and 1,2-epoxyhexahydrocannabinol: Mutagenicity investigation in the Ames test, *Mutat. Res.* **66**:329.

117. Stenchever, M. A., and Allen, H., 1972, The effect of delta-9-tetrahydrocannabinol on the chromosomes of human lymphocytes in vitro, *Am. J. Obstet. Gynecol.* **114**:819.

118. Greenland, S., Staish, D., Brown, N., *et al.*, 1982, The effects of marijuana use during pregnancy, *Am. J. Obstet. Gynecol.* **143**:408.

119. Fried, P. A., Watkinson, B., and Willan, A., 1984, Marijuana use during pregnancy and decreased length of gestation, *Am. J. Obstet Gynecol.* **150**:23.

120. Linn, S., Schoenbaum, S., Monson, R., *et al.*, 1984, The association of marijuana use with outcome of pregnancy, *Am. J. Publ. Health* **73**:1161.

121. Fried, P. A., 1980, Marijuana use by pregnant women: Neurobehavioral effects in neonates, *Drugs Alcohol Depend.* **6**:415.

122. Carr, J., 1975, Drug patterns among drug-addicted mothers: Incidence, variance in use and effects on children, *Pediatr. Ann.* **4**:408.

123. Salerno, L., 1977, Prenatal care, in: *Drug Abuse in Pregnancy and Neonatal Effects* (J. Rementeria, ed.), p. 19, C. V. Mosby, St. Louis.
124. Connaughton, J., Reeser, D., Schut, J., and Finnegan, L., 1977, Perinatal addiction: Outcome and management, *Am. J. Obstet. Gynecol.* **129:**679.
125. Ananth, J., 1978, Side effects from psychotropic agents excreted through breast feeding, *Am. J. Psychol.* **135:**801.
126. Zagon, I., and McLaughlin, P., 1977, Effect of chronic maternal methadone exposure on perinatal development, *Biol. Neonate* **31:**271.
127. Raye, J., Dubin, J., and Blechner, J., 1977, Fetal growth retardation following maternal morphine administration: Nutritional or drug effect?, *Biol. Neonate* **32:**222.
128. Lichtblau, L., and Sparber, S., 1984, Opioids and development: A perspective on experimental models and methods, *Neurobehav. Toxicol. Teratol.* **6:**3.
129. Markham, J., Emmerson, J., and Owen, N., 1971, Teratogenicity studies of methadone in rats and rabbits, *Nature (London)* **233:**342.
130. Hutchings, D., Towey, J., Gorinson, H., and Hunt, H., 1979, Methadone during pregnancy: Assessment of behavioral effects in the rat offspring, *J. Pharmacol. Exp. Ther.* **208:**106.
131. McGinty, J., and Ford, D., 1980, Effects of prenatal methadone on rat catecholamines, *Dev. Neurosci.* **3:**224.
132. Sandman, C., McGivern, R., Berka, C., *et al.*, 1979, Neonatal administration of β-endorphin produces chronic insensitivity to thermal stimuli, *Life Sci.*, **25:**1755.
133. Moldow, R., Kastin, A., Hollander, C., *et al.*, 1981, Brain beta-endorphin like immunoreactivity in adult rats given beta-endorphin prenatally, *Brain Res. Bull.* **7:**683.
134. Stimmel, B., and Adamson, K., 1976, Narcotic dependency in pregnancy, *J.A.M.A.* **235:**1121.
135. Zelson, C., Lee, S., and Casacino, M., 1973, Neonatal narcotic addiction, *N. Engl. J. Med.* **289:**1216.
136. Ostrea, E., Chavez, C., and Strauss, M., 1976, A study of factors that influence the severity of neonatal narcotic withdrawal, *J. Pediatr.* **88:**642.
137. Kandall, S., Albin, S., Lowinson, J., *et al.*, 1976, Differential effects of maternal heroin and methadone use on birthweight, *Pediatrics* 58:681.
138. Naeye, R., Blanc, W., Leblanc, W., and Khatamee, M., 1973, Fetal complications of maternal heroin addiction: Abnormal growth, infections and episodes of stress, *J. Pediatr.* **83:**1055.
139. Finnegan, L., 1981, The effects of narcotics and alcohol on pregnancy and the newborn, *Ann. N.Y. Acad. Sci.* **362:**136.
140. Householder, J., Hatcher, R., Burns, W., and Chasnoff, I., 1982, Infants born to narcotic-addicted mothers, *Psychol. Bull.* **92:**453.
141. Amarose, A., 1978, Chromosome aberrations in the mother and newborn from drug addiction pregnancies, *J. Reprod. Med.* **20:**323.
142. Gluck, L., and Kulovich, M., 1973, Lecithin/sphingomyelin ratios in amniotic fluid in normal and abnormal pregnancy, *J. Obstet. Gynecol.* **115:**541.
143. Zuspan, F., Gumpel, J., Mejia-Zelaya, A., *et al.*, 1975, Fetal stress and methadone withdrawal, *Am. J. Obstet. Gynecol.* **122:**43.
144. Rementaria, J., and Nuang, N., 1973, Narcotic withdrawal in pregnancy: Stillbirth incidence with a case report, *Am. J. Obstet. Gynecol.* **116:**1152.
145. Herzlinger, R., Kandall, S., and Vaughn, H., 1977, Neonatal seizures associated with narcotic withdrawal, *J. Pediatr.* **91:**638.
146. Burstein, Y., Giardina, P., Rausen, A., *et al.*, 1979, Thrombocytosis and increased platelet aggregates in newborn infants of polydrug users, *J. Pediatr.* **94:**895.

147. Hutchings, D., 1982, Methadone and heroin during pregnancy: A review of behavioral effects in human and animal offspring, *Neurobehav. Toxicol. Teretol.* **4:**429.
148. Strauss, M., Starr, R., Ostrea, E., *et al.*, 1979, Behavior of narcotics addicted newborns, *Child Dev.* **46:**887.
149. Strauss, M., Lessen-Firestone, J., Starr, R., and Ostrea, E., 1976, Behavioral concomitants of prenatal addiction to narcotics, *J. Pediatr.* **89:**842.
150. Dinges, D., Davis, M., and Glass, P., 1980, Fetal exposure to narcotics and neonatal sleep as a measure of nervous system disturbance, *Science* **209:**619.
151. Kron, R., Litt, M., Phoenix, M., and Finnegan, L., 1976, Neonatal narcotic abstinence and effects of pharmacotherapeutic agents and maternal drug use on nutritive sucking behavior, *J. Pediatr.* **88:**637.
152. Rajegowda, B., Kandall, S., and Falciglia, H., 1978, Sudden unexpected death in infants of narcotic-dependent mothers, *Early Human Dev.* **2:**219.
153. Chavez, C., 1979, Sudden infant death syndrome among infants of drug dependent mothers, *J. Pediatr.* **95:**407.
154. Johnson, H., Dian, A., and Rosen, T., 1983, 24 month neurobehavioral follow-up of children of methadone-maintained mothers, *Infant Behav. Dev.* **7:**115.
155. Wilson, G., Desmond, M., and Wait, R., 1981, Follow up of methadone treated and untreated narcotic-dependent women and their infants: Health developmental and social implications, *J. Pediatr.* **98:**716.
156. Rosen, T., and Johnson, H., 1982, Children of methadone-maintained mothers: Follow-up to 18 months of age, *J. Pediatr.* **101:**192.
157. Lifschitz, M., Wilson, G., Smith, E., and Desmond, M., 1983, Fetal and postnatal growth of children born to narcotic dependent women, *J. Pediatr.* **102:**686.
158. Milkovich, L., and Van den Berg, B., 1977, Effects of antenatal exposure to anorectic drugs, *Am. J. Obstet. Gynecol.* **129:**637.
159. Naeye, R., 1983, Maternal use of dextroamphetamine and growth of the fetus, *Pharmacology* **26:**117.
160. Steiner, E., Villen, T., Hallberg, M., and Rane, A., 1984, Amphetamine secretion in breast milk, *Eur. J. Clin Pharmacol.* **27:**123.
161. Shah, N., and Yates, J., 1978, Placental transfer and tissue distribution of dextroamphetamine in the mouse, *Arch. Int. Pharmacodyn. Ther.* **233:**200.
162. Kasirsky, G., and Tansy, M., 1971, Teratogenic effects of methamphetamine in mice and rabbits, *Teratology* **4:**131.
163. Cameron, R., Kolesari, G., and Kolbfleisch, J., 1983, Pharmacology of dextroamphetamine induced cardiovascular malformations in the chick embryo, *Teratology* **27:**253.
164. Middaugh, L., Blackwell, L., Santos, C., and Zemp, J., 1974, Effects of D-amphetamine sulfate given to pregnant mice on activity and catecholamines in the brains of the offspring, *Dev. Psychobiol.* **7:**429.
165. Adams, J., Buelke-Sam, J., Kimmel, C., and Laborde, J., 1982, Biobehavioral alterations in rats prenatally exposed to low doses of D-amphetamine, *Neurobehav. Toxicol. Teratol.* **4:**63.
166. Satinder, K., and Sterling, J., 1983, Differential effects of pre and/or postnatal D-amphetamine on avoidance response in genetically selected lines of rats, *Neurobehav. Toxicol. Teratol.* **5:**315.
167. Levin, J., 1971, Amphetamine ingestion with biliary atresia, *J. Pediatr.* **79:**130.
168. Nora, J., Vargo, T., Noca, A., 1970, Dextro-amphetamine: A possible environmental trigger in cardiovascular malformations, *Lancet* **1:**1290.
169. Eriksson, M., *et al.*, 1981, Amphetamine addiction and pregnancy, *Acta Obstet. Gynecol. Scand.* **60:**253.

170. Ramer, C., 1974, The case history of an infant born to an amphetamine addicted mother, *Clin. Pediatr.* **13**:597.
171. Eriksson, M., Larson, G., Winbladh, B., and Zetterström, R., 1978, The influence of amphetamine addiction on pregnancy and the newborn infant, *Acta Pediatr. Scand.* **67**:95.
172. Nicholi, A., 1984, Cocaine use among the college age group, *J. Am. Coll. Health* **32**:258.
173. Mahalik, M., Gautieri, R., and Mann, D., 1980, Teratogenic potential of cocaine hydrochloride in CFI mice, *J. Pharm. Sci.* **69**:703.
174. Fantel, A., and MacPhail, B., 1982, The teratogenicity of cocaine, *Teratology* **26**:17.
175. Asker, D., 1983, Abruptio placentai associated with cocaine use, *Am. J. Obstet. Gynecol.* **146**:220.
176. Chasnoff, I., Burns, W., Schnoll, S., and Burns, K., 1985, Cocaine use in pregnancy, *N. Engl. J. Med.* **313**(11):666.
177. Reinisch, J., and Sanders, S., 1982, Early barbiturate exposure: The brain, sexually dimorphic behavior and learning, *Neurosci. Biobehav. Rev.* **6**:331.
178. Cavaliere, A., Bacci, M., and Diflaviano, C., 1984, Prenatal phenobarbital provokes malformations but no brain tumors in mice, *Pathologica* **76**:47.
179. Karotkin, E., Kido, M., Redding, R., 1976, Inhibition of pulmonary maturation in the fetal rabbit by maternal treatment with phenobarbital, *Am. J. Obstet. Gynecol.* **124**:529.
180. Gupta, C., Yaffe, S., and Shapiro, B., 1982, Prenatal exposure to phenobarbital permanently decreases testosterone and causes reproductive dysfunction, *Science* **216**:994.
181. Ploman, L., and Persson, B., 1957, On the transfer of barbiturates to the human foetus and their accumulation in some of its vital organs, *J. Obstet. Gynaecol. Br. Commonw.* **64**:706.
182. Fredrick, J., 1973, Epilepsy and pregnancy: A report from the Oxford Linkage Study, *Br. Med. J.* **2**:442.
183. Speidel, B., and Meadow, S., 1972, Maternal epilepsy and abnormalities of the fetus and newborn, *Lancet* **2**:839.
184. Lowe, C., 1973, Congenital malformations among infants born to epileptic women, *Lancet* **1**:9.
185. Annegers, J., Elveback, L., Hauser, W., and Kurland, L., 1974, Do anticonvulsants have a teratogenic effect?, *Arch. Neurol.* **31**:364.
186. Shapiro, S., Hartz, S., Siskind, V., *et al.*, 1976, Anticonvulsants and parental epilepsy in the development of birth defects, *Lancet* **1**:272.
187. Desmond, M., Schwanecke, R., Wilson, G., *et al.*, 1972, Maternal barbiturate utilization and neonatal withdrawal symptomatology, *J. Pediatr.* **80**:190.
188. Blumenthal, I., and Lindsay, S., 1977, Neonatal barbiturate withdrawal, *Postgrad. Med. J.* **53**:157.
189. Bleyer, W., and Marshall, R., 1972, Barbiturate withdrawal syndrome in a passively addicted infant, *J.A.M.A.* **221**:185.
190. Davis, B., 1982, The PCP epidemic: A critical review, *Int. J. Addict.* **17**:1137.
191. Kaufman, K., Petrucha, R., Pitts, F., *et al.*, 1983, Phencyclidine in umbilical cord blood and preliminary date, *Am. J. Psychol.* **140**:451.
192. Golden, N., Kuhnert, B., Sokol, R., *et al.*, 1984, Phencyclidine use during pregnancy, *Am. J. Obstet. Gynecol.* **148**:254.
193. Jordan, R., Young, T., and Harry, G., 1978, Teratology of phencyclidine in rats: Preliminary studies, *Teratology* **17**:40A.
194. Nicholas, J., Lipshitz, J., and Schreiber, E., 1982, Phencyclidine: Its transfer across the placenta as well as into breast milk, *Am. J. Obstet Gynecol.* **143**:143.

195. Cooper, J., Cummings, A., and Jones, H., 1977, The placental transfer of phencyclidine in the pig, *J. Physiol.* **267**:17P.
196. Golden, N., Sokol, R., and Rubin, I., 1980, Angel dust: Possible effects on the fetus, *Pediatrics* **65**:18.
197. Chasnoff, L., Burns, W., Hatcher, R., and Burns, K., 1983, Phencyclidine: Effect on the fetus and neonate, *Dev. Pharmacol. Ther.* **6**:404.
198. Strauss, A., Modanlou, H., and Boser, S., 1981, Neonatal manifestations of maternal phencyclidine abuse, *Pediatrics* **68**:550.
199. Erkkola, R., Kangas, L., and Pekkarinen, A., 1973, The transfer of diazepam across the placenta during labor, *Acta Obstet. Gynecol. Scand.* **52**:167.
200. Mandelli, M., Morselli, M., Nordio, S., *et al.*, 1975, Placental transfer of diazepam and its disposition in the newborn, *Clin. Pharm. Ther.* **17**:564.
201. Scher, J., Hailey, D., and Beard, R., 1972, The effects of diazepam on the fetus, *J. Obstet. Gynaecol. Br. Commonw.* **79**:635.
202. Ridd, M., Brown, K., Nation, R., and Collier, C., 1983, Differential transplacental binding of diazepam: Causes and implications, *Eur. J. Clin. Pharmacol.* **24**:595.
203. Miller, R., and Becket, B., 1975, Teratogenicity of oral diazepam and DPH in mice, *Toxicol. Appl. Pharmacol.* **32**:53.
204. Shore, L., Voorhees, C., Bornschein, R., and Stemmer, K., 1983, Behavioral consequences of prenatal diazepam exposure in rats, *Neurobehav. Toxicol. Teratol.* **5**:565.
205. Simmons, R., Miller, R., and Kellog, C., 1984, Prenatal exposure to diazepam alters central and peripheral responses to stress in adult rat offspring, *Brain Res.* **307**:39.
206. Watanabe, Y., Shibuya, T., Salafsky, B., and Hill, H., 1983, Prenatal and postnatal exposure to diazepam: Effect on opioid receptor binding in rat brain cortex, *Eur. J. Pharmacol.* **96**:141.
207. Kellogg, C., Terno, D., Ison, J., *et al.*, 1980, Prenatal exposure to diazepam alters behavioral developmental in rats, *Science* **207**:205.
208. Safra, M., and Oakley, G., 1975, Association between cleft lip with or without cleft palate and prenatal exposure to diazepam, *Lancet* **2**:478.
209. Shiono, P., and Mills, J., 1984, Oral clefts and diazepam use during pregnancy, *N. Engl. J. Med.* **311**:919.
210. Rosenberg, L., Mitchell, A., Parsells, J., *et al.*, 1983, Lack of relation of oral clefts to diazepam use during pregnancy, *N. Engl. J. Med.* **309**:1282.
211. Cree, J., Meyer, J., and Hailey, D., 1973, Diazepam in labor: Its metabolism and effects on the clinical condition and thermogenesis of the newborn, *Br. Med. J.* **4**:251.
212. Flowers, C., Rudolph, A., and Desmond, M., 1969, Diazepam as an adjunct in obstetric analgesia, *Obstet. Gynecol.* **34**:68.
213. Owen, J., Rani, S., and Blair, A., 1972, Effect of diazepam administered to mothers during labour on temperature regulation of the neonate, *Arc. Dis. Child.* **47**:107.
214. McAllister, C., 1980, Placental transfer and neonatal effects of diazepam when administered to women just before delivery, *Br. J. Anaesth.* **52**:423.
215. Rementeria, J., and Bhatt, K., 1977, Withdrawal symptoms in neonates from intrauterine exposure to diazepam, *J. Pediatr.* **90**:123.

CHAPTER 5

Effect of Maternally Administered Drugs on the Fetus and Newborn

**ROBERT C. CHANTIGIAN and
GERARD W. OSTHEIMER**

1. Introduction

Many medications are available to the parturient to ease the pain associated with labor and delivery. These include barbiturates and tranquilizers that work by decreasing maternal anxiety and that may make the pain more manageable even though they have no intrinsic analgesic or pain-relieving properties. Parenteral analgesics (i.e., narcotics) are given by the intravenous or the intramuscular route and inhalation analgesics (i.e., nitrous oxide or enflurane) are given by inhalation for pain relief. General anesthesia is used not only to remove pain (analgesia) but also to remove all other perceptions as well, i.e., produce a loss of consciousness. Pain relief can be produced in specific parts of the body by the use of local anesthetics.

The drugs used can affect the fetus either directly or indirectly. The direct effect depends on the pharmacologic activity of the drug or its metabolites and the amount of drug that crosses the placenta. The indirect effect can occur through alterations in uteroplacental blood flow.

This chapter concentrates on the effects of maternally administered

ROBERT C. CHANTIGIAN and GERARD W. OSTHEIMER • Department of Anaesthesia, Harvard Medical School and Brigham and Women's Hospital, Boston, Massachusetts 02115. *Present address of Dr. Chantigian:* Department of Anesthesia, Mayo Clinic, Rochester, Minnesota 55905.

drugs on the fetus and subsequently, the newborn, during and after labor and delivery. We begin with a review of maternal cardiovascular and gastrointestinal (GI) changes and the anesthetic implications of these changes. How drugs affect the uteroplacental blood flow and how drugs cross the placenta follow. We then turn our attention to the evaluation of the fetus by fetal monitoring and the newborn by respiratory times, Apgar scores, umbilical cord blood-gas values, and neurobehavior tests. Methods of pain relief for vaginal and cesarean delivery are then presented. We conclude with a discussion of anesthesia for the compromised fetus and the possible long-term effects of anesthesia on the newborn.

2. Background Information

2.1. Maternal Physiologic Considerations

2.1.1. Cardiovascular System

2.1.1a. Maternal Physiologic Considerations including Aortocaval Compression. The cardiovascular changes that occur with pregnancy enable the parturient to deliver blood into the uterine arteries at a pressure needed to fulfill the demands of the uteroplacental circulation and to enable the parturient to handle the increased metabolic needs of pregnancy. These changes include a progressive increase in cardiac output that reaches a level of 30–50% above her nonpregnant state. This increase in cardiac output is the product of an increase in heart rate (12–15 beats/min in the last trimester compared with the nonpregnant state) and an increase in the heart's stroke volume. The plasma volume increases about 40–50% and the red blood cell (RBC) volume by about 20%, producing a net increase in total blood volume of about 25–40%.[1-4]

The gravid uterus can compress both the vena cava and the aorta when the parturient is in the supine position. Although vena cava compression was reported during the early 1940s[4], it was not until 1966 that aortic compression was demonstrated by Bieniarz et al.[5]

Compression of the vena cava decreases venous return, hence cardiac output. At term, about 10% of parturients will develop symptoms of supine hypotension if they lie supine for a period of about 5 min.[6] This can present as maternal hypotension along with symptoms of nausea, vomiting, pallor, sweating, and changes in cerebration.[3,6,7] Compression of the aorta is usually unassociated with maternal symptoms but may cause diminished blood flow below the compression of the aorta by the uterus, which may result in decreased uteroplacental perfusion.[3,5]

As a result of the decrease in venous return and cardiac output due to vena cava compression and the decrease in uteroplacental perfusion due to aortic compression, the parturient should not be placed supine from the early second trimester until after delivery to decrease the effects of aortocaval compression. The parturient should have her gravid uterus displaced off the great vessels by placing a blanket roll or wedge beneath the right hip. Occasionally, because of anatomic variation, the reverse must be used, i.e., blanket roll or wedge under the left hip.[2]

Early reports in obstetric anesthesia did not consider aortocaval compression. The fetuses in these earlier reports may have had decreased uteroplacental perfusion and may have developed acidosis. Since the 1970s, most clinical researchers have studied the parturient using left uterine displacement, so that blood flow to the uterus, placenta, and fetus is not compromised.

2.1.1b. Vasopressors. Blood flow to the uterus is approximately 700 ml/min and is determined by two factors: the force of blood flowing into the uterus or the perfusion pressure (uterine artery minus uterine vein pressures) and the resistance to flow through these vessels or uterine vascular resistance. The uterine vessels are thought to be maximally dilated in the normal pregnancy; therefore, uterine blood flow can fall when perfusion pressure decreases or when the uterine vascular resistance is increased.[3] Since it is not possible to measure the perfusion pressure directly during labor, efforts are made to maintain maternal blood pressure. This includes maintaining left uterine displacement when a regional block is performed, by acutely hydrating the parturient with crystalloid before initiating the block (1000 ml for a T10 block for vaginal delivery and 1500–2000 ml for a T4 block for a cesarean delivery).[2] As these methods are not always successful in preventing maternal hypotension, pharmacologic supplementation is commonly used.

Vasopressors can increase maternal blood pressure by four mechanisms: increasing preload (i.e., constriction of veins and venules or capacitance vessels), increasing afterload (i.e., constriction of arteries and arterioles or resistance vessels), increasing heart rate, or increasing myocardial contractility. The final result and cardiovascular response depends upon the contribution of each mechanism.

In 1964, Greiss et al.,[8] using pregnant ewes, noted an increase in both uterine vascular resistance and perfusion pressure when the ewes were given infusions of norepinephrine, phenylephrine, methoxamine, and angiotensin II. As the increase in resistance was greater than the increase in perfusion pressure, all four drugs decreased the blood flow to the uteroplacental unit.

In 1974, Ralston et al.,[9] using pregnant ewes, noted that when maternal blood pressure was increased by 50%, uterine blood flow was unchanged with ephedrine, was reduced 20% with mephentermine, 45% with metaraminol, and 62% with methoxamine.

The above studies were performed on normotensive unanesthetized ewes and suggested that ephedrine is the vasopressor of choice in obstetrics. Clinically ephedrine has become the prophylactic and therapeutic vasopressor of choice. However, is treating a hypotensive parturient with sympathetic blockade the same as giving a vasopressor to a normotensive parturient?

In 1984, Ramanathan et al.[10] investigated the treatment of maternal hypotension (systolic BP < 100 mm Hg) in human parturients undergoing cesarean delivery under epidural anesthesia with 15–20 ml 1.5% lidocaine with 1 : 200,000 epinephrine. Acute hydration with 1200 ml crystalloid and left uterine displacement was performed. Three groups were evaluated. Group 1 did not develop hypotension. Group 2 developed hypotension and was treated with 5-mg boluses of ephedrine (mean number of injections was three). Group 3 also developed hypotension but was treated with 100-μg boluses of phenylephrine (mean number of injections was three). Uterine incision to delivery, Apgar scores, maternal lactate, and pyruvate as well as umbilical vein and artery lactate, pyruvate, P_{O_2}, P_{CO_2}, and pH were similar in all three groups. Thus, when hypotension develops, phenylephrine or ephedrine can improve uterine blood flow toward normal as noted by umbilical blood studies. An observation on maternal heart rates showed a slower heart rate in group 3 compared with groups 1 and 2. Thus, phenylephrine may be advantageous in treating hypotension in parturients with cardiac disease who would not tolerate rapid heart rates.

2.1.2. Gastrointestinal System

2.1.2a. Maternal Physiologic Considerations.   The major risk for the parturient receiving anesthesia is aspiration of gastric contents. She is at greater risk to develop aspiration than is the nonpregnant patient because the parturient's gastric contents are more acidic (due to increased gastrin secretion) and larger in volume (due to decreased gastric emptying). Also, the gastroesophageal sphincter is more incompetent in the pregnant patient, and intragastric pressure is increased over the nonpregnant levels. Once labor begins, the pain that occurs increases catecholamine secretion, which can also decrease gastric emptying. Narcotic administration to alleviate pain has a side effect of decreasing gastric emptying.[11,12]

In 1946, Mendelson[13] reported two main types of aspiration syndromes: (1) the obstructive reactions that occur from the aspiration of solid foodstuffs, and (2) an asthmaticlike reaction that occurs from the aspiration of acidotic liquid material.

To decrease the chance of aspiration, several precautions are taken. First, attention is given to protect the airway when an anesthetic is administered. If general anesthesia is necessary, it is mandatory that an endotracheal tube be properly placed. Second, steps are taken to decrease the volume and acidity of the gastric contents. This includes rendering the patient NPO (nothing per os) when labor begins or on admission to the labor and delivery suite. However, in today's environment, many parturients wish to try "prepared childbirth." Therefore, when the parturient and the obstetrician decide on an anesthetic for pain relief during labor or for delivery the following steps must be taken:

1. An intravenous infusion is begun to prevent dehydration and to expand the intravascular volume.
2. Metoclopramide can be administered to increase gastric emptying.
3. Anticholinergic drugs, H_2-receptor antagonists, and/or oral antacids can be administered to raise gastric pH.

Although all antacids administered orally can raise gastric pH, current practice is to administer only soluble non-particulate antacids such as 0.3M sodium citrate or the commercially available Bicitra. This is because particulate antacids if aspirated can cause significant pulmonary damage, whereas the nonparticulate antacids cause less problems if aspirated.

2.1.2b. Anticholinergic Agents. Anticholinergics can decrease oropharyngeal, tracheal, and gastric secretions, increase gastric pH, and increase heart rate. However, they can also reduce lower esophageal sphincter tone, thus theoretically increasing the possibility of gastroesophageal reflux.[12]

Scopolamine. This drug crosses the blood–brain barrier and the placenta and may produce some maternal amnesia and sedation and a fetal loss of beat-to-beat variability that may be accompanied by tachycardia. It has been used with morphine for "twilight sleep." Scopolamine has no analgesic properties and often results in agitation, excitement, and loss of control in parturients experiencing pain. In modern obstetric care, scopolamine has no place, as maternal participation is desired in the delivery process. Although the drying effect of scopolamine is greater than with atropine, it has less vagolytic activities. Scopolamine is rarely used today even during the delivery of an intrauterine fetal death.

Atropine. This agent has been used to decrease maternal oropharyngeal and tracheal secretions. In 1977, Baraka *et al.*[14] showed that atropine does not significantly increase gastric pH when used as a premedicant for elective cesarean sections. Atropine does cross the placenta,[15] and some investigators report fetal tachycardia and a decrease in beat-to-beat variability,[16,17] whereas other investigators fail to show fetal heart rate changes.[15,18] In 1983, Abboud *et al.*[18] reported no significant fetal heart rate changes when doses of 0.01 mg/kg atropine were used. We believe that atropine should only be used when a specific indication exists, i.e., vagally induced maternal bradycardia.

Glycopyrrolate (Robinul). This quaternary ammonium compound displays limited placental transmission.[15] In 1977, Baraka *et al.*[14] demonstrated reasonable effectiveness in using glycopyrrolate as a premedicant for elective cesarean sections. They showed that 0.4 mg glycopyrrolate will produce a pH of >2.5 in two out of three parturients compared with a control group in which only one out of three subjects had a pH of >2.5. However, Manchikanti and Roush[19] in 1984 were unable to demonstrate an increase in gastric pH or a decrease in gastric volume in surgical outpatients. Glycopyrrolate is superior to atropine and scopolamine in reducing oropharyngeal secretions in the surgical patient.

2.1.2c. Antiemetics

Metoclopramide (Reglan). Metoclopramide can increase lower esophageal sphincter tone and increase gastric emptying—useful actions in decreasing the incidence of vomiting and aspiration of stomach contents.[11,12,20] The 10-mg dose administered intravenously has a half-life of about 4 hr.[20] Most of the drug is eliminated unchanged in the urine. Studies in surgical patients and parturients support the enhanced gastric emptying that occurs with metoclopramide.[21] Atropine and narcotics inhibit the action of metoclopramide.[20] This antagonism decreases the usefulness of metoclopramide in labor, as many patients receive narcotics.[12] Metoclopramide passes the placenta and achieves an umbilical/maternal blood concentration ratio of 0.59–0.88.[22,23] Newborns born by cesarean section under general anesthesia have similar Apgar scores and neurologic and adaptive capacity scores (NACS) when the mothers received metoclopramide or placebo.[21-23]

2.1.2d. H₂-Receptor Antagonists

Cimetidine (Tagamet). This drug inhibits gastric acid secretion and raises gastric pH. It has no effect on the lower esophageal sphincter tone or gastric emptying. The drug is primarily excreted unchanged in the urine and has a half-life of 1.5–2.5 hr.[24] Cimetidine has been evaluated as a premedicant before elective cesarean section and produces a significant decrease in gastric acidity and secretions. The umbilical cord/maternal blood ratio is about 0.5, with a range of 0.1–0.8, depending on the time from dose to delivery.[25-27] Apgar scores, Scanlon early neonatal neurobehavioral scale (ENNS) scores, and Brazelton scores are no different from control newborns whose mothers received an oral antacid.[25,27] No adverse effects on newborns have been reported from one or two doses. However, chronic maternal administration may cause transient problems. An interesting finding in one preliminary study was that newborns whose mothers had received cimetidine had a more alkaline gastric pH than that of control newborns. Dundee in Belfast (personal communication) has shown that the newborn begins to secrete acid immediately after birth, so this alkaline pH in the newborn appears to have no clinical significance. Consideration should be given to the utilization of cimetidine in patients undergoing elective cesarean delivery in doses of 300 mg PO the evening before and 300 mg IM 1 hr before surgery. Cimetidine has no immediate benefit for the emergency cesarean patient.[12]

Ranitidine (Zantac). This H₂-receptor antagonist has an elimination half-life of 2.5–3 hr and also inhibits gastric acid secretion. In 1984, Gillett *et al.*[28] found ranitidine effective in raising maternal gastric pH and found no difference in Apgar scores between the newborns whose mothers received ranitidine or placebo. In 1984, McAuley *et al.*[29] compared ranitidine with oral antacids. They found no difference in Apgar scores or in the time of achieving normal newborn gastric acidity. They did demonstrate low levels of ranitidine in some of the newborn blood up to 12 hr after birth.

In summary, our recommendations are as follows:

1. Rendering the parturient NPO except for medications.
2. Administration of a nonparticulate antacid before anesthesia.
3. Individual consideration for the use of cimetidine, ranitidine, and metoclopramide, as none has been approved by the Food and Drug Administration (FDA) for use in labor and delivery.

2.2. Drug Effects on the Uteroplacental Blood Flow

Blood flow to the placenta is by means of the uterine and ovarian arteries, which at term in the normal pregnancy are believed to be maximally dilated. Placental blood flow can be altered in a number of ways.[1]

First, blood flow to the uterus is related to uterine activity. An increase in tone or an increase in the number of contractions per unit time can decrease blood flow to the placenta. Occasionally, the uterus can become hypertonic and decrease blood flow to the placenta to the point of fetal distress. This can occur with overstimulation by oxytocin. If this occurs, oxytocin administration is stopped, oxygen is administered, and, if the parturient is supine, she is turned to displace the uterus off the aorta and vena cava. Administration of ritodrine, terbutaline, and, rarely, halothane has been used to decrease uterine tone and increase perfusion of the fetus.

Second, a decrease in the driving force of blood to the uterine and ovarian vessels can decrease blood flow to the placenta. This can occur either by a decrease in maternal cardiac output or by a decrease in maternal blood pressure. A decrease in maternal cardiac output can occur when the parturient develops supine hypotension. A decrease in maternal blood pressure below the gravid uterus can occur with aortic compression when the parturient is supine. Maternal blood pressure can also be decreased when a sympathetic block develops after the initiation of an epidural or spinal anesthetic. To limit the decrease in blood pressure due to the vasodilation that accompanies a sympathetic block, the parturient is acutely hydrated before the administration of the anesthetic. The parturient is given 1000 ml of a non-glucose-containing crystalloid solution before an epidural or spinal anesthetic for a vaginal delivery. For cesarean delivery, for which the sympathetic block is higher, 1500–2000 ml is administered before the regional anesthetic is initiated. Any significant decrease in blood pressure is treated with more fluid or ephedrine. Fetal heart rate monitoring is a useful adjunct to the aggressiveness of therapy.

Third, an increase in uterine artery tone can increase the resistance to blood flow and decrease flow to the placenta. A high concentration of local anesthetic can cause uterine artery vasoconstriction.[30,31] In the gravid ewe, a 25% mean reduction in uterine blood flow occurs with an uterine artery concentration of 7 μg/ml bupivacaine, 11.5 μg/ml of 2-chloroprocaine and 19.5 μg/ml lidocaine. These concentrations are similar to those obtained after paracervical block.[32]

2.3. Placental Transfer of Drugs

Many factors relate to drug transfer across the uteroplacental membrane. These factors include a diffusion constant for the drug, the surface area and the thickness of the placental membrane across which the drug will diffuse, and a diffusion gradient from maternal to fetal tissues.[1,3,24,33] This can be summarized by the following equation:

$$Q/t = \frac{KA\,(C_m - C_f)}{D}$$

where Q/t is the amount of drug diffuse per unit time, K is the diffusion coefficient or constant of the drug, A is the surface area of the placental membrane, D is the thickness of the placental membrane, and $(C_m - C_f)$ is the diffusion gradient (maternal drug concentration to fetal drug concentration).

The diffusion constant is dependent on several variables, including the molecular weight, lipid solubility, and protein binding of the drug. A molecular weight of 1000 appears to be the dividing line between drugs that can and cannot cross the placenta by simple diffusion.[3,24] As most drugs used in obstetrics have a molecular weight below 600 (see Table I), they may cross the placenta by simple diffusion. However, many drugs exist in both an ionized and a nonionized form. The nonionized form is more lipid soluble and can pass the placenta more readily. As the newborn's blood is more acidotic than mother's blood, basic drugs may achieve a blood concentration higher in the newborn than in the mother if enough time is given for equilibrium to occur. This is especially true if the fetus develops distress with a very low capillary pH. Protein binding may decrease drug transfer as only the unbound drug can pass the placenta. However, this may not be a very important factor, as binding is a reversible process and any unbound drug that crosses the placenta will promote drug release from the bound form.

Keep in mind the important factor of time when evaluating drug transfer. The more time allowed, the more drug transferred, all other factors being equal. That is one reason why general anesthesia is induced

Table I. Molecular Weights of Several Drugs Used in Obstetrics[a]

Induction agents	Local anesthetics
Thiopental (264)	Procaine (236)
Neuromuscular drugs	Chloroprocaine (271)
Succinylcholine (361)	Lidocaine (234)
Narcotics	Mepivacaine (246)
Morphine sulfate (285)	Prilocaine (220)
Meperidine hydrochloride (247)	Bupivacaine (288)
Methadone hydrochloride (309)	Tetracaine (264)
Fentanyl citrate (336)	Etidocaine (276)
Anticoagulants	Histamine H₂ antagonists
Warfarin (330)	Cimetidine (252)
Heparin (6000 +)	

[a] From refs. 3, 24, 26, and 34.

after the patient is prepared and drapped before the induction of anesthesia for delivery. Finally, one must bear in mind that placental transfer is a dynamic process that continues until birth.

2.4. Fetal Monitoring during Labor

2.4.1. Introduction

Continuous fetal monitoring during labor has only recently become a common and widespread practice. This practice has lead to early recognition of fetal compromise and permits active intervention by the obstetrician, with the result of healthier newborns, particularly in high-risk pregnancies.

The advantage of continuous monitoring can be seen when one compares unmonitored to monitored patients. One study reported that the unmonitored group had a fetal death rate of 3.3 in 1000 births compared with a rate of 1.3 in 1000 births in the monitored group. Intrapartum stillbirths decreased from 2.6 in 1000 in the unmonitored group to 0.02 in 1000 in the monitored group.[35]

Drugs as well as alterations in uteroplacental and fetal blood flow affect fetal heart rate (FHR). Fetal heart rate monitoring is best thought of as a screening technique to define a population at risk for the development of possible problems, such as acidosis. Fetal scalp blood testing for pH is performed to confirm or deny the presence of acidosis[3,36]. Normal fetal capillary blood pH is greater than 7.25, preacidosis occurs when the pH is 7.20–7.24, and acidosis occurs when the pH is below

7.20.[3,36-41] (When the pH is above 7.25, 92% of newborns will have an Apgar score of ≥7 whereas only 20% will have a score of ≥7 when the pH is below 7.16.[35]) Note that because fetal pH is relative to maternal pH, some authorities have suggested that a maternal venous sample be drawn at the same time as the fetal scalp sample, with fetal acidosis defined as 0.20 or more units below maternal pH.[36] By understanding the basic FHR patterns and the drug effects that may produce heart rate changes as well as knowing the scalp pH values when appropriately obtained, one can better understand which fetuses are in distress.

2.4.2. History of Fetal Heart Monitoring

Auscultation for fetal heart sounds dates back to around 1820.[35,36,39] The first fetal electrocardiogram (ECG) was obtained in 1906. Although obtainable, technical difficulties existed, and maternal ECG often interfered with the tracing. The first continuous FHR tracing was obtained in 1958 by Caldeyro-Barcia who implanted a transabdominal electrode into the fetus. It was then possible to record the FHR simultaneously with intrauterine pressure changes. However, the transabdominal approach is not very practical for routine use. In 1963, Hon developed a clip electrode that could be attached to the fetal scalp. The fetal membranes had to be ruptured and the cervix dilated 3 cm or more. In 1968, Bishop used the Doppler principle to develop an external fetal monitor that would permit noninvasive monitoring.[39] The continuous FHR monitor is still a relatively recent method for evaluating the fetus.

2.4.3. Evaluation of the Fetal Heart Rate

Both the FHR pattern and the uterine contraction pattern are evaluated simultaneously. For the FHR, the baseline rate between contractions, the heart rate variability, and the changes in the heart rate associated with uterine contractions are observed. For the uterine contractions, their frequency and amplitude are observed.

2.4.3a. Baseline Heart Rate Patterns. Fetal tachycardia or bradycardia refers to sustained baseline heart rate changes of >160 or <120 beats/min for more than 10 min[3,35-37,39,40,42]:

Marked tachycardia: >180 beats/min
Moderate tachycardia: 161–180 beats/min
Normal baseline rate: 120–160 beats/min
Moderate bradycardia: 100–119 beats/min
Marked bradycardia: <100 beats/min

The baseline heart rate can be elevated in a number of conditions,[16,35-37,42,43] including maternal fever, cigarette smoking, fetal infection, fetal paroxysmal atrial tachycardia, and by the maternal administration of drugs, such as sympathomimetics (ephedrine, epinephrine, isoxsuprine, ritodrine, and terbutaline) and the parasympatholytic drugs (atropine and scopolamine).

Fetal bradycardia may be due to fetal hypoxia, fetal acidosis, fetal heart block and to the action of some maternally administered drugs, such as propranolol and thiazides.[35,36] High levels of local anesthetics can cause uterine artery vasoconstriction and uterine hypertonus, resulting in decreased uterine blood flow and fetal bradycardia. This situation is often associated with paracervical blocks. Interestingly, hypoxia in the fetus is demonstrated by fetal bradycardia,[31,32] whereas an adult would manifest a tachycardia or an increase in pulse rate.

2.4.3b. Heart Rate Variability Patterns.   Fetal heart rate variability is evaluated between contractions and is equated with a functioning fetal autonomic nervous system.[35,36,39,44] Variability is considered a measure of fetal reserve and can be defined as follows[36]:

Marked or saltatory: >25 beats/min
Normal: 10–25 beats/min
Narrowed: 5–10 beats/min
Silent: 0–5 beats/min

Variability is significantly decreased when the fetal scalp pH is below 7.20.[35] Besides fetal acidosis, decreased variability is noted with a variety of conditions,[16,35,36,42-45] including maternal exposure to 12% oxygen, cigarette smoking, maternal fever, anemia, fetal immaturity, fetal sleep cycles, and various medications including local anesthetics, general anesthetics, diazepam, narcotics, atropine, and intravenous alcohol.

2.4.3c. Other Heart Rate Patterns

Early decelerations (type I dips). These are due to compression of the fetal head and are not associated with fetal distress.[3,35-37,39-43] The head compression causes an increase in intracranial pressure and results in a reflex bradycardia *via* the vagus nerve.[47] This pattern can be blocked with atropine. These decelerations begin within 18 sec of the onset of the uterine contraction and reflect the shape of the contractions. Generally the rate does not go below 90–100 beats/min. The frequency in the first stage of labor is 20%.[39]

Late decelerations (type II dips). These are due to uteroplacental insufficiency and are associated with fetal distress.[3,35–37,39–44] Uteroplacental insufficiency means a decrease in fetal blood flow and often fetal hypoxia and acidosis. These decelerations begin 18 sec or more after the onset of the uterine contractions and have a symmetrical pattern. The late timing of the deceleration may be related to the transit time of poorly oxygenated blood from the intervillous space to the fetus. Atropine may reduce the magnitude but will not mask the presence of late decelerations. These decelerations are mild if the decrease is less than 15 beats/min, moderate if the decrease is 15–45 beats/min, and severe if the decrease is more than 45 beats/min. The more severe the decelerations, the lower the fetal pH. When variability is decreased as well, the pH values are lower than when variability is normal. Anything that decreases uterine blood flow will make these decelerations more severe. This includes the supine position, hypotension, uterine hypertonus, abruptio placenta, and possibly placenta previa. Correction of the factors that impair uteroplacental perfusion as well as administering oxygen may improve the status of the fetus and diminish these decelerations. The frequency in the first stage of labor is 12%.[39]

Variable decelerations. These are due to umbilical cord compression and may be associated with fetal distress.[3,17,35–37,39–42] The cord compression causes an increase in fetal blood pressure and a reflex bradycardia by the vagus nerve via the baroreceptor mechanism. Less bradycardia exists if the mothers are given atropine. The deceleration wave is variable in shape and variable in timing with the uterine contractions. The duration of time needed to return the FHR to baseline is related to the severity of the fetal compromise, the longer the duration, the more severe the compression. The frequency in the first stage of labor is 25%.[39]

Prolonged decelerations and/or bradycardia. This pattern occurs when the FHR is less than 60 beats/min and lasts more than 4 min. It is indicative of acute fetal hypoxia and impending fetal demise.[37]

Note: Although atropine has been used to study the effects the vagus nerve may have on the deceleration pattern, the drug may mask the severity of the deceleration and its use cannot be recommended as a means of altering FHR patterns.

Acceleration patterns. These are transient increases in FHR greater than 10 beats/min and lasting 20–60 sec. Accelerations occur in 15% of first stage labors.[39] Spontaneous movements of the fetus are frequently associated with accelerations. When these accelerations are unassociated with uterine contractions, fetal well-being is thought to be present. However, when the transient accelerations are associated with uterine contractions, early signs of cord compression may be developing.

Sinusoidal pattern. This is an extremely regular undulating pattern with fluctuations in the range of 5–15 beats every 15–40 sec.[39] This pattern is often ominous even in the absence of acidosis in fetal capillary blood.[42] It has been associated with severe fetal anemia in newborns with erythroblastosis fetalis as well as with the maternal administration of alphaprodine.[35] The maternal administration of meperidine has been reported to induce this pattern and be reversed with naloxone.[48] The significance of this pattern after alphaprodine and meperidine administration is unclear.

2.5. Newborn Examinations

There are many ways to examine the newborn at birth to determine how well the newborn is adapting to extrauterine life and to determine whether drugs given to the mother during labor and delivery are affecting this adaptation. Early in the systematic evaluation of the newborn, time to the beginning of respiration was used. The Apgar score[49] was introduced in 1953 and continues to be widely used. Because extrinsic uterine events might affect uteroplacental blood flow, umbilical blood-gas data at the time of delivery can be examined. To detect more subtle changes in the newborn's adaptation to extrauterine life, several neurobehavioral tests were developed. This section presents an overview of these newborn examinations.

2.5.1. Respiratory Times

Breathing time: Time from delivery of the head to the first breath.

Time to sustained respiration (TSR): Occurs when breathing becomes sustained.

Crying time: Time until establishment of a satisfactory cry. (Breathing usually begins within 30 sec of life and is sustained by 90 sec of life.)

Apgar[49] pointed out some problems with breathing and crying times. She noted that breathing time can be difficult to interpret when the mother has received excessive amounts of depressant drugs in the antepartum period since the newborn may take a breath and then become apneic for several minutes. Crying time may also be difficult to interpret, as a satisfactory cry may not be established in all newborns by the time the infant leaves the delivery room. Because of the difficulty in interpreting the meaning of these times, they are not widely used today but are presented for historical interest.

2.5.2. Apgar Score

The Apgar score has been the traditional and most frequently used method for evaluating the well-being of the newborn and the effects of obstetric medications since Apgar[49] introduced the scoring system in 1953. Although subjective, her scoring system proved to be rapid and reproducible. A summary of her scoring system of five evaluations (heart rate, respiratory effort, reflex irritability, muscle tone, and color) and scoring of 0, 1, 2 are presented in Table II.

The five evaluations are essentially a set of vital signs that can be used not only to describe the healthly newborn's condition but as a guide to success during newborn resuscitation as well. Although she originally described the score to be performed 60 sec after birth, common usage now is to obtain the score at 1 and 5 min after birth. Table III shows typical percentages of scores of newborns.

The 1-min Apgar score is considered a reflection of the acid–base status of the newborn, whereas the 5-min score is more predictive of survival and neurologic abnormality. In 1966, Drage et al.[50] showed that a 5-min Apgar score of 0 or 1 was associated with a 49% incidence of neonatal death. They also reported[50,51] a correlation of neurologic abnormalities and the 5-min Apgar scores for infants at 1 year of age.

Table II. The Apgar Score[a]

Score	0	1	2
Heart rate	Absent	<100	>100
Respiratory effort	Absent	Irregular, shallow	Good, crying
Reflex irritability	No response	Grimace	Cough, sneeze
Muscle tone	Flaccid	Good tone	Spontaneous flexed arms/legs
Color	Blue, pale	Body pink, extremities blue	Entirely pink

[a] From ref. 49.

Table III. Normal Distribution of Apgar Scores[a]

Score	Description	1 min (%)	5 min (%)
0–3	Severely depressed	6.7	1.8
4–6	Moderately depressed	14.5	3.5
7–10	Normal	78.9	94.8

[a] From ref. 50.

They found that infants with a 5-min Apgar score of 0–3 had a higher incidence of neurologic abnormalities as compared with those infants with a score of 7–10 (7.4% vs. 1.7%). However, in 1969, Drage et al.[52] and in 1975, Niswander et al.[53] failed to show a correlation between Apgar score and neurologic abnormalities in 4-year-olds. Perhaps this is due to the enormous growth of nervous tissue that occurs after birth.

Of the five scores, Apgar[54] stated that heart rate and respiratory effort are much more important than reflex irritability and muscle tone. Color has the least significance. As a result, some researchers use an Apgar minus color (A − C) score.

It has been suggested that the person delivering the newborn not be the one to assign the Apgar score, as he or she is often unaware of being emotionally involved with the outcome of the delivery.[37,55] One problem with the Apgar score is that only the most severe neonatal narcotization from excessive or poorly timed maternal medications can be detected by the score at birth; thus the subtle effects of drugs will likely be overlooked. To improve evaluation of the subtle effects of medications, specific neurobehavior tests were developed (see Section 2.5.4).

2.5.3. Umbilical Blood-Gas Data

To appreciate placental perfusion, umbilical blood-gas studies are often performed. Newborn blood gases are sometimes performed to

Table IV. Normal Newborn Blood-Gas Data[a]

	Umbilical (vein)	at birth (artery)	−	arterial 8	(minutes after birth) 32	64
P_{O_2} =	27	17	−	60	68	69
P_{CO_2} =	38	47	−	40	35	35
pH =	7.32	7.25	−	7.25	7.33	7.36

[a] From ref. 56.

determine how well the newborn is adapting to the new environment (see Table IV).

2.5.4. Neurobehavior Tests

2.5.4a. Early Neurobehavior Examinations. Neurobehavioral assessment is not a standard part of the newborn examination but has been used to assess the newborn's response to its environment. In 1957, Graham et al.[57] developed one of the earliest neonatal behavioral assessments, which included an evaluation of motor strength, sensory responses to visual and auditory stimuli, tactile adaptive responses, pain thresholds, and irritability. The characteristic response of the infant was scored, whereas in the Rosenblith modification of the Graham's scale,[58] the best performance was noted and the pain threshold test was eliminated. In 1964, Prechtl and Beintema[59] called attention to the cycling of arousal states. These states and their changes provide the framework within which the neonate responds to its environment. Prechtl and Beintema evaluated the presence or absence of a series of reflexes including the sleep or awake state, postural movement, general activity, tremor, skin color, breathing, and twitching. This extensive test is still primarily neurological and not behavioral in its character.

In 1963, Desmond et al.[60] described a characteristic series of changes in the vital signs and behavior of term newborns during the first 6 hr of life. An initial period of reactivity was seen to occur immediately after birth, followed by an unresponsive interval, in turn followed by a second period of reactivity. The initial period of reactivity includes tachycardia, rapid and irregular breathing, decreased body temperature, increased body tone, and exploratory body behavior. Following this initial period of alertness, an unresponsive period occurs between 1 and 4 hr of age, characterized by a decrease in activity, heart rate, and breathing; the infant sleeps during this period. Upon awakening, the infant becomes responsive to its environment. Desmond et al. concluded that the effects of drugs given during labor and delivery might not be apparent during the first period of reactivity because of the stimulation associated with delivery but would become evident during the unresponsive interval. Thus, infants whose mothers have received anesthesia or analgesia are more accurately described as "recovering patients." Recovery from drug effects begins after delivery when placenta circulation to the fetus, now newborn, ceases and the newborn begins to eliminate the drugs directly or as metabolites. A good beginning characterized by a good Apgar score does not rule out the possibility of problems arising during the first few hours of life. These early examinations helped set the stage for the three neurobehavior examinations more commonly used today.

2.5.4b. Brazelton—Neonatal Behavior Assessment Scale (1973).
Brazelton[61] feels that "the neonate and his behavior cannot be assumed
to be purely of genetic origin. Intrauterine influences are powerful and
have already influenced the physiologic and behavioral reactions of the
baby at birth." Because intrauterine influence such as nutrition, infection,
hormones and medications may affect the fetus, a psychological scale to
evaluate the newborn was proposed.

The baby's state of consciousness or "state" (deep sleep, light sleep,
drowsy, alert, active, crying) is probably the most important element in
the behavior examination, as the newborn's responses to stimuli are
dependent on its state of consciousness. The neonatal behavior assessment scale includes 27 behavioral items scored on a nine-point scale as
well as 20 elicited responses scored on a three-point scale. The scales
are set so that the midpoint of the scale is the norm. The mean is set
for an average 7 + -pound, 40-week-gestation, normal Caucasian infant
whose mother has received no more than 100 mg of barbiturate and no
more than 50 mg of other sedatives before delivery, who has an Apgar
score of ≥7 at 1 min and ≥8 at 5 min, and whose intrauterine experience
was considered normal. The score is based on the newborn's best—not
average—performance. Repeated tests on several days in the newborn
period are of more value than any one examination. Because many
infants are discoordinated for the first 48 hr of life, the behavior on the
third day is the expected norm (see Table V).

A period of 3–4 weeks of training is needed in order to become
adequately trained to perform the Brazelton examination. About 45 min
is required to perform each test.[62] As a result of the amount of training
needed and the time to perform this test, the Brazelton examination is
not widely used today in the clinical evaluation of the effects of maternally administered drugs on the newborn, but, is the "gold standard"
for neurobehavioral evaluations, particularly in the research setting.

Although Brazelton designed his assessment for the normal infant,
its use in comparing in and across cultures has been demonstrated. Its
potential for evaluating the abnormal newborn gives the examination a
broad spectrum of applicability. The Brazelton examination has been
used to study a variety of perinatal influences including maternal medication, narcotic withdrawal syndrome, neonatal hyperbilirubinemia and
phototherapy, intrauterine malnutrition, and subsequent neonatal performance after maternal oxytocin challenge testing. Data comparing the
Brazelton scale as a predictor of 1-year neurologic outcome with the
Standard National Institutes of Health Collaborative Study Neurologic
Examination have been reported.[63] The Brazelton scale detected equal
numbers of neurologically impaired children and had far fewer false-
positive results (i.e., fewer subsequently normal children were considered

Table V. Brazelton Examination[a]

Behavior items (9-point scale)	Elicited responses (3-point scale)
1. Response decrement to light	1. Plantar grasp
2. Response decrement to rattle	2. Hand grasp
3. Response decrement to bell	3. Ankle clonus
4. Response decrement to pinprick	4. Babinski reflex
5. Orientation inanimate visual	5. Standing
6. Orientation inanimate auditory	6. Automatic walking
7. Orientation animate visual	7. Placing
8. Orientation animate auditory	8. Incurvation
9. Orientation animate visual and auditory	9. Crawling
10. Alertness	10. Glabella
11. General tonus	11. Tonic deviation of head and eyes
12. Motor maturity	12. Nystagmus
13. Pull-to-sit	13. Tonic neck reflex
14. Cuddliness	14. Moro
15. Defensive movements	15. Rooting (intensity)
16. Consolability	16. Sucking (intensity)
17. Peak of excitement	17. Passive movement, right arm
18. Rapidity of buildup	18. Passive movement, left arm
19. Irritability	19. Passive movement, right leg
20. Activity	20. Passive movement, left leg
21. Tremulousness	
22. Startle	
23. Lability of skin color	
24. Lability of states	
25. Self-quieting activity	
26. Hand–mouth facility	
27. Smiles	

[a]From ref. 61.

suspect in the neonatal period). The Brazelton scale also correlated well with the Bayley Mental Quotient at 10 weeks of age.[62,64]

2.5.4c. Scanlon—Early Neonatal Neurobehavioral Scale (1974). In an attempt to simplify neurobehavior testing and to assess the neonatal effects of epidural anesthesia, Scanlon et al.[64,65] developed a neurobehavior examination based on the neurologic examination of Prechtl and Beintema and the neurobehavioral examination of Brazelton. The main advantage of this examination is that it is simple to perform and rapid (takes only 5–10 min), and personnel can be trained to 85% reliability in only 2–3 days.

The examination begins with the evaluation of the newborn's state of consciousness (four awake and two sleep states). It is then followed by specific tests. Tests 1–9 are scored on a 0, 1, 2, 3 scale. Test 10 is scored as either abnormal, borderline, normal, or superior. Again, an

Table VI. Early Neonatal Neurobehavioral Scale (ENNS)[a]

1. Response to pinprick
2. Resistance against passive motion (muscle power and tone)
    Pull to sitting
    Arm recoil
    Truncal tone
    General body tone
3. Rooting
4. Sucking
5. Moro reflex
6. Response decrement to light in eyes
7. Response to sound
8. Placing
9. Alertness
10. General assessment
State
Lability of state

[a] From ref. 65.

important aspect of the ENNS is the assessment of state and its changes during the examinations (see Table VI).

In regard to statistical analysis for the ENNS, it should be noted that none of the items are continuous scales. For several scores (tone particularly), both extreme high and low scores may be abnormal; a summation of "total score" can therefore be misleading. Statistical techniques should attempt to measure differences in median scores. Several nonparametric tests are useful, such as χ^2 and the Fisher exact test. F-testing and matched-pair median subtest covariance analysis are also appropriate.[62]

2.5.4d. Amiel-Tison, Barrier, and Shnider—Neonatal Neurologic and Adaptive Capacity Score (1982).   Recently Amiel-Tison et al.[66] introduced another neurobehavior test called the neonatal neurologic and adaptive capacity score (NACS), also the ABS score. This examination takes less time than the ENNS (4.4 min vs. 7.2 min); it places greater emphasis on motor tone and avoids the use of noxious stimuli. This examination is divided into five sections and includes 20 criteria. Each criterion is scored 0, 1, or 2. The score of each criterion can be added together, for a maximum score of 40. A score of 35–40 denotes a vigorous newborn (see Table VII).

Tronick[67] raised doubt as to the value of the NACS. He criticized the statistical analysis used to compare the NACS and ENNS. He also stated that the "examination fails to adequately conceptualize the capabilities of the neonate and the process of early development, and so it is unlikely to detect the effects of drugs or other variables in neonatal performance."

Table VII. Neonatal Neurologic and
Adaptive Capacity Score (NACS)[a]

Adaptive capacity
  1. Response to sound
  2. Habituation to sound
  3. Response to light
  4. Habituation to light
  5. Consolability
Passive tone
  6. Scarf sign
  7. Recoil of elbows
  8. Popliteal angle
  9. Recoil of lower limbs
Active tone
  10. Active contraction of neck flexors
  11. Active contraction of neck extensors
  12. Palmar grasp
  13. Response to traction
  14. Supporting reaction
Primary reflexes
  15. Automatic walking
  16. Moro reflex
  17. Sucking
General assessment
  18. Alertness
  19. Crying
  20. Motor activity

[a] From ref. 66.

2.5.4e. Interpretation of Neurobehavior Assessments. One must realize that the neurobehavior assessments are only designed to screen newborns' early activity. Only a few long-term studies are available that determine whether the findings on these screening neurobehavioral examinations have any significant correlation with later mental and neurologic developments of the newborn. Additional work needs to be done in defining the normal newborn. For the high-risk newborn, evaluation of what is normal has only recently begun.

3. Methods of Pain Relief

3.1. Vaginal Delivery

At our hospital 6544 vaginal deliveries were performed between October 1, 1983 and September 30, 1984. Anesthetic techniques used were 2755 epidural anesthetics (42.1%), 149 spinal anesthetics (2.3%), and 7 general anesthetics (0.1%); the remaining 3633 (55.5%) may have received parenteral medications and/or local anesthetics such as infiltration and pudendal nerve blocks.

3.1.1. Prepared Childbirth and Its Variations

The concept of natural childbirth was first proposed during the early 1930s by Dick-Read. He claimed that the pain of childbirth was induced by "fear and tension" and could be completely relieved by antepartum preparation and intrapartum care. During the 1940s, Velvovski, a Russian neuropsychiatrist, developed the psychoprophylaxis method popularized by Lamaze. The sensations of labor are felt but, with training, are not construed as painful.[1,40,68]

To reduce the anxiety and fear of labor and delivery, education concerning the childbirth process is given. Maternal stress during labor has been demonstrated to raise the level of circulating catecholamines, especially norepinephrine, and to diminish uterine blood flow.[69] To decrease the pain and stress during labor, the parturient breathes in a specific pattern until the contraction is over. Unfortunately, this approach may be taught by overzealous "prepared childbirth" educators who believe that all medications are hazardous.[1,40] The end result can be excessive maternal hyperventilation, which not only decreases maternal P_{CO_2} but also decreases fetal P_{O_2}.[70] In addition, "bearing down" in the second stage of labor can also diminish uterine blood flow.[71] Thus, excessive hyperventilation in a stressed parturient who "pushes" for a prolonged period of time can biochemically jeopardize the fetus even though "no medications" are administered.

Melzack et al.[72] recently demonstrated that parturients perceive pain over a range, but all experience pain. Controversy over when to use or not to use pain medication will continue. It has been established from well-controlled studies that good results can be achieved with or without medications for vaginal delivery.[73,74]

The present authors prefer that all parturients attend prepared childbirth classes for an orientation to the labor and delivery process and that they become acquainted with the methods of pain relief available at that particular institution. The possibility of operative obstetrics (forceps delivery or cesarean delivery) should also be mentioned within the context of patient education. Individualization is the key in every case, and it is the responsibility of the obstetric care provided to educate the parturient and her significant other in the methods of pain relief used in each particular practice.

3.1.2. Parenteral Medications

3.1.2a. Narcotics and Narcotic Antagonists.   Narcotics are still the primary form of pain relief used in obstetrics. The effects of narcotics for the parturient include analgesia, decreased gastric motility, nausea and vomiting, orthostatic hypotension, respiratory depression, and inhibition of labor during the latent phase. Fetal effects include a loss of beat-to-beat variability. Newborn effects include respiratory depression and neurobehavioral alterations.[1]

Morphine was the first narcotic isolated from opium (1803). It was first used in labor in 1837. In 1906, Gauss reported his use of "twilight sleep," a procedure by which the parturient received a single dose of morphine and scopolamine, followed by repeated doses of scopolamine alone. Twilight sleep was often accompanied by protracted labor, restlessness in the parturient, and respiratory depression of the newborn. This narcotic was commonly used until World War II.[40] Dosage was 5–10 mg IM or 2–3 mg IV. At equianalgesic doses, morphine appears to produce more neonatal respiratory depression than meperidine; therefore, it is not as popular[33,75] since the introduction of the latter. However, a truly equianalgesic comparison with other narcotics has never been satisfactorily attempted.

Meperidine or pethidine (Demerol), was synthesized in 1939 and was first used in obstetrics in 1940.[40] Today, it is the most popular narcotic administered during labor. A dose of 80–100 mg meperidine is equal to 10 mg morphine in analgesic effect. Dosage is 50–100 mg IM and 25–50 mg IV. The peak analgesia effect occurs 40–50 min after intramuscular injection and 5–10 min after intravenous administration. The duration of maternal analgesia is 2–4 hr.[24] Significantly more drug gets into the fetus after intravenous administration as compared with intramuscular administration of equal amounts. Meperidine reaches the fetus within 2 min of maternal intravenous administration and has a fetal to maternal blood concentration ratio of about 1 : 3 in the early minutes, later approaching 1 : 1.[76] The half-life of meperidine is about 3 hr in the parturient and 23 hr in the newborn.[77] Although meperidine has been found in the neonate for up to 6 days after maternal administration for labor,[78] it may influence the ENNS scores for only the first 2–3 days of life.[79,80] Arterial pH is lower, and PCO_2 is higher in newborns whose mothers received 50–100 mg meperidine within 3.5 hr of delivery as compared with a control group of newborns.[81] It has recently been suggested that the metabolites of meperidine, principally normeperidine, may cause more neonatal respiratory depression than meperidine itself.[82] This might explain why maximal depression of Apgar scores and breathing time occurs when delivery occurs 1–3 hr after intramuscular injection, whereas if delivery occurs within 1 hr or after 3 hr of administration, these evaluations do not appear to be affected.[83,84]

Alphaprodine (Nisentil) is popular in obstetrics because of its rapid onset and short duration of action.[33,85] A dose of 30 mg alphaprodine is equal to 10 mg morphine in analgesic effect. Dosage is 20–40 mg IM and 10–20 mg IV. The duration of analgesia is 1–2 hr.[86]

Fentanyl (Sublimaze) is a short-acting narcotic. A dose of 100 μg of fentanyl is equal to 10 mg morphine in analgesic effect.[24] Dosage is 50–100 μg IM and 25–50 μg IV. The duration of analgesia intravenously is only 30–60 min. It is not widely used because of the rapid onset of respiratory depression and its short duration of analgesia compared with meperidine.[87]

Pentazocine (Talwin) is a narcotic agonist with some weak antagonist activity. A dose of 30 mg pentazocine is equal to 10 mg morphine in analgesic effect.[88] Dosage is 20–30 mg IM and 10–20 IV. It is mainly metabolized in the liver and has an elimination half-life of about 2 hr.[24] Like other narcotics, pentazocine passes the placenta. Umbilical to maternal blood concentration is 0.4 : 0.7 and is less than that of meperidine if time from injection to delivery is the same.[89]

Butorphanol (Stadol) is a narcotic agonist-antagonist. A dose of 2–3 mg butorphanol is equal to 10 mg morphine in analgesic effect. Dosage is 1–2 mg IM or IV. Excretion of butorphanol is primarily in the urine (70%), and the elimination half-life is 2.5–3.5 hr.[24] In 1979, Hodgkinson *et al.*[90] looked at 200 parturients in labor and compared intravenous butorphanol 1 mg and 2 mg with IV meperidine 40 and 80 mg. These workers reported no significant differences in maternal analgesia in FHR during labor, in the Apgar scores, or in ENNS neurobehavioral scores. They did find fewer side effects with butorphanol (2%) as compared with meperidine (13%). When larger doses are needed, butorphanol may be better than meperidine because less respiratory depression is seen to occur with butorphanol.[91] At our institution, 1 mg IM and 1 mg IV given together produces good analgesia and some sedation for 2–3 hr.

Nalbuphine (Nubain) is a narcotic agonist-antagonist. A dose of 10 mg nalbuphine is considered to equal 10 mg morphine in analgesic effect. Dosage is 10–20 mg IM and 10–15 mg IV. The duration of analgesia is 3–6 hr.[24] Maximal respiratory depression occurs after administration of 30 mg nalbuphine.[92] Our experience has shown that nalbuphine can be used in doses of 1–2 mg/kg after cesarean delivery, under general anesthesia, of the baby without the parturient requiring naloxone at the end of the operation. Few studies of nalbuphine in labor are available.

Naloxone is a pure narcotic antagonist. The question has been raised as to whether naloxone should be given before delivery in order to avert the possible respiratory depression in the newborn seen with narcotics given during labor. Naloxone should not be administered to the mother just before delivery in an attempt to prevent neonatal depression from maternal narcotic administration. This will only reverse the analgesia at a time when it is needed most. Second, reversal of neonatal narcotic depression will be unpredictable at best and may not even be necessary. Thus, naloxone should be administered to the neonate after delivery only if clinically needed. Dosage of neonatal naloxone is 0.01 mg/kg IM. After naloxone administration, the newborn must be observed for at least 4 hr before transfer to the regular nursery, since the longer-acting narcotics may outlast the antagonist.[1,41]

3.1.2b. Barbiturates. These drugs have continued to lose popularity, since it has become increasingly apparent that they have prolonged depressant effects on the newborn.[38] These sedative/hypnotics, i.e., pentobarbital (Nembutal) and secobarbital (Seconal), possess no analgesic properties and in agitated parturients with pain may produce an antianalgesic effect that makes management more difficult.[1] The only use we see is overnight sedation of a parturient who is undergoing a stepwise induction of labor that may take 2 or 3 days. The doses commonly used are 100–200 mg pentobarbital or secobarbital orally. Intramuscular injection is painful.

3.1.2c. Tranquilizers. Tranquilizers have been used in obstetrics to decrease the anxiety experienced by parturients during labor and delivery as well as to potentiate the analgesic properties of narcotics. They fall into three groups: benzodiazepines, hydroxyzine, and phenothiazines. Diazepam, the most studied of the tranquilizers, also has anticonvulsant activity and has been used to prevent and treat toxemic seizures.

Diazepam (Valium), introduced in the early 1960s, has proved an effective antianxiety agent for the parturient. This benzodiazepine also has the advantage of decreasing the need for and the total dosage of narcotics during labor.[93–96] Effects on the duration of labor are minimal.[93,95] However, the drug rapidly crosses the placenta and achieves fetal/maternal blood levels often exceeding 1.[45,46,97–102] With the use of 5–10 mg doses, fetal monitoring shows a slight increase in baseline heart rate and a significant decrease in beat-to-beat variability. This decrease in variability is not associated with changes in fetal pH, Po_2, Pco_2, or base deficit and thus does not signify fetal asphyxia.[46] The metabolism of diazepam in the newborn is slow, with a mean half-life of about 31 hr.[101] Diazepam and its active metabolites have been detected in the newborn for up to 1 week after birth.[98,103] Thus, effects of this drug on the newborn are likely to last several days. When mothers receive ≤20 mg diazepam, the Apgar scores are not affected.[45,93,96,97,100] Neonates whose mothers have received large doses of diazepam demonstrate lethargy, apnea, hypotonia, hypothermia, poor feeding, and inability to respond to their environment, as demonstrated by neurobehavioral assessments.[94,98,102,103]

Lorazepam (Ativan) has pharmacologic actions similar to those of diazepam. Although lorazepam has a shorter elimination half-life as compared with diazepam, its clinical effects are longer lasting. This is related to its less rapid and less extensive drug distribution phase. Pharmacologic action after intravenous administration of this benzodiazepine takes 20–40 min.[24] Lorazepam crosses the placenta and the fetal/maternal blood values are usually less than 1. However, the depressant effects are similar to diazepam, namely, depressed respiration, hypothermia, and poor feeding. These effects are more pronounced in the preterm neonate.[104]

Hydroxyzine (Vistaril) is rapidly transmitted across the placenta. When used as a premedicant (doses of 1.5 mg/kg up to a maximum of 100 mg IM) for elective cesarean sections under spinal anesthesia, Apgar scores and NACS neurobehavior tests were normal.[105] Hydroxyzine has been used in conjunction with narcotics during labor to reduce anxiety and potentiate the effect of the narcotic in a similar manner as diazepam and promethazine.

Promethazine (Phenergan) has been commonly used in conjunction with meperidine during labor to relieve anxiety and provide sedation in labor. This phenothiazine also has antihistaminic, antiemetic and anticholinergic effects.

Promazine (Sparine), *chlorpromazine* (Thorazine), and *prochlorperazine* (Compazine) are not widely used in obstetrics, as they have significant α-adrenergic blocking properties that may result in maternal hypotension.[3]

3.1.2d. Ketamine.   Ketamine is an intravenous anesthetic that produces intense analgesia and a dissociative state regarded as sleep.[106] Its use for vaginal delivery is controversial. It has the advantage of being both a powerful analgesic as well as a good induction agent for general anesthesia in cesarean delivery (see Section 3.2.3b). Once thought to preserve laryngeal or pharyngeal reflexes in the anesthetized patient, this has proved not to be the case.[24,107,108] Another disadvantage is the production of unpleasant dreams. If ketamine is given in a dose of 2 mg/kg for anesthesia for forceps delivery, more than 50% of parturients will report unpleasant dreams that could adversely affect the mother–child relationship.[109]

In 1974, Akamatsu et al.[110] reported the use of low-dose ketamine (12.5–25 mg or 0.2–0.4 mg/kg repeated, as needed, for a total of 100 mg) for vaginal delivery in 80 patients. Excellent results were reported in 78 patients who had complete analgesia and amnesia for delivery. Apgar scores were ≥7 for all newborns.

In 1974, Janeczko et al.[111] reported the use of higher doses of ketamine (0.7 mg/kg and 2.2 mg/kg) with many women who also received nitrous oxide analgesia by mask for vaginal delivery. In the 0.7 mg/kg group, 9.4% of newborns had low Apgar scores (≤6). In the 2.2-mg/kg group, 29% had low Apgar scores. This was compared with a group who delivered under epidural or spinal anesthesia with 6% low Apgar scores and a group delivered under general endotracheal anesthesia with 13.5% low Apgar scores. These workers did report one patient in their 0.7-mg/kg ketamine group who vomited and aspirated.

Thus, low doses of ketamine are not overly depressant to the newborn, whereas large doses may be. One must always keep in mind the ever-present risk of aspiration when this drug is administered intravenously to a parturient who subsequently becomes unresponsive. The induction dose for general anesthesia is 1 mg/kg.[1] In our practice, ketamine is only used in the parturient for an emergency cesarean delivery—usually in the circumstances of maternal hypotension from hemorrhage, since sympathetic tone will be maintained.

3.1.3. Regional Analgesia and Anesthesia

3.1.3a. Local Anesthetics. Local anesthetics are commonly divided into three groups according to their duration of action[112] (see Table VIII). Local anesthetics may affect the neonate directly or indirectly.[113] The direct mechanism is related to the amount of local anesthetic that crosses the placenta to the newborn. The indirect effects of local anesthetics are related to a decrease in maternal blood pressure (driving force) or to an increase in uterine artery tone (resistance) that can occur with high levels of local anesthetic, as in paracervical block.[30,114]

The direct effects of the drug can be assessed by measuring the amount of drug in the newborn. Many studies have measured the blood concentration; this is an indirect measurement of the amount of drug in the newborn, since we are unable to measure the drug directly in the fetal/neonatal tissue. The toxic blood levels that produce a higher incidence of depressed newborns have been determined for several drugs. For lidocaine[115] and mepivacaine,[116] the toxic levels above which newborns appear depressed are thought to be 3 μg/ml. Because chloroprocaine is broken down so rapidly in the maternal and fetal blood (about 21 sec in the mother and 43 sec in the fetus[117]), direct effects with this

**Table VIII. Common Local
Anesthetics Used Today[a]**

Short duration of action
  1. Procaine (Novacaine)
  2. 2-Chloroprocaine (Nesacaine)
Intermediate duration of action
  1. Lidocaine (Xylocaine)
  2. Mepivacaine (Carbocaine)
  3. Prilocaine (Citanest)
Long duration of action
  1. Bupivacaine (Marcaine)
  2. Tetracaine (Pontocaine)
  3. Etidocaine (Duranest)

[a] From ref. 112.

drug probably do not occur. As local anesthetics cross the placenta by passive diffusion, attempts have been made to see whether some drugs pass the placenta more slowly than others and thus produce less direct effects on the fetus/newborn. Early attempts looked at the ratio of drug in the fetus (umbilical vein) to drug in the mother (maternal vein), or the UV/M ratio. The UV/M ratio does not appear to depend on the route of administration, except for paracervical block (see Table IX). In the latter case, the local anesthetic is deposited near the uterine arteries; this permits diffusion of the drug directly into the vessels, producing a high blood level in the placental intervillous space.[118]

If the fetus becomes acidotic, ion trapping of the local anesthetic is possible and may produce a high fetal/maternal ratio.[119,120] For example, Brown et al.[120] reported a UV/M ratio of 2.91 for a parturient who received a mepivacaine epidural anesthetic and whose child showed a fetal pH of 7.03.

The lower UV/M ratio for bupivacaine and etidocaine as compared with lidocaine and mepivacaine may be related to the higher maternal protein binding that exists with these long-acting agents. As a result of

**Table IX. Fetal/Maternal (UV/M) Ratio for
Amide Local Anesthetics**

Mepivacaine ≅ 0.45–0.7[112,113,121,122]
Lidocaine ≅ 0.45–0.7[112,113,115,121,123–126]
Prilocaine is the highest ≅ 1.0–1.2[112,113,127]
Bupivacaine ≅ 0.20–0.45[112,113,118,122,124,125,128]
  (Paracervical bupivacaine ≅ 0.60)[118]
Etidocaine ≅ 0.15–0.40[112,113,128,129]

this finding, many believe that the effects on the newborn may be less with bupivacaine and etidocaine as compared with lidocaine or mepivacaine. However, recent studies suggest that this may not be the case. The lower UV/M ratios may be related to the higher lipid solubility of these long-acting agents making distribution greater to some fetal lipid tissues, such as the brain.[37,112] The duration of effects of any local anesthetic that exists in the newborn will depend on the half-life of the drug (see Table X).

Because the metabolic product of prilocaine is *o*-toluidine, which can cause methemoglobinemia in the mother and the fetus/newborn, this drug is not commonly used today, even though the maternal cyanosis caused by methemoglobin can be reversed with methylene blue and produce no adverse effects on the newborn.[127,130]

3.1.3b. Routes of Administration for Local Anesthetics.
Infiltration. Infiltration of the perineum can affect the fetus by the direct mechanism of drug. In 1974, Brown *et al.*[131] noted rapid maternal absorption and fetal transmission following perineal infiltration of lidocaine in the parturient. The mean umbilical vein concentration was 0.73 μg/ml, not unlike that seen with epidural anesthesia. Since the injection to delivery time is usually much less with perineal infiltration as compared with an epidural anesthetic, the total amount of drug transferred is less, and presumably the direct newborn effects would also be less.

Pudendal block. In 1974, Brown *et al.*[131] noted rapid absorption and transmission of lidocaine after pudendal nerve block. They also found that when pudendal nerve block and perineal infiltration was performed, maternal blood levels actually exceeded levels obtained after epidural anesthesia. The fetal to maternal ratio increased with longer injection to delivery intervals from 0.42 under 9 min to 0.69 over 9 min.

In 1980, Merkow *et al.*[132] compared chloroprocaine 3% (900 mg) with mepivacaine 1% (300 mg) and bupivacaine 0.5% (150 mg) in parturients having a pudendal block for delivery; 36 of 54 of the parturients were also given 20–30 mg alphaprodine, a mean of 2 hr before delivery. Umbilical vein level of mepivacaine was 0.94 μg/ml and for bupivacaine

**Table X: Half-Life of Local
Anesthetics in the Newborn**

Chloroprocaine	43 sec[117]
Lidocaine	3–4 hr[65,121]
Mepivacaine	9–10 hr[121]
Bupivacaine	9 hr[65]

was 0.35 μg/ml. No difference was found in Apgar scores or blood-gas data in the newborn between the different drug groups. When the ENNS examination was performed at 4 and 24 hr of age, all tests were similar except that infants who received mepivacaine scored better at 4 hr in the response decrement to pinprick (noxious stimuli). Thus, pudendal nerve block performed shortly before delivery does not adversely affect the newborn if reasonable doses are administered.

Paracervical block. A paracervical block involves the injection of local anesthetic around the rim of the cervix for relief of pain of the first stage of labor. It is easy to perform and has an almost immediate onset of analgesia. It has the advantage of not producing sympathetic blockade; thus, maternal hypotension is not associated with paracervical block. However, fetal bradycardia and sometimes fetal death have occurred.[133]

In 1981 Morishima et al.[114] demonstrated that the fetal bradycardia is not due to a direct toxic effect from a high fetal blood concentration of local anesthetic, as the fetal levels obtained are much lower than the levels needed for direct cardiovascular toxicity. However, the bradycardia is due to a decrease in the oxygen availability to the fetus, which is secondary to an increase in uterine activity and a reduction in uterine blood flow. The resultant decrease in oxygen delivery to the fetus produces fetal hypoxia and acidosis. The uterine artery vasoconstriction that reduces uterine blood flow is caused by the high concentration of local anesthetic that exists near the arteries (see Section 2.2).

Typically when a bradycardia occurs, the heart rate decreases between 2 and 10 min after the block and persists for 3–30 min.[37] The bradycardia can be associated with fetal asphyxia. The incidence of bradycardia is less with chloroprocaine than with lidocaine or mepivacaine.[134]

Continuous FHR monitoring is now considered mandatory if paracervical block is administered.[37] If signs of fetal distress appear, capillary blood sampling from the fetal scalp should be done to evaluate the capillary blood pH of the fetus.[133] If deterioration is progressive, delivery is indicated.

Epidural block. Epidural anesthesia with local anesthetics can affect the fetus by a direct effect of the anesthetic and also by an indirect effect if maternal blood pressure decreases secondary to sympathetic blockade resulting in decreased uteroplacental perfusion. Lidocaine[115] and bupivacaine have been detected in the maternal bloodstream within 3 min of epidural injection, and peak concentrations occur between 10 and 30 min after injection.

In 1974, Scanlon et al.[65] compared newborns of women who received epidural lidocaine (9 patients) and mepivacaine (19 patients) with a control group of newborns whose mothers did not receive an epidural block (13 patients). Alphaprodine and/or secobarbital was given to 11 of 28 of the epidural group and 4 of 13 of the control group 6 or more hours prior to delivery. The mean dose of lidocaine was 423 mg and for mepivacaine, 374 mg. The mean time from last dose of local anesthetic to delivery was 22 min for lidocaine and 27 min for mepivacaine. They found Apgar scores of ≥7 in all newborns. Using the ENNS test, the newborns in the epidural group demonstrated a decrease in motor strength and tone during the first few hours of life and they characterized these newborns as "floppy but alert."

In 1976, Scanlon et al.[135] compared newborns of women who received epidural bupivacaine (20 patients) with the control group infants in the 1974 study. The mean dose of bupivacaine during labor was 112 mg. The time from last dose of local anesthetic to delivery was 71 min, which was well into the redistribution phase of bupivacaine. Umbilical vein blood levels were 0.11 μg/ml. Apgar scores, umbilical blood pH values and ENNS scores between 2 and 4 hr of life were all normal.

In 1976, Tronick et al.,[136] using the ENNS, compared newborns whose mothers received minimal medication (no analgesia, spinal, or infiltration anesthesia) with an analgesic group (alphaprodine and/or promazine) to an epidural group (lidocaine or mepivacaine). They found a transient (less than 12 hr) diminution of motor tone in the newborns whose mothers had received an epidural anesthetic. A recent reanalysis of their data showed that the differences were present when nonoptimal obstetric factors were assessed, particularly in the skinny baby (low ponderal index) who was the product of a less optimal obstetric history. The ponderal index is a ratio of body weight to length estimating lean body mass. A low value correlates with a thin baby, a large value with a fat baby.

In 1977, Corke et al.[137] compared newborns of women who received sedation with meperidine and promazine (22 newborns), epidural analgesia with 0.25–0.5% bupivacaine (15 newborns), and a control group (14 newborns) that received no analgesics. Utilizing the ENNS test within 4 hr of birth, the newborns whose mothers received meperidine and promazine scored significantly worse than the newborns in the epidural or control groups. Although not statistically significant, it is interesting to note the better ENNS scores in newborns in the epidural group than in the control group in all scores except motor tone.

In 1981, Rosenblatt et al.[138] reported significant neurobehavioral alterations after the use of maternal epidural analgesia with bupivacaine.

They make several statements including "infants with greater exposure to bupivacaine *in utero* were more likely to be cyanotic and unresponsive to their surroundings." We have never seen cyanosis directly attributed to the use of bupivacaine. A careful look at their paper is essential for two reasons. First, advocates of no pain relief during childbirth will take such material as evidence to further their cause. Second, one must realize that some papers are printed that have not undergone adequate peer review. Significant problems with their report include misquoting other papers such as that of Tronick *et al.*, lack of any obstetric information (Were the newborns born vaginally or by cesarean delivery?), absence of any information on the fetus during labor (Was fetal monitoring used?), no neonatal information such as gestational age or weight, and no information on the common newborn examinations such as Apgar scores or acid–base data. Furthermore, their technique of epidural anesthesia is questionable, as they made no attempt to prevent maternal hypotension (i.e., no use of acute hydration) and did not mention whether hypotension occurred and, if so, how it was treated. We also do not know whether this study was double-blind. We have included this paper as an example to point out that one must read not only the summary but must analyze the contents of papers as well. Interestingly, no anesthetist is included among the eight authors.

In 1982, Abboud *et al.*[139] compared newborns of women who received epidural chloroprocaine 2% (50 patients), lidocaine 1.5% (50 patients), and bupivacaine 0.5% (50 patients) with a control group (20 patients) who received no maternal analgesics. Fetal heart rate monitoring showed no significant changes in baseline FHR or variability. However, they noted late decelerations in 0 of 34 of the chloroprocaine-treated group, in 3 of 47 of the lidocaine-treated group, and in 8 of 42 of the bupivacaine-treated group. Umbilical vein levels of chloroprocaine was 10 ng/ml, for lidocaine 0.80 μg/ml, and for bupivacaine 0.10 μg/ml. Apgar scores, umbilical vein and arterial blood gas values, and ENNS scores at 2 and 24 hr of life were all normal and showed no significant differences among the groups.

In 1983, Abboud *et al.*[140] compared newborns of women who received epidural lidocaine 1.5% (22 patients) with a control group (17 patients). The mean dose of lidocaine in this study was larger (mean 446 mg) compared with 240 mg in the previous study. The umbilical vein lidocaine level was 1.25 μg/ml. Apgar scores, cord acid–base values, and ENNS scores were normal.

In summary, epidural analgesia is commonly performed for obstetric analgesia during labor and delivery. Of the local anesthetics currently available, mepivacaine is not widely used due to adverse newborn neurobehavior tests and the long half-life in the newborn. Prilocaine is seldom used because of the potential for methemoglobinemia in the newborn. Etidocaine and tetracaine are not commonly used because they produce marked maternal motor block. Procaine is rarely used today for epidural analgesia. Chloroprocaine, lidocaine, and bupivacaine are the primary agents for epidural use in obstetrics. Adverse neurobehavior results have not been seen with chloroprocaine or with bupivacaine. For lidocaine, some studies show decreased motor tone for the first few hours of life, while other studies do not show decreased motor tone. Since the clinical significance of neurobehavior examinations is lacking, all three drugs (chloroprocaine, lidocaine, and bupivacaine) appear safe for the fetus/newborn.

Note that the interpretation of studies evaluating the neurobehavioral effects of local anesthetics administered epidurally for pain relief during labor and delivery—vaginal or cesarean—is difficult with the best-designed studies and impossible with less well-constructed studies.

Neurobehavioralists expend a great deal of time and effort in designing studies to define the population to be assessed. For example, in the original Brazelton (BNBAS) study, the mean is set for an average 7 + -pound, 40-week-gestation, normal Caucasian infant, whose mother has received no more than 100 mg barbiturate and no more than 50 mg of other sedatives prior to delivery, who has an Apgar score of ≥7 at 1 min and ≥8 at 5 min and whose intrauterine experience was considered normal.[61]

Neurobehavioralists are skeptical of the studies performed by anesthesiologists, particularly when using the screening ENNS and NACS, since the maternal and neonatal populations are poorly defined (if at all) and generalizations are made on questionable statistical analysis. The population to be assessed must include ethnic origin and sex for an objective study. In a mixed population, equal numbers must be evaluated. The reader must therefore carefully evaluate the results of studies in which the characteristics of the population are not distinctly spelled out. Only when we use the same rigid criteria as the neurobehavioralists will our studies gain the respect of the behavioral scientists.

Spinal (subarachnoid block). Spinal anesthesia can affect the fetus by the indirect effect of a decrease in maternal blood pressure secondary to sympathetic block producing a decrease in intervillous blood flow (see Section 3.2.1). The lack of a direct effect is attributed to the small amounts of local anesthetic injected and the negligible blood levels measured in the mother.[37]

3.1.3c. Narcotics (Spinal and Epidural). The intrathecal and epidural use of narcotics in humans began in 1979. Advantages include localized and prolonged pain relief without blocking proprioception, light touch, or autonomic or motor function. Disadvantages include respiratory depression, nausea and vomiting, pruritus, and urinary retention.[34,141]

In obstetrics, spinal and epidural narcotics are used in two settings: for postcesarean analgesia and for labor pain. As this chapter deals with effects on the newborn, our discussion is limited to labor analgesia.

For labor pain, intrathecal narcotics appear more effective than epidural narcotics but only give adequate analgesia for the first stage of labor. Second-stage labor pain requires local anesthetic supplementation. Recently the combination of local anesthetics and narcotics administered epidurally together has been shown to decrease the total dose of each drug needed to produce adequate analgesia. Further study is needed to find the best combination for use in labor.

Intrathecal narcotics. Intrathecal narcotics can produce prolonged analgesia with a small dose of narcotic (i.e., 1–2 mg morphine). The blood levels obtained are very small and are unlikely to produce systemic analgesia.[142] These small blood levels most likely would have no significant effect on the fetus/newborn.

In 1981, Srinivasan[143] reported results in 16 parturients using 1.5 mg morphine for labor. Onset occurred in 10 min with a maximal duration of 19 hr. Analgesia was adequate for all first-stage labor pain but inadequate in three cases for second-stage pain. Apgar scores were excellent in all newborns.

In 1981, Baraka *et al.*[144] reported excellent maternal analgesia in 20 primiparous women with 1–2 mg morphine and no adverse effects on the newborn assessed by Apgar scores and neurobehavioral testing. The average onset of pain relief was 32–36 min and lasted 8–11 hr. Lidocaine was needed as a supplement (14 infiltration, 2 pudendal, 4 epidural) for the second stage of labor and delivery.

In 1982, Bonnardot *et al.*[145] reported results in 25 parturients with 1–1.75 mg intrathecal morphine. These workers confirmed effective labor analgesia for the parturient. They measured maternal and fetal plasma levels of morphine and found levels below 6 ng/ml (sedation is noted when levels are greater than 30 ng/ml). Apgar scores were ≥7 in all newborns, except one who had a "misplaced umbilical cord" and an Apgar score of 5.

Although spinal narcotics can produce adequate first-stage analgesia, most parturients have inadequate perineal pain relief for the second stage. Even though the results of spinal narcotics are encouraging, the possibility of delayed maternal respiratory depression occurring up to 10–12 hr after injection of morphine makes spinal narcotic use difficult to recommend for routine obstetric practice at this time.[146]

Epidural narcotics. Epidural narcotics have given varying degrees of analgesia for the first stage of labor but are not as effective as local anesthetics.[147,148] Blood levels obtained after epidural morphine are similar to those obtained after intramuscular administration of morphine.[149] In the parturient, absorption is faster with epidural than with intramuscular administration. One might suspect similar effects on the newborn with similar doses of intramuscular and epidural morphine.

In 1981, Nybell-Lindahl *et al.*[150] reported rapid absorption and rapid placental transfer after 4–6 mg morphine was injected epidurally and found a close correlation between the fetal and maternal blood concentrations. They also reported a case of a newborn who may have been depressed by the epidural morphine (delivery occurred 110 min after 5 mg morphine).

In 1984, Hughes *et al.*[147] compared the epidural administration of 0.5% bupivacaine with 2, 5, and 7.5 mg morphine. Better analgesia was obtained with bupivacaine. Two and 5 mg morphine proved inadequate for labor pain, although 7.5 mg was adequate. A period of 20–45 min was needed for the onset of analgesia. All patients required local anesthetic if instrumentation or episiotomy was needed. No effects on the FHR monitor were noted with epidural morphine. The newborns were normal with respect to Apgar scores, umbilical blood-gas data, and evaluation by the NACS at 2 and 24 hr of life.

Recent evidence suggests that low levels of fentanyl appear in the blood after maternal epidural administration. This may be related to the faster penetration of the dura by fentanyl as compared with morphine due to the shape and higher lipid solubility of fentanyl.[34,151] Further study is needed on all available preservative free narcotics.

Thus, the use of epidural narcotics for labor may not be as advantageous as intrathecal narcotics due to the varying degrees of analgesia obtained and the larger dose required. Perhaps the combination of epidural narcotic and local anesthetics may prove to be useful.[141]

3.1.4. Inhalation Anesthetics

The use of inhalation anesthetics in obstetrics dates back to January 1847, when Dr. Simpson of Edinburgh "administered the vapour [ether] in a case of labour, and ascertained that it was capable of removing the sufferings of the patient without interfering with the process of parturition." Since then several other agents have been used in obstetrics.

These included chloroform (November, 1847), nitrous oxide (1880), cyclopropane (1935), trichloroethylene (1942), methoxyflurane (1962), and recently halothane, enflurane, and isoflurane.[40]

Volatile agents have dose-related uterine muscle relaxant properties. At levels of 0.5 minimal alveolar concentration (MAC) of the anesthetic gas that produces immobility in 50% of patients exposed to a noxious stimulus, spontaneous uterine activity is depressed. At 0.8–0.9 MAC the oxytocin response is suppressed. The MAC for nonpregnant adult patients is 0.76% for halothane, 1.12% for isoflurane, and 1.68% for enflurane. The MAC is decreased about 40% for the pregnant patient.

The use of inhalation anesthetics falls into two categories: inhalation analgesia and inhalation anesthesia. Inhalation analgesia is the administration of a low concentration of the inhalation anesthetic either continuously or intermittently with contractions to provide partial relief of pain. The parturient remains awake and has intact laryngeal reflexes so that the risk of aspiration is minimized. Inhalation anesthesia is the administration of higher concentrations of inhalation agents to produce maternal unconsciousness. With the loss of consciousness, there is the ever present risk of maternal aspiration unless the larynx is protected. Thus, if inhalation anesthesia is needed, a rapid sequence induction with the placement of an endotracheal tube is mandatory.[1,3]

In 1982, Stefani et al.[152] investigated the administration of inhalation analgesia during the second stage of labor. They compared enflurane 0.3–0.8% in oxygen with nitrous oxide 30–50% in oxygen and with a control group that received no inhalation agent. Thirty to 50% also received meperidine or alphaprodine. Two-thirds of these patients received local anesthetic (pudendal block and/or infiltration) just before delivery. They found no differences in time to sustained respiration, Apgar score, blood-gas data, the ENNS neurobehavioral score performed at 2 and 24 hr after birth, or the NACS neurobehavioral score performed at 15 min, 2 hr, and 24 hr after birth. Stefani et al. conclude that inhalation analgesia with enflurane and nitrous oxide does not adversely affect the newborns. However, there have been criticisms of the study, since other medications were administered and the ENNS was designed to evaluate epidural anesthesia. Further testing will determine whether the NACS will be a significant tool for neurobehavioral testing.

3.2. Cesarean Delivery

Cesarean delivery is becoming a common mode of delivery. Fifteen years ago, the incidence was 3–8%, whereas the rate is now 9–30%

throughout the United States, depending on the geographic location and population characteristics.[1,153]

At our hospital, a tertiary referral center, from October, 1, 1983 to September 30, 1984 (our reporting year), the cesarean delivery rate was 24.3% (2103 sections for the 8647 total deliveries). Spinal anesthesia was performed in 760 cases (36.1%), epidural anesthesia in 844 cases (40.1%), and general anesthesia in 499 cases (23.7%)

With the current management of spinal, epidural, and general anesthesia, newborns will do well with each technique as long as adequate uteroplacental perfusion is maintained.

Each of these techniques is reviewed with emphasis placed on the important points that make each technique safe for the fetus-soon-to-be-newborn.

3.2.1. Spinal Anesthesia (Subarachnoid Block)

Spinal anesthesia is commonly performed for cesarean delivery. Direct effect of the local anesthetic injected is not likely to contribute to newborn depression, as the total dose is small and the maternal blood level is insignificant. However, indirect effects of the spinal anesthetic may influence newborn behavior if maternal hypotension decreases the uteroplacental blood flow.[153]

Hypotension, defined as a maternal systolic blood pressure below 100 mm Hg or a fall in maternal systolic blood pressure of 30 mm Hg or more, occurs in about 80% of parturients if measures are not taken to prevent hypotension due to sympathetic blockade in the mother with resultant increase in the intravascular space and to the aortocaval compression that occurs if the woman is in the supine position. By acutely hydrating the mother with intravenous fluid and placing her on the table with her uterus displaced off the aorta and inferior vena cava, the incidence of hypotension can be reduced to about 50%. Vasopressors are commonly employed to treat and prevent maternal hypotension.

In 1981, Datta et al.[154] looked at parturients who underwent spinal anesthesia with tetracaine for cesarean delivery. They noted that in the absence of hypotension, a prolonged uterine incision-to-delivery interval (UI–D) of more than 3 min was associated with an increase in neonatal acidosis and depressed Apgar scores when compared with neonates whose maternal UI–D interval was less than 3 min.

In 1982, Corke et al.[155] looked at blood gases and ENNS between 2 and 4 hr of birth in a group of 18 newborns whose mothers had hypotension for less than 2 min and at a group of 13 newborns whose mothers remained normotensive. Although the ENNS was similar in both groups, newborns whose mothers developed hypotension were more acidotic than were those whose mothers had remained normotensive. It was concluded that short periods of hypotension (less than 2 min) were not harmful to the neonate.

In 1982, Datta et al.[156] looked at the blood gases of parturients and their newborns under spinal anesthesia. They evaluated three groups: Group A (22 parturients) did not develop hypotension and received no vasopressors; group B (18 parturients) developed hypotension and were rapidly treated with ephedrine and more intravenous fluid, and group C (20 parturients) had a decrease in blood pressure of 10 mm Hg or more as an indication for ephedrine (aggressive management). The parturients in group C did not develop hypotension as previously defined. The induction to delivery and the uterine incision to delivery intervals were similar between the three groups. Infants in group B had lower 1-min Apgar scores and lower average pH values of the umbilical artery and vein as compared with groups A and C (no hypotension). Thus, lower Apgar scores and poorer blood-gas data develop when maternal hypotension occurs.

We recently compared two spinal anesthetic solutions for elective cesarean delivery.[157] Group I (10 parturients) received tetracaine made hyperbaric with dextrose, and group II (11 parturients) received tetracaine made hyperbaric with procaine. All parturients received 1500–2000 ml Ringer's lactated solution, all had left uterine displacement, and all parturients received oxygen by face mask. Ephedrine was used in eight patients in each group as their blood pressure fell 10 mm Hg or more. Two parturients in group I and three parturients in group II developed hypotension (BP < 100 mm Hg) and were rapidly given more fluid and ephedrine. The induction to delivery and the uterine incision to delivery times were similar. We found the newborns to do equally well between the groups as assessed by Apgar scores and umbilical blood-gas data. Mothers, however, were significantly more comfortable with the tetracaine–procaine mixture as assessed by the amount of narcotics needed for maternal comfort.

In summary, direct effects of intrathecal local anesthetics on the fetus/newborn are not significant. Indirect effects occur when maternal blood pressure and uteroplacental perfusion are decreased but are not significant if the blood pressure is rapidly corrected in less than 2 min or if prevented by early infusion of ephedrine when blood pressure starts to fall. However, we postulate that if maternal hypotension is permitted to persist, newborn CNS changes may develop (see Section 3.2.2, on epidural anesthesia).

Maternal administration of oxygen to increase maternal and fetal PO_2 and a uterine incision-to-delivery interval of less than 3 min is recommended (see Table XI and Table XII).

Table XI. Spinal Anesthetic Technique for Cesarean Delivery at the Brigham and Women's Hospital

1. Preinduction
   A. Antacid—30 ml (nonparticulate)
   B. Large bore intravenous line with Lactated Ringer's Solution
   C. Administer 1500–2000 ml in the 15–20 min before anesthesia
   D. Monitors attached (EKG, blood pressure)
2. Induction
   A. Right side down with back parallel to the floor (or sitting if patient is obese)
   B. Prepare the patient's back
   C. Insert a 26 gauge spinal needle at the L2-3 or L3-4 interspace
   D. Determine dose of local anesthetic according to Table XII (If patient is obese or has a larger than normal uterus, i.e., twins at term, consider decreasing the dose slightly; if patient is preterm and has a small uterus consider increasing the dose slightly)
   E. Inject the local anesthetic slowly
3. Maintenance
   A. Turn patient supine and immediately place blanket roll under right hip to effect left uterine displacement
   B. Administer oxygen by face mask
   C. Check blood pressure frequently. Any fall in blood pressure of 10 mmHg or more is treated with ephedrine (10 mg boluses) and more fluid (200 ml boluses)
   D. If needed, administer small doses of diazepam (2 mg doses up to 10 mg) for maternal anxiety, if necessary
4. At delivery
   A. Add oxytocin to the intravenous fluid (20 units of oxytocin/liter of fluid)
5. After delivery
   A. Give small doses of narcotic or tranquilizer as needed

3.2.2. Epidural Anesthesia

Epidural anesthesia is commonly performed for cesarean delivery. The effects that may be produced on the newborn can be either direct (effects of the local anesthetic) or indirect (altered uteroplacental blood flow from a decrease in maternal blood pressure). Most studies evaluate parturients who are at term and are for elective cesarean delivery and therefore are not in labor. This eliminates the effects of labor on the fetus.

Note that the common belief is that the neurobehavioral examinations will reveal alterations attributable to drug effect more frequently in cesarean-delivered babies whose mothers received epidural anesthesia than in babies born vaginally under the same conditions because of the higher dose of local anesthetic. This may not be true because the time the local anesthetic has to pass the placenta may be shorter; elective cesarean-delivered babies are delivered within minutes after the local anesthetic is injected, whereas vaginally delivered babies may be exposed to the local anesthetic for several hours. Thus, the total amount of drug transferred may be less, even though the peak maternal level may be greater. Further work is needed to clarify this situation.

In 1977, Lund et al.[129] evaluated etidocaine for cesarean section. All 40 newborns assessed by the ENNS examination at 2–4 hr of age were normal.

In 1977, Rolbin et al.[158] compared two groups of patients undergoing cesarean section under epidural anesthesia. One group had up to 10 mg diazepam prior to delivery; the other group received no diazepam. Rolbin et al. found no differences in high Apgar scores (7–10), although the 1-min scores demonstrated a decrease in muscle tone in the diazepam group. No differences existed in umbilical cord blood gas data. The ENNS showed a decrease in muscle tone at 4 hr of age in the diazepam-treated group, but by 24 hr of age no differences were seen.

In 1980, Datta et al.[128] compared chloroprocaine 3% (16 ± 1 ml) with bupivacaine 0.75% (17 ± 1 ml) and etidocaine 1% (22 ± 1 ml). Mean umbilical vein levels of bupivacaine was 0.12 µg/ml and for etidocaine 0.15 µg/ml. Apgar scores, blood-gas data, and the ENNS scores performed at 2–4 hr after birth demonstrated no significant differences.

In 1980, James et al.[159] compared chloroprocaine 3% (23 ± 2 ml) with bupivacaine 0.5% (26 ± 2 ml); they also demonstrated similar values for time to sustained respiration, Apgar scores, and blood-gas data.

In 1982 Higuchi et al.[160] compared 145 infants delivered by cesarean section under epidural anesthesia, utilizing chloroprocaine, lidocaine, mepivacaine, and bupivacaine. They found no differences in Apgar scores or umbilical blood-gas data. Substantially lower ENNS scores were found when lidocaine or mepivacaine was used as compared with chlorprocaine and bupivacaine and tetracaine spinal anesthesia.

In 1982, Ramanathan et al.[161] demonstrated that by increasing the inspired maternal oxygen concentration from 0.21–0.47 to 0.74–1.0 in parturients undergoing epidural anesthesia with bupivacaine, umbilical vein PO_2 increased from 28–36 to 41–47, and the umbilical artery PO_2 increased from 15–19 to 21–25. Although Apgar scores were similar in their groups, oxygen administration can improve fetal oxygen stores and is recommended at the time of cesarean delivery.

In 1983, Abboud et al.[162] compared chloroprocaine 3% (21.5 ml), lidocaine 2% (21.5 ml), lidocaine 2% with epinephrine 1 : 200,000 (20 ml), and bupivacaine 0.75% (17 ml). Umbilical vein level was 2.74 ng/ml for chloroprocaine, 1.43 µg/ml for lidocaine without epinephrine, 1.15 µg/ml for lidocaine with epinephrine, and 0.21 µg/ml for bupivacaine. Apgar scores, blood-gas data, and the ENNS scores at 2 and 24 hr after birth demonstrated no significant differences.

In 1984, Kileff *et al.*[124] compared lidocaine 2% (29 ± 5 ml) with bupivacaine 0.5% (29 ± 6 ml). Mean umbilical vein levels of lidocaine were 1.82 μg/ml and for bupivacaine were 0.27 μg/ml. No differences were found in Apgar scores, blood-gas data, or ENNS scores performed at 4 and 24 hr of age, except for a higher score in the lidocaine-treated group at 24 hr for the sucking response. It is interesting to note that several women in the lidocaine-treated group had some evidence of elevated levels of local anesthetic as evidenced by CNS symptoms of dizziness or diaphoresis. No women in the bupivacaine group had CNS symptoms suggestive of a high local anesthetic level.

In summary, chloroprocaine, lidocaine, and bupivacaine are the most commonly used epidural drugs. All three appear to have minimal

Table XII. Medication for a T-2 to T-4 Sensory Level Spinal Anesthetic

	Patient's height				
Local anesthetic	5 ft	5 ft 3 inches	5 ft 6 inches	5 ft 9 inches	6 ft
Lidocaine 5% in 7.5% dextrose in water (premixed)	60 mg (1.2 ml)	65 mg (1.3 ml)	70 mg (1.4 ml)	75 mg (1.5 ml)	80 mg (1.6 ml)
Tetracaine 1% mixed with equal volume of 10% procaine	6 mg− (0.6 ml)	7 mg− (0.7 ml)	8 mg− (0.8 ml)	9 mg− (0.9 ml)	10 mg− (1.0 ml)
	60 mg (0.6 ml)	70 mg (0.7 ml)	80 mg (0.8 ml)	90 mg (0.9 ml)	100 mg (1.0 ml)
Total volume =	(1.2 ml)	(1.4 ml)	(1.6 ml)	(1.8 ml)	(2.0 ml)
Tetracaine 1% mixed with equal volume of 10% dextrose[a]	7 mg− (0.7 ml) (0.7 ml)	8 mg− (0.8 ml) (0.8 ml)	9 mg− (0.9 ml) (0.9 ml)	10 mg− (1.0 ml) (1.0 ml)	11 mg− (1.1 ml) (1.1 ml)
Total volume =	(1.4 ml)	(1.6 ml)	(1.8 ml)	(2.0 ml)	(2.2 ml)
Bupivacaine 0.5% in 8% dextrose in water (premixed)[b]	8 mg (1.6 ml)	9 mg (1.8 ml)	10 mg (2.0 ml)	11 mg (2.2 ml)	12mg (2.4ml)
Bupivacaine 0.75% in 8.25% dextrose in water (premixed)[b]	9 mg (1.2 ml)	10 mg (1.3 ml)	11 mg (1.5 ml)	12 mg (1.6 ml)	13 mg (1.7 ml)

[a] At our hospital, the tetracaine–dextrose mixture is largely replaced with the tetracaine–procaine mixture (see text).
[b] Doses of bupivacaine are only approximate doses as this drug has only recently been introduced. The 0.75% bupivacaine preparation is FDA approved, the 0.5% bupivacaine preparation is investigational at present.

effects on neonatal behavior, provided uteroplacental perfusion (i.e., maternal blood pressure) is maintained. Etidocaine, although safe, is rarely used today because of its marked maternal motor block.

Oxygen administration is recommended during all cesarean deliveries, and small amounts of diazepam can help alleviate some maternal anxiety and produce minimal effects in the newborn.

Epidural anesthesia is becoming more popular, as narcotics can be injected into the epidural space at the end of the cesarean section to provide prolonged postpartum maternal analgesia (see Table XIII).

Table XIII. Epidural Anesthetic Technique for Cesarean Delivery at the Brigham and Women's Hospital

1. Preinduction
   A. Antacid—30 ml (nonparticulate)
   B. Large bore intravenous line with Lactated Ringer's Solution
   C. Administer 1500–2000 ml in the 15–20 min before anesthesia
   D. Monitors attached (EKG, Blood Pressure)
2. Induction
   A. Lateral or sitting position
   B. Prepare the patient's back
   C. Insert an epidural needle at the L2-3 or L3-4 interspace
   D. After identifying the epidural space, insert the epidural catheter 2 cm[a]
3. Maintenance
   A. Turn patient supine and immediately place a blanket roll under the right hip for left uterine displacement
   B. Administer oxygen by face mask
   C. Perform a test dose of 2–3 ml of local anesthetic
   D. Wait 4–5 minutes, if no signs of subarachnoid block exists, inject the dose of local anesthetic in incremental doses of 3–5 ml waiting 30–60 seconds between injections (aim for a T-2 to T-4 sensory level)
   E. Check blood pressure frequently. Any fall in blood pressure of 10 mmHg or more is treated with ephedrine (10 mg boluses) and more fluid (200 ml boluses)
   F. If needed, administer small doses of diazepam intravenously (2 mg doses up to 10 mg) for maternal anxiety
4. At delivery
   A. Add oxytocin to the intravenous fluid (20 units of oxytocin/liter of fluid)
5. After delivery
   A. Give small doses of tranquilizer and/or narcotic intravenously as needed
   B. Reinject local anesthetic as needed (With chloroprocaine, reinject at 35–45 minutes, with lidocaine reinject at 45–60 minutes)
   C. Consider administering fentanyl 50–100 ug (See Narcotics—epidural and spinal) in 10 ml of saline through the epidural catheter after delivery of the fetus/newborn for postoperative maternal analgesia

[a] Medications for epidural anesthesia: (1) 2-chloroprocaine 3%, (2) lidocaine 2% with or without epinephrine, (3) bupivacaine 0.5%. (Note: In 1983 the FDA no longer approved the use of 0.75% bupivacaine in obstetrics. We have found 0.5% bupivacaine to be unsatisfactory for most patients.)

3.2.3. General Anesthesia

Many variables can affect the newborn during a general anesthetic for cesarean delivery. This section reviews the variables, so that we can appreciate how general anesthesia is administered today.

3.2.3a. Preparations for General Anesthesia. The parturient is placed on the operating table with left uterine displacement to decrease the deleterious effects of aortocaval compression. This practice grew out of such investigations as Crawford et al.,[163] who in 1972 demonstrated better Apgar scores, less neonatal acidosis, and less hypercarbia in newborns whose mothers were operated upon in the right lateral position as compared with parturients operated upon in the supine position, and Buley et al.,[164] who in 1977 noted better newborn results when the parturients were in the left lateral position as compared with parturients in the right lateral position.

All parturients receive supplemental oxygen before induction. In 1974, Archer et al.[165] demonstrated that after preinduction oxygenation, 1 min of apnea will decrease maternal PO_2 from 473 to 334 and will increase PCO_2 from 31 to 40. This study confirmed the increase in oxygen consumption at term and emphasized the need for preinduction oxygenation.

Although the importance of giving preinduction supplemental oxygen is established, the traditional technique of giving 100% oxygen for 3–5 min has been questioned. In 1981, Gold et al.[166] compared a group of nonpregnant patients who had 5 min of preinduction oxygenation with a similar group who took four deep breaths of oxygen and found similar oxygen levels. In 1984, Norris et al.[167] found similar results in parturients undergoing elective cesarean delivery.

Induction of anesthesia is performed after the patient's abdomen is prepared and draped. This decreases the time between induction of anesthesia and delivery of the newborn and may decrease the total amount of drugs that reach the fetus.

3.2.3b. Induction Agents. Although many drugs have been used to induce general anesthesia for cesarean delivery, thiopental is today the most frequently used drug, with ketamine second. Because thiopental is the standard, many drugs are compared with it.

Thiobarbiturates. Clinical research of the effects of thiobarbiturates includes both thiopental (Pentothal), introduced in 1931, and thiamylal (Surital), introduced in 1948. They are commonly grouped together, as there are no significant clinical differences in these drugs.[86,168,169]

For the parturient, the mean dose and standard deviation of thiopental needed to induce sleep is 3.5 ± 0.5 mg/kg pregnant body weight (PBW).[170] For the nonpregnant young woman, the dose of thiopental is

5.4 ± 0.6 mg/kg.[171] The lower dose needed to induce sleep in the parturient may be related to the lower serum albumin levels in the parturient, i.e., 75% of the nonparturient (thiobarbiturates are bound predominantly to albumin),[172] or to the lower concentration of the drug needed to anesthetize the parturient's brain due to the hormonal effects of pregnancy.

Thiamylal and thiopental rapidly cross the placenta with levels detected within 45 sec of induction and peak fetal blood levels occur 1.5 to 3 min after induction.[168,173] The concentration then rapidly decreases.[172,174] Although the thiobarbiturates pass the placenta rapidly, the newborn is not asleep when the mother is asleep after the induction of anesthesia (with low doses of barbiturates). Several factors may explain why the fetal brain appears to be protected from the maternal dose. These factors include a rapid decline in maternal and fetal blood levels due to the rapid distribution of drug,[172] uptake of the drug by the fetal liver as the drug passes from the placenta into the fetal circulation[175] (although this has recently been challenged[176]), progressive dilution of the drug in the fetal circulation due to shunting, and the higher relative water content of the fetal brain.

At an induction dose of 4 mg/kg PBW of thiobarbiturate followed by succinylcholine, intubation, and 100% oxygen, about 90% of newborns have a 1-min Apgar score of 7–10, whereas with an 8 mg/kg PBW induction dose only about 60% have a score of 7–10.[168]

Thus, because the fetal outcome as measured by Apgar score does not appear to be affected by a dose of 4 mg/kg PBW, and anesthesia is reliably induced in the parturient at this dose, it is the most commonly used dose for induction today. In addition, delivery should not be delayed in an attempt to allow redistribution to occur, as the fetal brain appears to be exposed only to a small concentration of drug as compared with the exposure sustained by the maternal brain.

Methohexital. Methohexital (Brevital), introduced in 1954, is 2.5–3 times as potent as thiopental.[24] Because it has a shorter half-life as compared with thiopental, its use has been suggested for obstetrics. In 1962, Sliom et al.[177] compared 100 mg methohexital with 250 mg thiopental, followed by succinylcholine, intubation, and maintenance with 70% nitrous oxide in oxygen. They found no significant difference in breathing times or Apgar scores between the two groups. In 1974, Holdcroft et al.[178] compared two doses of methohexital (1.0 mg/kg vs 1.4 mg/kg). Although they found no significant difference in the umbilical cord pH, PO_2, or PO_2, a marked difference in Apgar scores existed. Fifty percent of the newborns in the 1.4 mg/kg group had Apgar scores of ≤ 4, whereas only 7% of the newborns in the 1.0 mg/kg group scored ≤ 4.

Note that these studies were performed more than 10 years ago with the parturient in the supine position and utilizing 70% nitrous oxide in oxygen.

Diazepam. Diazepam (Valium), introduced in 1961, is a benzodiazepine; it has an adult half-life of 15–25 hr and a newborn half-life of 25–100 hr.[24] To induce anesthesia in the unmedicated nonpregnant patient, doses of up to 0.8 mg/kg may be required.[86] As hypotonia, hypothermia, and respiratory depression have been noted in the neonate after use of diazepam, the current recommendation is to limit maternal dose before delivery to 10 mg. This makes its use as an induction agent for general anesthesia unadvisable, although in 1974 Stover *et al.*[179] compared 20 mg diazepam with 200 mg thiopental as induction agents and found no significant difference in Apgar scores or clinical observation of the newborns in the postnatal period. Perhaps the short induction to delivery interval (3–6 min) permitted only a small amount of the drug to cross the placenta.

Ketamine. Ketamine (Ketalar, Ketaject), introduced in 1965, is an intravenous anesthetic agent that produces intense analgesia and a dissociate state regarded as sleep. When used alone for vaginal delivery, ketamine produces unpleasant dreams in more than 50% of parturients.[109] But when ketamine is combined with other drugs for cesarean delivery, the incidence of unpleasant dreams is about the same as with induction with thiopental—less than 16%.[180,181]

Ketamine rapidly crosses the placenta and achieves peak levels in 1–2 min.[182] In the parturient, a 1-mg/kg PBW dose is sufficient to induce general anesthesia.[181] In doses of ≤1 mg/kg, ketamine does not appear to be a depressant to the fetus.[181] In doses of ≥2 mg/kg, ketamine produces significant neonatal depression.[111]

Because of the cardiovascular stimulation that occurs with ketamine and the cardiovascular depression that occurs with thiopental, ketamine is recommended when maternal intravascular volume is decreased (i.e., antepartum hemorrhage). When fetal distress exists (i.e., acidotic fetus), ketamine appears to preserve fetal cerebral blood flow better than thiopental.[183] Because of the cardiovascular stimulation, ketamine is not recommended for use in parturients with preeclampsia or eclampsia.[182]

Since ketamine produces its dissociative state by CNS excitation, is it not possible that the newborn also experiences some CNS effects? In studies that compare thiopental with ketamine for induction of general anesthesia, infants who receive ketamine scored better on the ENNS than infants who received thiopental.[184] The authors believe that the pharmacologic effect of ketamine on the CNS may be responsible for the apparent "better" score in the ENNS.

Althesin. Althesin, introduced in 1971, is a combination of two steroid anesthetics; it comes in a solution of 9 mg/ml alphaxalone and 3 mg/ml alphadolone. Because it is a mixture, the dose is reported in microliters per kilogram; 60–80 μl/kg equals 4 mg/kg thiopental.[24] This agent has a short duration of action primarily by redistribution but also by its rapid metabolism. It has a half-life of only 6–8 min.[106] Because of its rapid distribution and rapid metabolism, althesin theoretically could be a better induction agent than thiopental. However, in a comparison study performed in 1974 by Downing *et al.*[185] in which althesin (60–70 μl/kg) or thiopental (4 mg/kg) was followed by succinylcholine, intubation, and 60–65% nitrous oxide in oxygen, the newborns of mothers who received althesin had lower oxygen levels and more acidosis than did those newborns whose mothers received thiopental. Thus, althesin does not appear to offer advantages over thiopental.

3.2.3c. Neuromuscular Blockers. Neuromuscular relaxants are used to facilitate intubation and to obtain abdominal relaxation and a relaxed patient for cesarean section. Placental transfer at first was thought to be absent because the mothers were relaxed and the newborns were not relaxed; with improved assays, however, it has been noted that transmission exists, but at a very reduced rate. This probably is related to the low lipid solubility of the drugs and high degree of ionization. Placental transfer has been noted for the short-acting agent succinylcholine;[186,187] for the intermediate-acting agents, atracurium,[188] and vecuronium;[189] and for the long-acting agents, *d*-tubocurarine,[174,190–192] metocurine,[193] gallamine,[174] and pancuronium.[189,194–198]

Under some abnormal conditions in which a large gradient between the mother and the fetus exists, the newborn can be clinically paralyzed. Baraka *et al.*[186] reported the administration of succinylcholine to a mother with homozygote atypical serum cholinesterase whose newborn also was homozygote atypical for serum cholinesterase; the result was the need for 6 hr ventilatory support for the newborn and for 2½ hr ventilatory support for the mother. Both mother and infant had dibucaine numbers below 30. A second example, reported by Older *et al.*,[192] was the administration of 245 mg *d*-tubocurarine over 16 hr to a woman in status epilepticus. Her newborn made no effort to breathe until edrophonium was given.

3.2.3d. Inhalation Agents. *Oxygen.* Maternal arterial oxygen tension during cesarean section is an important determinant of fetal oxygenation and the clinical condition of the newborn at birth.[199–201] In 1970, Baraka[199] varied the inspiratory oxygen concentrations and looked at both maternal and fetal (umbilical vein) Po_2. Anesthesia was induced with thiopental, followed by succinylcholine and intubation. The maintenance anesthetic was different in each of four groups. Group 1 had 20% oxygen and 80% nitrous oxide, group 2 had 33.3% oxygen and 66.7% nitrous oxide, group 3 had 50% oxygen and 50% nitrous oxide, and group 4 had 100% oxygen and 0.5% halothane. Results are shown in Table XIV.

Thus, increasing the maternal inspired oxygen concentration from 20 to 50% increased maternal and fetal Po_2. Increasing the maternal oxygen concentration from 50 to 100% increased maternal but not fetal Po_2.

Nitrous oxide. In 1970, Marx *et al.*[202] demonstrated rapid placental transfer of N_2O during parturition. The maternal N_2O level rose rapidly during the first 4 min of anesthesia. After 4 min, the increase was small. The umbilical vein–maternal artery concentration ratio was 0.8 after 3 min of anesthesia. The umbilical artery–umbilical vein ratio rose progressively with increased duration of anesthesia from 0.6 at 2–4 min to 0.9 after 15–19 min of anesthesia. After an induction to delivery interval of 15–19 min, further increase in the level of N_2O was small. Thus, N_2O is rapidly taken up by the mother, rapidly crosses the placenta and is rapidly taken up by the fetus.

If neonatal depression occurs at birth, one must consider the anesthetic effect of N_2O as well as the possibility of diffusion hypoxia as the N_2O is excreted by the newborn. Thus, oxygen should be available for the neonate and used especially when the I–D interval is prolonged.[203]

Because of the narcoticlike effects of N_2O, some anesthesiologists decreased the level of N_2O from 70 to 50% and found less narcosis of the newborn. But maternal awareness rose from about 5 to 20%. Now that the addition of a small amount of a volatile agent can be added to keep the N_2O concentration at 50%, maternal awareness approaches zero.

Volatile agents. After induction of anesthesia, maintenance of the anesthetic state is required. Oxygen with the addition of N_2O does not

Table XIV. Maternal and Fetal Oxygenation[a]

Group	Oxygen concentration (%)	Maternal pO_2 (mm Hg)	Fetal umbilical vein pO_2 (mm Hg)
1	20	78–100	20–26
2	33	115–157	28–35
3	50	200–300	38–65
4	100	440–500	43–65

[a] From ref. 199.

always provide adequate anesthesia. The addition of small amounts of volatile agents permits the use of a higher oxygen concentration, i.e., 50% oxygen, with N_2O and a decrease in the incidence of maternal recall of intraoperative events.[204–207] Because volatile agents cause a dose-related decrease in uterine contractility, it has been claimed that they might also cause an increase in postpartum hemorrhage. However, no increased blood loss has been demonstrated with small amounts of halothane (Fluothane),[205–207] enflurane (Ethrane),[204,207] or isoflurane (Forane),[207] when used for cesarean section.

In 1983, Warren et al.[207] using the standard anesthetic induction, which consisted of preinduction oxygenation for 3 min followed by thiopental and succinylcholine, intubation, and ventilation with a tidal volume of 10 ml/kg PBW at a rate of 10 breaths/min, compared four maintenance groups: 50% O_2–50% N_2O alone, 50% O–50% N_2O combined with 0.5% halothane, 0.75% isoflurane, and 1.0% enflurane. The recall rate was 17% in the 50% O_2–50% N_2O group. None of the patients with the added volatile agent had recall. Blood loss was similar in all groups. No differences were noted in induction to delivery and uterine incision-to-delivery intervals, Apgar scores, maternal and fetal blood-gas values, lactate values, or the ENNS at 2–4 hr.

3.2.3e. Ventilation. In 1983, Burger et al.[208] compared controlled maternal ventilation under general anesthesia at 8 ml/kg, 9 ml/kg, and 10 ml/kg PBW at a respiratory rate of 10 breaths/min. They found no differences in Apgar scores or fetal oxygenation but did find less fetal acidosis in the 10-mg/kg group. This group also showed more normal maternal PCO_2 values. Thus, 10 ml/kg at 10 breaths/min is the suggested maternal minute ventilation.

3.2.3f. Timing of Delivery. In evaluating newborn outcome under anesthesia, two times are commonly evaluated. They are the induction to delivery time (I–D) and the uterine incision to delivery time (UI–D).[153] Recent investigations have demonstrated that the UI–D interval is equally as important as the I–D interval. When the uterine incision to delivery time is greater than 3 min, a greater proportion of newborns will demonstrate depressed Apgar scores and will have more acidosis than newborns delivered with uterine incision to delivery times of less than 3 min[154] (see Table XV).

3.2.4. Comparison of Anesthetic Techniques for Cesarean Delivery

In 1953, Apgar[49] compared different anesthetic techniques for cesarean section. She found that despite frequent maternal hypotension,

Table XV. General Anesthetic Technique for Cesarean Delivery at the Brigham and Women's Hosptial

1. Preinduction
   A. Antacid—30 ml (nonparticulate)
   B. Large bore intravenous line with Lactated Ringer's Solution
   C. Left uterine displacement
   D. Monitors (EKG, Blood Pressure)
   E. Preinduction oxygenation with 100% oxygen
2. Rapid sequence induction
   A. Thiopental 4 mg/kg or ketamine 1 mg/kg of pregnant body weight
   B. Cricoid pressure as sleep occurs
   C. Succinylcholine 1.5 mg/kg of pregnant body weight
   D. Intubate the trachea with a cuffed endotracheal tube[a]
   E. Inflate cuff
   F. Check for bilateral breath sounds
   G. If all checks out, say "cut" and release cricoid pressure
3. Maintenance anesthesia until delivery
   A. Oxygen–nitrous oxide at 50%–50%
   B. Volatile agent (0.5% halothane, 0.75% isoflurane, or 1% enflurane)
   C. Succinylcholine drip as needed (or depolarizing agent)
   D. Ventilator setting of 10 ml/kg at 10 breaths per min
4. At delivery
   A. Add oxytocin to the intravenous fluid (20 units of oxytocin/liter of fluid)
5. Maintenance anesthesia after delivery
   A. Oxygen–nitrous oxide at 30%–70%
   B. Narcotic (i.e., morphine at 0.1 mg/kg or fentanyl at 1 μg/kg)
   C. Tranquilizer (i.e., diazepam 5 mg)
   D. Discontinue volatile agent
   E. Suction stomach with an oral suction catheter or gastric tube and remove tube
6. End of surgery
   A. Reverse nondepolarizers if used or discontinue succinylcholine drip
   B. Discontinue nitrous oxide when muscle tone returns to normal
   C. Extubate patient when the patient is responsive and awake
   D. Give supplemental oxygen in the recovery room

[a] If intubation fails or is not possible, every anesthesiologist must have a "failed intubation protocol" to follow!

newborns performed best under spinal anesthesia. The 1-min mean score under spinal anesthesia (nupercaine or tetracaine) was 8, for general anesthesia (cyclopropane and oxygen) 5, and for epidural anesthesia (0.75% lidocaine) 6.3. Needless to say, several changes have occurred during the last 30-plus years, making all three techniques quite safe for the newborn.

In 1978, McGuinness et al.[209] compared epidural anesthesia with 0.75% bupivacaine (22.5 ml) with spinal anesthesia with tetracaine (10 mg). They found no significant difference in Apgar scores, blood-gas data or ENNS scores performed at 4 and 24 hr of age.

In 1978, Hodgkinson et al.[210] compared general anesthesia using a thiopental or ketamine induction with 50% O_2 and 50% N_2O as maintenance anesthesia versus spinal anesthesia with tetracaine. Apgar scores were similar in their groups. Using the ENNS they found spinal anesthesia was associated with the greatest percentage of high scores on the first and second day for most items. There was a statistically significant difference between all the scores for the spinal group compared with the ketamine and thiopental groups. The scores were lowest following a thiopental induction and intermediate with ketamine, although the differences between these two groups were not statistically significant.

In 1978, Hollmen et al.[211] compared epidural anesthesia (1.5% lidocaine with 1 : 200,000 epinephrine) with general anesthesia (thiopental, succinylcholine, and N_2O-O_2). Apgar scores, neonatal acid–base values and neurologic activity were similar between the groups. They also looked at a subset of the epidural group, newborns whose mothers had a mean blood pressure at one time of ≤70 mm Hg. In four of these six newborns, the pH values 15 min after delivery were below 7.20. There was also a significant correlation between the maternal hypotension and weak rooting and sucking reflexes in the newborns at 1 and 2 days after birth. This work emphasizes that if maternal hypotension is not corrected, alterations in the infant's neurobehavioral status are possible. Perhaps the newborn changes would have been more apparent if ephedrine was not used to correct the hypotension.

In 1982, Zagorzycki et al.[212] compared 90 parturients who underwent general anesthesia with 105 parturients who underwent epidural anesthesia. Both groups had left uterine displacement. The general anesthesia sequence included preinduction oxygenation, thiopental 4 mg/kg PBW, succinylcholine, intubation, and maintenance with 50% $O_2-50\%$ N_2O and 0.5% halothane. The epidural group received 15–20 ml 0.75% bupivacaine and received O_2 by face mask. There was no significant difference in Apgar score at 1 or 5 min.

In summary, many studies compare the different anesthetic techniques used for cesarean section, of which we have reviewed a few. It becomes obvious that the key to maintaining the best possible intrauterine environment for the fetus—soon to become newborn—is to maintain adequate uteroplacental perfusion and thus prevent fetal acidosis and hypoxia. If uteroplacental blood flow is maintained and the induction to delivery and the uterine incision to delivery intervals are not excessive, neonatal outcome as noted by Apgar scores are equally good with epidural, spinal, or general anesthesia.

4. Anesthesia and the Compromised Fetus

The anesthesiologist may be confronted with two types of situations of fetal compromise for which anesthesia is necessary. The first situation involves acute fetal distress and impending fetal demise. Here delivery is urgent and, if rapid vaginal delivery is possible, it should be performed. If not, cesarean delivery is accomplished. If cesarean delivery is urgent, i.e., "emergency" or "STAT," we prefer to administer general anesthesia because maintenance of maternal blood pressure and uteroplacental perfusion is more probable than with regional anesthesia and the parturient's abdomen can be prepared as induction of anesthesia is performed. (The only exception to this rule occurs when an epidural anesthetic is functioning for labor. In that instance, we would attempt to raise the level of block without interfering with the delivery. Obviously, if this is *not* possible, general anesthesia is initiated without delay.) The abdomen cannot be prepared if the parturient is on her side or in the sitting position for an induction of a spinal anesthetic. General anesthesia always permits surgery to be performed, whereas regional techniques may be inadequate.

In the second situation, the fetus is potentially at greater risk. The fetus may be postdates, or the parturient could have diabetes or toxemia, conditions in which the uteroplacental circulation is more tenuous. In these cases, uteroplacental perfusion must be maintained as the fetal reserve is less. Close fetal monitoring can diagnose situations of uteroplacental insufficiency (severe variable or late decelerations) and fetal capillary pH values performed as needed. In these "emergent" situations, individualization is the key, provided that adequate uteroplacental perfusion is preserved.

5. Relationship of Obstetric Anesthesia to Long-Term Neonatal Effects

Several investigators have demonstrated that obstetric anesthesia does not produce adverse long-term neonatal effects. In 1980, Ounsted *et al.*[213] reported a prospective study of 570 infants who were examined within 3 days of delivery and at regular intervals for 4 years. At 4 years of age, medical, behavioral, and developmental assessments were performed. These tests evaluated gross-motor, fine-motor, visuomotor, language, and comprehension. Strong associations were made between emergency cesarean sections, fetal distress during labor, and asphyxia at birth. They also examined the impact of obstetric anesthesia.[214] Methods of pain relief were categorized as general anesthesia, epidural (or caudal) anesthesia, systemic analgesia (usually meperidine), or none which included local infiltration. Some patients received a combination of pain-relief methods. No significant differences were found in the development status of the children at 4 years of age according to the method of maternal pain relief.

In 1980, Van de Berg et al.[215] reported the association of obstetric medications with scores of cognitive development at age 5 using the Peabody Picture Vocabulary Test (PPVT) and the Coloured Raven Progressive Matrices. The PPVT is a language-based achievement test that correlates with scholastic ability. The Raven test is not based on vocabulary but rather on logic; it consists of sets of configuration problems arranged in order of increasing difficulty. There were no significant effects of obstetric anesthesia or analgesia on child development.

In summary, our effort has been to give the reader an up-to-date overview of the effects of analgesics and anesthetics on the mother and the soon-to-be-newborn fetus. Our mission in obstetric anesthesia is the same today as the objective stated by Walter Channing in A Treatise on Etherization in Childbirth, published in 1848:[216]

> My great, I had almost said my sole, object in this circular,—in short, in my whole efforts,—was to ascertain here at home, in the birthplace of etherization, what had been the precise results of many experiments, made by physicians, of the employment of the remedy of pain. My object was to learn if this use of it has been *safe*, safe both to *mother* and to *child*; and thus, as far as such results might reach, to contribute something towards settling the most important point concerning its further use, namely, that of its *safety*.

References

1. Ostheimer, G. W. (ed.), 1984, *Manual of Obstetric Anesthesia*, Churchill Livingstone, New York.
2. Ostheimer, G. W., 1984, Anesthetic considerations in complicated obstetrics, *1984 ASA Annual Refresher Course Lectures*, Section 304.
3. Shnider, S. M., and Levinson, G. (eds.), 1979, *Anesthesia for Obstetrics*, Williams & Wilkins, Baltimore.
4. Skaredoff, M. N., and Ostheimer, G. W., 1981, Physiologic changes during pregnancy—Effects of major regional anesthesia, *Reg. Anesth.* **6:**28.
5. Bieniarz, J., Maqueda, E., and Caldeyro-Barcia, R., 1966, Compression of aorta by the uterus in late human pregnancy, *Am. J. Obstet. Gynecol.* **95:**795.
6. Howard, B. K., Goodson, J. H., and Mengert, W. F., 1953, Supine hypotensive syndrome in late pregnancy, *Obstet. Gynecol.* **1:**371.
7. McRoberts Jr., W. A., 1951, Postural shock in pregnancy, *Am. J. Obstet. Gynecol.* **62:**627.

8. Greiss Jr., F. C., and VanWilkes, D., 1964, Effects of sympathomimetic drugs and angiotensin on the uterine vascular bed, *Obstet. Gynecol.* **23:**925.

9. Ralston, D. H., Shnider, S. M., and deLorimier, A. A., 1974, Effects of equipotent ephedrine, metaraminol, mephentermine, and methoxamine on uterine blood flow in the pregnant ewe, *Anesthesiology* **40:**354.

10. Ramanathan, S., Friedman, S., Moss, P., *et al.*, 1984, Phenylephrine for the treatment of maternal hypotension due to epidural anesthesia. *Anesth. Analg.* **63:**262 (abs.).

11. Biehl, D. R., 1981, Prevention of aspiration pneumonitis in the parturient, *Curr. Rev. Clin. Anesth.* **1:**187.

12. Cohen, S. E., 1982, The aspiration syndrome, *Clin. Obstet. Gynecol.* **9:**235.

13. Mendelson, C. L., 1946, The aspiration of stomach contents into the lungs during obstetric anesthesia, *Am. J. Obstet. Gynecol.* **52:**191.

14. Baraka, A., Saab, M., Salem, M. R., *et al.*, 1977, Control of gastric acidity by glycopyrrolate premedication in the parturient, *Anesth. Analg.* **56:**642.

15. Murad, S. H. N., Conklin, K. A., Tabsh, K. M. A., *et al.*, 1981, Atropine and glycopyrrolate—Hemodynamic effects and placental transfer in the pregnant ewe, *Anesth. Analg.* **60:**710.

16. Hellman, L. M., Johnson, H. L., Tolles, W. E., *et al.*, 1961, Some factors affecting the fetal heart rate, *Am. J. Obstet. Gynecol.* **82:**1055.

17. Hon, E. H., Bradfield, A. H., and Hess, O. W., 1961, The electronic evaluation of the fetal heart rate, *Am. J. Obstet. Gynecol.* **82:**291.

18. Abboud, T., Raya, J., Sadri, S., *et al.*, 1983, Fetal and maternal cardiovascular effects of atropine and glycopyrrolate. *Anesth. Analg.* **62:**426.

19. Manchikanti, L., and Roush, J. R., 1984, Effect of preanesthetic glycopyrrolate and cimetidine on gastric fluid pH and volume in outpatients, *Anesth. Analg.* **63:**40.

20. Schulze-Delrieu, K., 1981, Metoclopramide, *N. Engl. J. Med.* **305:**28.

21. Bylsma-Howell, M., Riggs, K. W., McMorland, G. H., *et al.*, 1983, Placental transport of metoclopramide—Assessment of maternal and neonatal effects, *Can. Anaesth. Soc. J.* **30:**487.

22. Cohen, S. E., and Barrier, G., 1983, Does metoclopramide decrease gastric volume in cesarean section patients?, *Anesthesiology* **59:**A403.

23. Cohen, S. E., Jasson, J., Talafre, M-L., *et al.*, 1984, Does metoclopramide decrease the volume of gastric contents in patients undergoing cesarean section?, *Anesthesiology* **61:**604.

24. Wood, M., and Wood, A. J. J., 1982, *Drugs and Anesthesia—Pharmacology for Anesthesiologists*, Williams & Wilkins, Baltimore.

25. Hodgkinson, R., Glassenberg, R., Joyce, T. H. III, *et al.*, 1983, Comparison of cimetidine (Tagamet®) with antacid for safety and effectiveness in reducing gastric acidity before elective cesarean section, *Anesthesiology* **59:**86.

26. Howe, J. P., McGowan, W. A. W., Moore, J., *et al.*, 1981, The placental transfer of cimetidine, *Anaesthesia* **36:**371.

27. Ostheimer, G. W., Morrision, J. A., Lavoie, C., *et al.*, 1982, The effect of cimetidine on mother, newborn and neonatal neurobehavior, *Anesthesiology* **57:**A405.

28. Gillett, G. B., Watson, J. D., and Langford, R. M., 1984, Ranitidine and single-dose antacid therapy as prophylaxis against acid aspriation syndrome in obstetric practice, *Anaesthesia* **39:**638.

29. McAuley, D. M., Moore, J., Dundee, J. W., *et al.*, 1984, Oral ranitidine in labour, *Anaesthesia* **39:**433.

30. Cibils, L. A., 1976, Response of human uterine arteries to local anesthetics, *Am. J. Obstet. Gynecol.* **126:**202.

31. Greiss Jr., F. C., Still, J. G., and Anderson, S. G., 1976, Effects of local anesthetic agents on the uterine vasculatures and myometrium, *Am. J. Obstet. Gynecol.* **124**:889.
32. Fishburne, Jr., J. I., Greiss Jr., F. C., Hopkinson, R., *et al.*, 1979, Responses of the gravid uterine vasculature to arterial levels of local anesthetic agents, *Am. J. Obstet. Gynecol.* **133**:753.
33. Conklin, K. A., 1981, The effects of drugs on the fetus and newborn, *Curr. Rev. Clin. Anesth.* **2**:51.
34. Cousins, M. J., and Mather, L. E., 1984, Intrathecal and epidural administration of narcotics, *Anesthesiology* **61**:276.
35. Fishburne, J. I., 1982, Fetal monitoring in high risk pregnancy, in: *Obstetric Anesthesia: The Complicated Patient* (F. M. James III and A. S. Wheeler, eds.), pp. 1–37, F. A. Davis, Philadelphia.
36. Hill, L. M., 1979, Diagnosis and management of fetal distress, *Mayo Clin. Proc.* **54**:784.
37. Albright, G. A., 1978, *Anesthesia in Obstetrics—Maternal, Fetal, and Neonatal Aspects*, Addison-Wesley, Menlo Park, Calif.
38. Brazelton, T. B., 1970, Effect of prenatal drugs on the behavior of the neonate, *Am. J. Psychiatry* **126**:1261.
39. Cibils, L. A., 1981, *Electronic Fetal–Maternal Monitoring: Antepartum, Intrapartum*, PSG, Boston.
40. Marx, G. F., and Bassell, G. M. (eds.), 1980, *Obstetric Analgesia and Anaesthesia*, Elsevier, New York.
41. Ostheimer, G. W., 1981, Newborn resuscitation, *Clin. Obstet. Gynecol.* **24**:635.
42. McCrann, D. J., Jr., and Schifrin, B. S., 1974, Fetal monitoring in high-risk pregnancy, *Clin. Perinatol.* **1**:229.
43. Mendez-Bauer, C., Poseiro, J. J., Arellano-Hernandez, G., *et al.*, 1963, Effects of atropine on the heart rate of the human fetus during labor, *Am. J. Obstet. Gynecol.* **85**:1033.
44. Paul, R. H., Suidan, A. K., Yeh, S-Y., *et al.*, 1975, Clinical fetal monitoring. VII. the evaluation and significance of intrapartum baseline FHR variability, *Am. J. Obstet. Gynecol.* **123**:206.
45. Scher, J., Hailey, D. M., and Beard, R. W., 1972, The effects of diazepam on the fetus, *J. Obstet. Gynaecol. Br. Commonw.* **79**:635.
46. Yeh, S-Y., Paul, R. H., Cordero, L., *et al.*, 1974, A study of diazepam during labor, *Obstet. Gynecol.* **43**:363.
47. Mocsary, P., Gaal, J., Komaromy, B., *et al.*, 1970, Relationship between fetal intracranial pressure and fetal heart rate during labor, *Am. J. Obstet. Gynecol.* **106**:407.
48. Epstein, H., Waxman, A., Gleicher, N., *et al.*, 1982, Meperidine-induced sinusoidal fetal heart rate pattern and reversal with naloxone, *Obstet. Gynecol.* **59**:22S.
49. Apgar, V., 1953, A proposal for a new method of evaluation of the newborn infant, *Anesth. Analg.* **32**:260.
50. Drage, J. S., and Berendes, H., 1966, Apgar scores and outcome of the newborn, *Pediatr. Clin. North Am.* **13**:635.
51. Drage, J. S., Kennedy, C., Berendes, H., *et al.*, 1966, The apgar score as an index of infant morbidity—A report from the collaborative study of cerebral palsy, *Dev. Med. Child Neurol.* **8**:14.
52. Drage, J., Berendes, H., and Fisher, P., 1969, The Apgar scores and four-year psychological examination performance, *Pan Am. Health Org. Sci. Publ.* **185**:222.
53. Niswander, K. R., Gordon, M., and Drage, J. S., 1975, The effects of intrauterine hypoxia on the child surviving to 4 years, *Am. J. Obstet. Gynecol.* **121**:892.

54. Apgar, V., Holaday, D. A., James, L. S., *et al.*, 1958, Evaluation of the newborn infant—Second report, *JAMA* **168**:1985.
55. Apgar, V., 1966, The newborn (Apgar) scoring system—Reflections and advice, *Pediatr. Clin. North Am.* **13**:645.
56. Modanlou, H., Yeh, S-Y., and Hon, E. H., 1974, Fetal and neonatal acid–base balance in normal and high-risk pregnancies—During labor and the first hour of life, *Obstet. Gynecol.* **43**:347.
57. Graham, F. K., Pennayer, M. M., Caldwell, B. M., *et al.*, 1957, Relationship between clinical status and behavior test performance in a newborn group with histories suggesting anoxia, *J. Pediatr.* **50**:177.
58. Rosenblith, J. F., 1961, The modified Graham behavior test for neonates—Test–retest reliability, normative data and hypotheses for future work, *Biol. Neonate* **3**:174.
59. Prechtl, J. F. R., and Beintema, D., 1964, *Clinics in Developmental Medicine*, Vol 12: *The Neurologic Examination of the Full Term Infant*, Spastics International Medical Publishers, London.
60. Desmond, M. M., Franklin, R. R., Vallbona, C., *et al.*, 1963, The clinical behavior of the newly born. I. The term baby, *J. Pediatr.* **62**:307.
61. Brazelton, T. B., 1973, *Clinics in Developmental Medicine*, Vol 50: *Neonatal Behavioral Assessment Scale*, Spastics International Medical Publishers, London.
62. Ostheimer, G. W., 1981, Neurobehavioral effects of local anesthesia and fetal resuscitation, *Reg. Anaesth.* **6**:136.
63. Tronick, E., and Brazelton, T. B., 1975, Clincial uses of the Brazelton neonatal behavioral assessment scale, in: *Exceptional Infant*, Vol. III: *Assessments and Intervention* (B. Z. Friedlander, *et al.*, eds.), Brunner/Mazel, New York.
64. Scanlon, J. W., 1979, Clinical neonatal neurobehavioral assessments—Methods and significance, in: *Clinical Management of Mother and Newborn* (G. Marx, ed.), pp. 65–83, Springer-Verlag, New York.
65. Scanlon, J. W., Brown, W. U., Jr., Weiss, J. B., *et al.*, 1974, Neurobehavioral responses of newborn infants after maternal epidural anesthesia, *Anesthesiology* **40**:121.
66. Amiel-Tison, C., Barrier, G., Shnider, S. M., *et al.*, 1982, A new neurologic and adaptive capacity scoring system for evaluating obstetric medications in full-term newborns, *Anesthesiology* **56**:340.
67. Tronick, E., 1982, A critique of the neonatal neurologic and adaptive capacity score (NACS) (Editorial), *Anesthesiology* **56**:338.
68. Bonica, J., 1967, *Principles and Practice of Obstetric Analgesia and Anesthesia*, FA Davis, Philadelphia.
69. Shnider, S. M., Wright, R. G., Levinson, G., *et al.*, 1979, Uterine blood flow and plasma norepinephrine changes during maternal stress in the pregnant ewe, *Anesthesiology* **50**:524.
70. Motoyama, E. K., Rivard, G., Acheson, F., *et al.*, 1966, Adverse effect of maternal hyperventilation on the foetus, *Lancet* **1**:286.
71. Bassell, G. M., Humayun, S. G., and Marx, G. F., 1980, Maternal bearing down efforts—Another fetal risk? *Obstet. Gynecol.* **56**:39.
72. Melzack, R., Taenzer, P., Feldman, P., *et al.*, 1981, Labour is still painful after prepared childbirth training, *Can. Med. Assoc. J.* **125**:357.
73. Nelson, N. M., Enkin, M. W., Saigal, S., *et al.*, 1980, A randomized clinical trial of the Leboyer approach to childbirth, *N. Engl. J. Med.* **302**:655.
74. Scott, J. R., and Rose, N. B., 1976, Effect of psychoprophylaxis (Lamaze preparation) on labor and delivery in primiparas, *N. Engl. J. Med.* **294**:1205.
75. Way, W. L., Costley, E. C., and Way, E. L., 1965, Respiratory sensitivity of the newborn infant to meperidine and morphine, *Clin. Pharmacol. Ther.* **6**:454.

76. Crawford, J. S., and Rudofsky, S., 1965, The placental transmission of pethidine, *Br. J. Anaesth.* **37**:929.

77. Caldwell, J., Wakile, L. A., Notarianni, L. J., *et al.*, 1978, Maternal and neonatal disposition of pethidine in childbirth—A study using quantitative gas chromatograph–mass spectrometry, *Life Sci.* **22**:589.

78. Cooper, L. V., Stephen, G. W., and Aggett, P. J. A., 1977, Elimination of pethidine and bupivacaine in the newborn, *Arch. Dis. Child.* **52**:638.

79. Hodgkinson, R., Bhatt, M., and Wang, C. N., 1978, Double-blind comparison of the neurobehavior of neonates following the administration of different doses of meperidine to the mother, *Can. Anaesth. Soc. J.* **25**:405.

80. Hodgkinson, R., and Husain, F. J., 1982, The duration of effect of maternally administered meperidine on neonatal neurobehavior, *Anesthesiology* **56**:51.

81. Koch, G., and Wendel, H., 1968, The effect of pethidine on the postnatal adjustment of respiration and acid–base balance, *Acta Obstet. Gynecol. Scand.* **47**:27.

82. Morrison, J. C., Whybrew, W. D., Rosser, S. I., *et al.*, 1976, Metabolites of meperidine in the fetal and maternal serum, *Am. J. Obstet. Gynecol.* **126**:997.

83. Morrison, J. C., Wiser, W. L., Rosser, S. I., *et al.*, 1973, Metabolites of meperidine related to fetal depression, *Am. J. Obstet. Gynecol.* **115**:1132.

84. Shnider, S. M., and Moya, F., 1964, Effects of meperidine on the newborn infant, *Am. J. Obstet. Gynecol.* **89**:1009.

85. Forrest, W. H., Jr., and Bellville, J. W., 1968, Respiratory effects of alphaprodine in man, *Obstet. Gynecol.* **31**:61.

86. Collins, V. J., 1976, *Principles of Anesthesiology*, 2nd ed., Lea and Febiger, Philadelphia.

87. Downes, J. J., Kemp, R. A., and Lambertsen, C. J., 1967, The magnitude and duration of respiratory depression due to fentanyl and meperidine in man, *J. Pharmacol. Exp. Ther.* **158**:416.

88. Paddock, R., Beer, E. G., Bellville, J. W., *et al.*, 1969, Analgesic and side effects of pentazocine and morphine in a large population of postoperative patients, *Clin. Pharmacol. Ther.* **10**:355.

89. Beckett, A. H., and Taylor, J. F., 1967, Blood concentrations of pethidine and pentazocine in mother and infant at time of birth, *J. Pharm. Pharmacol. (Suppl.)* **19**:50S.

90. Hodgkinson, R., Huff, R. W., Hayashi, R. H., *et al.*, 1979, Double-blind comparison of maternal analgesia and neonatal neurobehaviour following intravenous butorphanol and meperidine, *J. Int. Med. Res.* **7**:224.

91. Quilligan, E. J., Keegan, K. A., and Donahue, M. J., 1980, Double-blind comparison of intravenously injected butorphanol and meperidine in parturients, *Int. J. Gynaecol. Obstet.* **18**:363.

92. Romagnoli, A., and Keats, A. S., 1980, Ceiling effect for respiratory depression by nalbuphine, *Clin. Pharmacol. Ther.* **27**:478.

93. Bepko, F., Lowe, E., and Waxman, B., 1965, Relief of the emotional factor in labor with parenterally administered diazepam, *Obstet. Gynecol.* **26**:852.

94. Flowers, C. E., Rudolph, A. J., and Desmond, M. M., 1969, Diazepam (Valium®) as an adjunct in obstetric analgesia, *Obstet. Gynecol.* **34**:68.

95. Friedman, E. A., Niswander, K. R., and Sachtleben, M. R., 1969, Effect of diazepam on labor, *Obstet. Gynecol.* **34**:82.

96. Niswander, K. R., 1969, Effect of diazepam on meperidine requirements of patients during labor, *Obstet. Gynecol.* **34**:62.

97. Cavanagh, D., and Condo, C. S., 1964, Diazepam—A pilot study of drug concentrations in maternal blood, amniotic fluid and cord blood, *Curr. Ther. Res.* **6**:122.

98. Cree, J. E., Meyer, J., and Hailey, D. M., 1973, Diazepam in labour—Its metabolism and effect on the clinical condition and thermogenesis of the newborn, *Br. Med. J.* 4:251.

99. DeSilva, J. A. F., D'Arconte, L., and Kaplan, J., 1964, The determination of blood levels and the placental transfer of diazepam in humans, *Curr. Ther. Res.* 6:115.

100. Kanto, J., Erkkola, R., and Sellman, R., 1973, Accumulation of diazepam and n-demethyldiazepam in the fetal blood during the labour, *Ann. Clin. Res.* 5:375.

101. Mandelli, M., Morselli, P. L., Nordio, S., *et al.*, 1975, Placental transfer of diazepam and its disposition in the newborn, *Clin. Pharmacol. Ther.* 17:564.

102. Owen, J. R., Irani, S. F., and Blair, A. W., 1972, Effect of diazepam administered to mothers during labour on temperature regulation of neonate, *Arch. Dis. Child.* 47:107.

103. McCarthy, G. T., O'Connell, B., and Robinson, A. E., 1973, Blood levels of diazepam in infants of two mothers given large doses of diazepam during labour, *J. Obstet. Gynaecol. Br. Commonw.* 80:349.

104. Whitelaw, A. G. L., Cummings, A. J., and McFadyen, I. R., 1981, Effect of maternal lorazepam on the neonate, *Br. Med. J.* 282:1106.

105. Abouleish, E. I., and Pan, P., 1984, Placental transfer of hydroxyzine hydrochloride and its effect on the human neonate, *Anesth. Analg.* 63:176 (abs.).

106. Vickers, M. D., Wood-Smith, F. G., and Stewart, H. C., 1978, *Drugs in Anaesthetic Practice*, 5th ed., Butterworths, London.

107. Carson, I. W., Moore, J., Balmer, J. P., *et al.*, 1973, Laryngeal competence with ketamine and other drugs, *Anesthesiology* 38:128.

108. Penrose, B. H., 1972, Aspiration pneumonitis following ketamine induction for general anesthesia, *Anesth. Analg.* 51:41.

109. Ellingson, A., Haram, K., and Sagen, N., 1977, Ketamine and diazepam as anaesthesia for forceps delivery, a comparative study, *Acta Anaesthesiol. Scand.* 21:37.

110. Akamatsu, T. J., Bonica, J. J., Rehmet, R., *et al.*, 1974, Experiences with the use of ketamine for parturition. I. Primary anesthetic for vaginal delivery, *Anesth. Analg.* 53:284.

111. Janeczko, G. F., El-Etr, A. A., and Younes, S., 1974, Low-dose ketamine anesthesia for obstetrical delivery, *Anesth. Analg.* 53:828.

112. Covino, B. G., and Vassallo, H. G., 1976, *Local Anesthetics—Mechanisms of Action and Clinical Use*, Grune & Stratton, New York.

113. Ralston, D. H., and Shnider, S. M., 1978, The fetal and neonatal effects of regional anesthesia in obstetrics, *Anesthesiology* 48:34.

114. Morishima, H. O., Covino, B. G., Yeh, M. N., *et al.*, 1981, Bradycardia in the fetal baboon following paracervical block anesthesia, *Am. J. Obstet. Gynecol.* 140:775.

115. Shnider, S. M., and Way, E. L., 1968, Plasma levels of lidocaine (Xylocain®) in mother and newborn following obstetrical conduction anesthesia—Clinical applications, *Anesthesiology* 29:951.

116. Morishima, H. O., Daniel, S. S., Finster, M., *et al.*, 1966, Transmission of mepivacaine hydrochloride (Carbocaine®) across the human placenta, *Anesthesiology* 27:147.

117. O'Brien, J. E., Abbey, V., Hinsvark, O., *et al.*, 1979, Metabolism and measurement of chloroprocaine, an ester-type local anesthetic, *J. Pharm. Sci.* 68:75.

118. Hyman, M. D., and Shnider, S. M., 1971, Maternal and neonatal blood concentrations of bupivacaine associated with obstetrical conduction anesthesia, *Anesthesiology* 34:81.

119. Biehl, D., Shnider, S. M., Levinson, G., *et al.*, 1978, Placental transfer of lidocaine—Effects of fetal acidosis, *Anesthesiology* 48:409.

120. Brown, W. U., Jr., Bell, G. C., and Alper, M. H., 1976, Acidosis, local anesthetics, and the newborn, *Obstet. Gynecol.* **48:**27.
121. Brown, W. U., Jr., Bell, G. C., Lurie, A. O., *et al.*, 1975, Newborn blood levels of lidocaine and mepivacaine in the first postnatal day following maternal epidural anesthesia, *Anesthesiology* **42:**698.
122. Tucker, G. T., Boyes, R. N., Bridenbaugh, P. O., *et al.*, 1970, Binding of anilide-type local anesthetics in human plasma. II. Implications in vivo, with special reference to transplacental distributions, *Anesthesiology* **33:**304, 1970.
123. Blankenbaker, W. L., DiFazio, C. A., and Berry, F. A., Jr., 1975, Lidocaine and its metabolites in the newborn, *Anesthesiology* **42:**325.
124. Kileff, M. E., James, F. M., III, Dewan, D. M., *et al.*, 1984, Neonatal neurobehavioral responses after epidural anesthesia for cesarean section using lidocaine and bupivacaine, *Anesth. Analg.* **63:**413.
125. Reynolds, F., and Taylor, G., 1970, Maternal and neonatal blood concentrations of bupivacaine—A comparison with lignocaine during continuous extradural analgesia, *Anaesthesia* **25:**14.
126. Shnider, S. M., and Way, E. L., 1968, The kinetics of transfer of lidocaine (Xylocaine®) across the human placenta, *Anesthesiology* **29:**944.
127. Poppers, P. J., and Finster, M., 1968, The use of prilocaine hydrochloride (Citanest®) for epidural analgesia in obstetrics, *Anesthesiology* **29:**1134.
128. Datta, S., Corke, B. C., Alper, M. H., *et al.*, 1980, Epidural anesthesia for cesarean section—A comparison of bupivacaine, chloroprocaine and etidocaine, *Anesthesiology* **52:**48.
129. Lund, P. C., Cwik, J. C., Gannon, R. T., *et al.*, 1977, Etidocaine for caesarean section—Effects on mother and baby, *Br. J. Anaesth.* **49:**457.
130. Poppers, P. J., Vosburgh, G. J., and Finster, M., 1966, Methemoglobinemia following epidural analgesia during labor, *Am. J. Obstet. Gynecol.* **95:**630.
131. Brown, W. U., Jr., Scanlon, J. W., Ostheimer, G. W., *et al.*, 1974, Levels of lidocaine in mother and baby following pudendal and local blocks, *Abstracts of Annual Meeting of the Society for Obstetric Anesthesia and Perinatology*, San Francisco.
132. Merkow, A. J., McGuinness, G. A., Erenberg, A., *et al.*, 1980, The neonatal neurobehavioral effects of buivacaine, mepivacaine, and 2-chloroprocaine used for pudendal block, *Anesthesiology* **52:**309.
133. Teramo, K., and Widholm, O., 1967, Studies of the effect of anaesthetics on foetus. Part I. The effect of paracervical block with mepivacaine upon foetal acid–base values, *Acta Obstet. Gynecol. Scand. (Suppl.)* **46(2):**3.
134. Philipson, E. H., Kuhnert, B. R., Syracuse, C. B., *et al.*, 1983, Intrapartum paracervical block anesthesia with 2-chloroprocaine, *Am. J. Obstet. Gynecol.* **146:**16.
135. Scanlon, J. W., Ostheimer, G. W., Lurie, A. O., *et al.*, 1976, Neurobehavioral responses and drug concentrations in newborns after maternal epidural anesthesia with bupivacaine, *Anesthesiology* **45:**400.
136. Tronick, E., Wise, S., Als, H., *et al.*, 1976, Regional obstetric anesthesia and newborn behavior—Effect over the first ten days of life, *Pediatrics* **58:**94.
137. Corke, B. C., 1977, Neurobehavioural responses of the newborn—The effect of different forms of maternal analgesia, *Anaesthesia* **32:**539.
138. Rosenblatt, D. B., Belsey, E. M., Lieberman, B. A., *et al.*, 1981, The influence of maternal analgesia on neonatal behaviour. II. epidural bupivacaine, *Br. J. Obstet. Gynaecol.* **88:**407.
139. Abboud, T. K., Khoo, S. S., Miller, F., *et al.*, 1982, Maternal, fetal, and neonatal responses after epidural anesthesia with bupivacaine, 2-chloroprocaine, or lidocaine, *Anesth. Analg.* **61:**638.

140. Abboud, T. K., Sarkis, F., Blikian, A., *et al.*, 1983, Lack of adverse neonatal neurobehavioral effects of lidocaine, *Anesth. Analg.* **62**:473.

141. Bromage, P. R., 1983, Epidural and spinal narcotics, *Semin. Anesth.* **2**:75.

142. Nordberg, G., Hedner, T., Mellstrand, T., *et al.*, 1984, Pharmacokinetic aspects of intrathecal morphine analgesia, *Anesthesiology* **60**:448.

143. Srinivasan, T., 1981, Intrathecal morphine for obstetric analgesia, *Anesthesiology* **55**:A298.

144. Baraka, A., Noueihid, R., and Hajj, S., 1981, Intrathecal injection of morphine for obstetric analgesia, *Anesthesiology* **54**:136.

145. Bonnardot, J. P., Maillet, M., Colau, J. C., *et al.*, 1982, Maternal and fetal concentration of morphine after intrathecal administration during labor. *Br. J. Anaesth.* **54**:487.

146. Crawford, J. S., 1981, Intrathecal morphine in obstetrics (Letter to the editor), *Anesthesiology* **55**:487.

147. Hughes, S. C., Rosen, M. A., Shnider, S. M., *et al.*, 1984, Maternal and neonatal effects of epidural morphine for labor and delivery, *Anesth. Analg.* **63**:319.

148. Writer, W. D. R., James, F. M., III, Wheeler, A. S., 1981, Double-blind comparison of morphine and bupivacaine for continuous epidural analgesia in labor, *Anesthesiology* **54**:215.

149. Nordberg, G., Hedner, T., Mellstrand, T., *et al.*, 1983, Pharmacokinetic aspects of epidural morphine analgesia, *Anesthesiology* **58**:545.

150. Nybell-Lindahl, G., Carlsson, C., Ingemarsson, I., *et. al.*, 1981, Maternal and fetal concentrations of morphine after epidural administration during labor, *Am. J. Obstet. Gynecol.* **139**:20.

151. Wolfe, M. J., and Davies, G. K., 1980, Analgesic action of extradural fentanyl, *Br. J. Anaesth.* **52**:357.

152. Stefani, S. J., Hughes, S. C., Shnider, S. M., *et al.*, 1982, Neonatal neurobehavioral effects of inhalation analgesia for vaginal delivery, *Anesthesiology* **56**:351.

153. Datta, S., and Alper, M. H., 1980, Anesthesia for cesarean section, *Anesthesiology* **53**:142.

154. Datta, S., Ostheimer, G. W., Weiss, J. B., *et al.*, 1981, Neonatal effect of prolonged anesthetic induction for cesarean section, *Obstet. Gynecol.* **58**:331.

155. Corke, B. C., Datta, S., Ostheimer, G. W., *et al.*, 1982, Spinal anaesthesia for caesarean section—The influence of hypotension on neonatal outcome, *Anaesthesia* **37**:658.

156. Datta, S., Alper, M. H., Ostheimer, G. W., *et al.*, 1982, Method of ephedrine administration and nausea and hypotension during spinal anesthesia for cesarean section, *Anesthesiology* **56**:68.

157. Chantigian, R. C., Datta, S., Burger, G. A., *et al.*, 1984, Anesthesia for cesarean delivery utilizing spinal anesthesia—Tetracaine versus tetracaine and procaine, *Reg. Anaesth.* **9**:195.

158. Rolbin, S. H., Wright, R. G., Shnider, S. M., *et al.*, 1977, Diazepam during cesarean section—Effects on neonatal Apgar scores, acid–base status, neurobehavioral assessment and maternal and fetal plasma norepinephrine levels, *Abstracts of Scientific Papers, Annual Meeting of the American Society of Anesthesiologists* **449**.

159. James, F. M. III, Dewan, D. M., Floyd, H. M., *et al.*, 1980, Chloroprocaine vs. bupivacaine for lumbar epidural analgesia for elective cesarean section, *Anesthesiology* **52**:488.

160. Higuchi, M., and Takeuchi, S., 1982, Studies on neurobehavioral response (Scanlon test) in newborns after epidural anesthesia with various anesthetic agents for cesarean section, *Acta. Obstet. Gynaecol. Jpn.* **34**:2143.

161. Ramanathan, S., Gandhi, S., Arismendy, J., *et al.*, 1982, Oxygen transfer from mother to fetus during cesarean section under epidural anesthesia, *Anesth. Analg.* **61**:576.

162. Abboud, T. K., Kim, K. C., Noueihed, R., et al., 1983, Epidural bupivacaine, chloroprocaine, or lidocaine for cesarean section—Maternal and neonatal effects, Anesth. Analg. 62:914.

163. Crawford, J. S., Burton, M., and Davies, P., 1972, Time and lateral tilt at caesarean section, Br. J. Anaesth. 44:477.

164. Buley, R. J. R., Downing, J. W., Brock-Utne, J. G., et al., 1977, Right versus left lateral tilt for caesarean section, Br. J. Anaesth. 49:1009.

165. Archer, G. W., Jr., and Marx, G., 1974, Arterial oxygen tension during apnoea in parturient women, Br. J. Anaesth. 46:358.

166. Gold, M. I., Duarte, I., and Muravchick, S., 1981, Arterial oxygenation in conscious patients after 5 minutes and after 30 seconds of oxygen breathing, Anesth. Analg. 60:313.

167. Norris, M. C., and Dewan, D. M., 1984, Preoxygenation for cesarean section—Two techniques, Abstracts of Annual Meeting of the Society for Obstetric Anesthesiology and Perinatalogy, San Antonio.

168. Kosaka, Y., Takahashi, T., and Mark, L. C., 1969, Intravenous thiobarbiturate anesthesia for cesarean section, Anesthesiology 31:489.

169. Tovell, R. M., Anderson, C. C., Sadove, M. S., et al., 1955, A comparative clinical and statistical study of thiopental and thiamylal in human anesthesia, Anesthesiology 16:910.

170. Christensen, J. H., Andreasen, F., and Jansen, J. A., 1981, Pharmacokinetics of thiopental in caesarean section, Acta Anaesthesiol. Scand. 25:174.

171. Christensen, J. H., Andreasen, F., and Jansen, J. A., 1980, Pharmacokinetics of thiopentone in a group of young women and a group of young men, Br. J. Anaesth. 52:913.

172. Morgan, D. J., Blackman, G. L., Paull, J. D., et al., 1981, Pharmacokinetics and plasma binding of thiopental. II. Studies at cesarean section, Anesthesiology 54:474.

173. McKechnie, F. B., and Converse, J. G., 1955, Placental transmission of thiopental, Am. J. Obstet. Gynecol. 70:639.

174. Crawford, J. S., Kane, P. O., and Gardiner, J. E., 1956, Some aspects of obstetric anaesthesia, Br. J. Anaesth. 28:146.

175. Finster, M., Morishima, H. O., Mark, L. C., et al., 1972, Tissue thiopental concentrations in the fetus and newborn, Anesthesiology 36:155.

176. Woods, W. A., Stanski, D. R., Curtis, J., et al., 1982, The role of the fetal liver in the distribution of thiopental from mother to fetus, Anesthesiology 57:A390.

177. Sliom, C. M., Frankel, L., and Holbrook, R. A., 1962, A comparison between methohexitone and thiopentone as induction agents for caesarean section anaesthesia, Br. J. Anaesth. 34:316.

178. Holdcroft, A., Robinson, M. J., Gordon, H., et al., 1974, Comparison of effect of two induction doses of methohexitone on infants delivered by elective caesarean section, Br. Med. J. 2:472.

179. Stovner, J., and Vangen, O., 1974, Diazepam compared to thiopentone as induction agent for caesarean sections, Acta Anaesthesiol. Scand. 18:264.

180. Dich-Nielsen, J., and Holasek, J., 1982, Ketamine as induction agent for caesarean section, Acta Anaesthesiol. Scand. 26:139.

181. Peltz, B., and Sinclair, D. M., 1973, Induction agents for caesarean section—A comparison of thiopentone and ketamine, Anaesthesia 28:37.

182. Ellingson, A., Haram, K., Sagen, N., et al., 1977, Transplacental passage of ketamine after intravenous administration, Acta Anaesthesiol. Scand. 21:41.

183. Pickering, B. G., Palahniuk, R. J., Cote, J., et al., 1982, Cerebral vascular responses to ketamine and thiopentone during foetal acidosis, Can. Anaesth. Soc. J. 29:463.

184. Hodgkinson, R., Marx, G. F., Kim, S. S., *et al.*, 1977, Neonatal neurobehavioral tests following vaginal delivery under ketamine, thiopental, and extradural anesthesia, *Anesth. Analg.* **56:**548.

185. Downing, J. W., Mahomedy, M.C., Coleman, A. J., *et al.*, 1974, Anaesthetic induction for cesarean section-althesin versus thiopentone, *Anaesthesia* **29:**689.

186. Baraka, A., Haroun, S., Bassili, M., *et al.*, 1975, Response of the newborn to succinylcholine injection in homozygotic atypical mothers. *Anesthesiology* **43:**115.

187. Kvisselgaard, N., and Moya, F., 1961, Investigation of placental thresholds to succinylcholine, *Anesthesiology* **22:**7.

188. Flynn, P. J., Frank, M., and Hughes, R., 1982, Evaluation of atracurium in caesarian section using train-of-four responses, *Anesthesiology* **57:**A286.

189. Dailey, P. A., Fisher, D. M., Shnider, S. M., *et al.*, 1984, Pharmacokinetics, placental transfer, and neonatal effects of vecuronium and pancuronium administered during cesarean section, *Anesthesiology* **60:**569.

190. Cohen, E. N., 1962, Thiopental–curate–nitrous oxide anesthesia for cesarean section 1950–1960, *Anesth. Analg.* **41:**122.

191. Finster, M., Poppers, P. J., Horowitz, P. E., *et al.*, 1973, Placental transfer of d-tubocurarine, *Abstracts of Scientific Papers, Annual Meeting American Society of Anesthesiologists* **43.**

192. Older, P. O., and Harris, J. M., 1968, Placental transfer of tubocurarine, Case report, *Br. J. Anaesth.* **40:**459.

193. Kivalo, I., and Saarikoski, S., 1976, Placental transfer of ^{14}C-dimethylcurarine during caesarean section, *Br. J. Anaesth.* **48:**239.

194. Abouleish, E., Wingard, L. B., Jr., De La Vega, S., *et al.*, 1980, Pancouronium in caesarean section and its placental transfer, *Br. J. Anaesth.* **52:**531.

195. Booth, P. N., Watson, M. J., and McLeod, K., 1977, Pancuronium and the placental barrier, *Anaesthesia* **32:**320.

196. Duvaldestin, P., Demetriou, M., Henzel, D., *et al.*, 1978, The placental transfer of pancuronium and its pharmacokinetics during caesarean section, *Acta Anaesthesiol. Scand.* **22:**327.

197. Heaney, G. A. H., 1974, Pancuronium in maternal and fetal serum, *Br. J. Anaesth.* **46:**282.

198. Speirs, I., and Sim, A. W., 1972, The placental transfer of pancuronium bromide, *Br. J. Anaesth.* **44:**370.

199. Baraka, A., 1970, Correlation between maternal and foetal pO_2 and pCO_2 during caesarean section, *Br. J. Anaesth.* **42:**434.

200. Marx, G. F., and Mateo, C. V., 1971, Effect of different oxygen concentrations during general anaesthesia for elective caesarean section, *Can. Anaesth. Soc. J.* **18:**587.

201. Rorke, M. J., Davey, D. A., and Du Toit, H. J., 1968, Foetal oxygenation during caesarean section, *Anaesthesia* **23:**585.

202. Marx, G. F., Joshi, C. W., and Orkin, L. R., 1970, Placental transmission of nitrous oxide, *Anesthesiology* **32:**429.

203. Mankowitz, E., Borck-Utne, J. G., and Downing, J. W., 1981, Nitrous oxide elimination by the newborn, *Anaesthesia* **36:**1014.

204. Coleman, A. J., and Downing, J. W., 1975, Enflurane anesthesia for cesarean section, *Anesthesiology* **43:**354.

205. Galbert, M. W., and Gardner, A. E., 1972, Use of halothane in a balanced technique for cesarean section, *Anesth. Analg.* **51:**701.

206. Moir, D. D., 1970, Anaesthesia for caesarean section—An evaluation of a method using low concentrations of halothane and 50 per cent oxygen, *Br. J. Anaesth.* **42:**136.

207. Warren, T. M., Datta, S., Ostheimer, G. W., *et al.*, 1983, Comparison of the maternal and neonatal effects of halothane, enflurane, and isoflurane for cesarean delivery, *Anesth. Analg.* **62:**516.

208. Burger, G. A., Datta, S., Chantigian, R. C., *et al.*, 1983, Optimal ventilation in general anesthesia for cesarean delivery, *Anesthesiology* **59:**A420.

209. McGuinness, G. A., Merkow, A. J., Kennedy, R. L., *et al.*, 1978, Epidural anesthesia with bupivacaine for cesarean section—Neonatal blood levels and neurobehavioral responses, *Anesthesiology* **49:**270.

210. Hodgkinson, R., Bhatt, M., Kim, S. S., *et al.*, 1978, Neonatal neurobehavioral tests following cesarean section under general and spinal anesthesia, *Am. J. Obstet. Gynecol.* **132:**670.

211. Hollmen, A. I., Jouppila, R., Koivisto, M., *et al.*, 1978, Neurologic activity of infants following anesthesia for cesarean section, *Anesthesiology* **48:**350.

212. Zagorzycki, M. T., and Brinkman, C. R. III, 1982, The effect of general and epidural anesthesia upon neonatal Apgar scores in repeat cesarean section, *Surg. Gynecol. Obstet.* **155:**641.

213. Ounsted. M., Scott, A., and Moar, V., 1980, Delivery and development—To what extent can one associate cause and effect?, *J. R. Soc. Med.* **73:**786.

214. Ounsted, M., Scott, A., and Moar, V., 1981, Pain relief during childbirth and development at 4 years (Letters to the editor), *J. R. Soc. Med.* **74:**629.

215. Van den berg, B. J., Levinson, G., Shnider, S. M., *et al.*, 1980, Evaluation of long-term effects of obstetric medication on child development, *Abstracts of Annual Meeting of the Society for Obstetric Anesthesia and Perinatology,* Boston.

216. Channing, W. B., 1948, *A Treatise on Etherization in Childbirth,* Illustrated by 581 cases, Ticknor and Company, Boston.

CHAPTER 6

Chlamydial Infection

DAVID A. ESCHENBACH

1. Introduction

The organism now known as *Chlamydia trachomatis* was first discovered in 1907 from the eye scrapings of adults with trachoma.[1] The organism that formed inclusions within conjunctival cells of adults was also noted in 1909 to be present in the conjunctiva of neonates with nongonococcal ophthalmia neonatorium,[2] and by the 1930s the organism was a well-established cause of neonatal conjunctivitis. It was also recognized by the 1940s that similar inclusions were present in the urethral discharge of men with nongonococcal urethritis and that discharge could infect the cervix of pregnant female partners who in turn infected the eyes of neonates during delivery.[3] However, at this date, the organism had not been cultured, and it could only be identified by smear. The subsequent ability to culture *Chlamydia*—first in embryonated hen's eggs and then in tissue culture—permitted what has now become a tremendous expansion of knowledge about both the organism and the diseases it causes. Prior cytologic methods used to detect *C. trachomatis* in the eye were too insensitive to identify the organism in genital tract secretions. Direct cytologic smears from the cervix, such as Giemsa stain, will detect only 20–40% of cervical culture-positive women. The ability to culture *Chlamydia* has led to the identification of many new infections and syndromes caused by *C. trachomatis* that would not have been recognized by using cytology. In fact, it is now known that *C. trachomatis* causes a wide spectrum of disease virtually identical to that of *Neisseria gonorrhoeae* (Table

DAVID A. ESCHENBACH • Department of Obstetrics and Gynecology, University of Washington, Seattle, Washington 98195.

I). The ability to culture the organism also led to information about its physiology. It was established that the organism is a small intracellular bacteria and not a virus as first believed. An understanding of its intracellular life cycle was an important step in explaining many of the clinical peculiarities of *C. trachomatis* to be discussed in this chapter.

2. Organism

The genus *Chlamydia* comprises two species, *C. psittaci* and *C. trachomatis*. *Chlamydia psittaci* is transmitted by birds, although it causes minimal infection in birds, it produces a respiratory infection, psittacosis, in humans and arthritis and conjunctivitis and abortion in other mammals. *C. trachomatis* causes endemic and epidemic trachoma, still the leading cause of blindness throughout the world. It also causes lymphogranuloma venerum, an ulcerative genital infection found in developing countries and in a small number of patients living in the southern region of the United States. The remaining oculo–respiratory–genital infections in Table I are usually caused by D-K immunotypes[4]; they are spread by oculogenital contact.

Chlamydia are bacteria that contain both RNA and DNA. They have a cell wall similar to that of gram-negative bacteria, and they replicate by binary fission. However, similar to viruses, they are obligate intracellular organisms that require cell culture techniques for recovery. Chlamydia are isolated either on McCoy or HeLa tissue culture lines pre-

Table I. Spectrum of Clinical Illness Caused by *Chlamydia trachomatis*

Infected site	Disease	Immunotype
Eye	Trachoma	A-C
	Adult inclusion conjunctivitis	A-C
	Neonatal ophthalmia	D-K
Respiratory tract	Neonatal pneumonia	D-K
	Nasopharyngeal discharge	D-K
Urethra	Nongonococcal urethritis (male)	D-K
	Urethral syndrome (female)	D-K
Male genital tract	Epididymitis	D-K
	Lymphogranuloma venereum	L
Female genital tract	Cervicitis	D-K
	Endometritis, salpingitis	D-K
	Late postpartum endometritis	D-K
	Adverse pregnancy outcome	D-K
	Lymphogranuloma venereum	L

treated with irradiation or 5-iodo-2-deoxyuridine to depress cellular metabolism and to prevent replication of the host tissue culture cell. Enhanced infectivity is obtained by centrifuging *Chlamydia* onto a monolayer of the host cells. The organism is then identified by iodine staining or more recently, by a monoclonal fluorescein chlamydial antibody spread across the monolayer.[5]

The 15 serotypes of *C. trachomatis* have been broadly grouped strains that cause endemic trachoma (A-C), LGV (L_{1-3}), and oculo–respiratory–genital infection, the largest group (D-K).[4] Trachoma and oculo–respiratory–genital strains have similar *in vitro* virulence and attack only columnar epithelial cells, while LGV strains are more pathogenic in tissue culture systems and *in vivo* attack even squamous epithelium.

Chlamydia has a slow developmental cycle relevant to the understanding of why chlamydial infection often has an insidious onset. There are two forms of *Chlamydia*. The first form is the elementary body, the infectious chlamydial particle. The elementary body of oculogenital strains attaches only to columnar epithelium. Once attachment has occurred, it is incorporated into the host cell by a process of pinocytosis that surrounds the organism with a membrane.[6] Chlamydial particles remain within this phagosome membrane throughout their existence within the host cell. This membrane isolates the organism from the cellular immune system, protecting it from recognition and attack by cellular defense mechanisms. The organism adapts well in its intracellular environment. After being present for a few hours within the cell, the elementary body is transformed into a noninfectious reticular body. Protected by the phagosome membrane from destruction, the reticular body directs virtually all the ATP produced by the host cell for its own growth. In this stage, the organism becomes metabolically active and begins to synthesize new protein. The reticular bodies eventually divide by binary fission. This noninfectious reticular stage lasts 18–24 hr, after which new infectious elementary bodies are formed. The multiplication process repeats itself until a chlamydial inclusion body is formed that eventually nearly replaces the host cell.[7] At this point, the numerous new infectious elementary bodies are released back into the extracellular environment to infect adjacent epithelium, and the host cell is destroyed.

The oculo–respiratory–genital serotypes attach only to columnar epithelium. Thus, the conjunctiva, cervix, endometrium, endosalpinx, urethra, and rectum are targets of infection, but the stratified squamous epithelium that exists on the external genitalia and vagina is not susceptible to the D-K serotypes. The 24-hr replication process required for *Chlamydia* is rather slow compared with the 2–4 hr division time of most classic bacteria. It is not surprising to find a characteristically long latency period between the time *Chlamydia* is acquired and symptoms are produced. As an example, *N. gonorrhoeae* and *C. trachomatis* are often acquired at the same time in the urethra of males. *Neisseria gonorrhoeae* usually produces urethral symptoms in males within 3–7 days after acquisition. Symptoms caused by the gonococcus disappear when the patient is treated with penicillin. However, 2–4 weeks later, a second discharge (postgonococcal urethritis) occurs caused by *C. trachomatis*. Due in part to the slow growth of the organism, the leukocyte response and tissue response such as edema develop slowly. Thus it is understandable that a second characteristic of chlamydial infection is the insidious onset of symptoms, and often infection occurs without producing recognizable symptoms. In fact, LGV and trachoma strains can exist for years and produce few or no symptoms.

3. Epidemiology

Chlamydia trachomatis can be vertically acquired during birth from infected maternal cervical secretions or it can be acquired by sexual contact. Direct hand-to-eye spread also occurs in trachoma. Congenital infection has not been documented. A significant number of neonates are exposed to *Chlamydia* at birth. Approximately two-thirds of infants exposed to maternal *C. trachomatis* will develop an antibody response (Table IV). Microimmunofluorescence (IF) antibodies are present in about 2–3% of pediatric patients under the age of 6, presumably as a result of vertical transmission from the mother.[8] Exposure to *Chlamydia* subsequently occurs as the population becomes sexually active and the prevalence of *C. trachomatis* antibody increases to 20–30% in the 9–15-age group.[8] From 20 to 40% of sexually active women have been exposed to *Chlamydia* based on the presence of chlamydial antibody.[9,10]

Infants first acquire maternal *C. trachomatis* in the eye and nasopharynx. The organism can be recovered from the eye of infants in whom conjunctivitis develops, usually within the first 2–3 weeks of life.[11,12] Among asymptomatic infants, *Chlamydia* is most frequently isolated from the nasopharynx, but cultures usually do not become positive until the fourth week of life.[11] Thereafter, rectal cultures become positive. The organism is spontaneously cleared from the nasopharynx by 6 months of life,[11] but persistent rectal colonization can occur for longer periods of time.[12]

Several factors have been associated with an increased frequency of chlamydia in teenagers. Active chlamydial infection demonstrated by culture is present in as many as 15–25% of selected sexually active adolescents.[13–15] Since chlamydia is sexually transmitted, among adolescents, the organism has been present most often among women with multiple current partners,[14] among women who had their first intercourse at a younger age, and among women with an increased number of years of sexual activity.[13] For reasons that are not entirely clear, the organism is also associated with oral contraceptive use.[13,15] The association between oral contraceptive use and the presence of cervical ectopy and between chlamydia and ectopy[13] could explain the increased chlamydia rate among oral contraception users. Women exposed to chlamydia who have a larger cervical columnar cell surface area caused by the cervical ectopy may be at an increased risk of acquiring the organism. Chlamydia is also frequently associated with other lower genital tract infection,[13,16] particularly with gonorrhea. C. trachomatis has been isolated from about one-half the women with gonorrhea attending sexually transmitted disease clinics. In fact, chlamydia is three to four times more common than gonorrhea among many populations of sexually active women.[13,16] Although some studies have indicated higher infection rates among women in lower socioeconomic groups,[16] at least among adolescents, the organism is also prevalent in middle socioeconomic groups.

4. Perinatal Infections

Chlamydia trachomatis is a frequent infection among pregnant women. Although recovery rates vary widely depending on the population studied, usually *C. trachomatis* is isolated in 10–20% of pregnant women. However, isolation rates of 30–40% have been reported (Table II). As with nonpregnant women, pregnant women usually have *C. trachomatis* three to four times more frequently than they do *N. gonorrhoeae*.

Female urethritis (acute urethral syndrome) is one of the newly described syndromes caused by *C. trachomatis*.[17] Women typically complain of acute dysuria and urinary frequency. Bacteriuria causes the symptoms in most women, but approximately 20% of women with these symptoms have sterile pyuria ($\geq$8 leukocytes/mm^3 of urine) caused by chlamydia. Several characteristics were associated with chlamydial infection—long duration of symptoms, high frequency of new sexual partners in the previous month, low frequency of prior urinary tract infection, and a low rate of hematuria.[17] Symptomatic women with sterile pyuria need to be scrutinized for chlamydial infection.

Chlamydia has been shown to cause a well-described cervicitis among nonpregnant women. This cervicitis is defined either by the yellow color

Table II. Prevalence of *Chlamydia trachomatis* and Neonatal Outcome among Pregnant Women

Study	Population	Weeks of pregnancy	No. studied	Prevalence of *C. trachomatis* N	%	Prevalence of IgG chlamydial antibody (%)	*Chlamydia* positive N	%	*Chlamydia* negative N	%
Chandler et al.[36]	Mixed SES	36–40	142	18	13	—	—	—	—	—
Frommell et al.[38]	Inner city	<32	340	30	9	—	—	—	—	—
Schachter et al.[37]	Inner city	First visit	900	36	4	—	—	—	—	—
Hammerschlag et al.[39]	Inner city	First visit	322	6	2	73	—	—	—	—
Hammerschlag et al.[40]	Mixed SES	First visit	572	67	12	48	—	—	—	—
Mårdh et al.[41]	Prior to abortion	8–13	231	14	6	25	—	—	—	—
	Swedish	Puerperal	273	23	8	—	—	—	—	—
Heggie et al.[29]	Inner city	8–12	451	73	16	—	—	—	—	—
Martin et al.[24]	Mixed SES	35–37	1007	184	18	—	12/214	6	16/214	7[b]
Thompson et al.[30]	Inner city	<19	268	18	7	—	6/18	33	20/238	8[c]
Grossman et al.[31]	Inner city	First visit	433	71	16	—	10/71	14	45/362	12
Harrison et al.[25]	Mixed SES	First visit	4218[a]	155	4	—	6/71	8	31/362	9
Harrison et al.[42]	American indian	First visit	1185	95	8	81	4/17	24	52/793	7[d]
Ismail et al.[32]	Inner city	3rd trimester	201	44	21	—	—	—	—	—
Khurana et al.[43]	Phillipino	1–3 trimester	363	61	17	—	—	—	—[e]	—
	Low SES									
Hardy et al.[23]	Inner city	3rd trimester	105	39	37	—	5/39	13	7/65	11

[a] Second report, which included patients in ref. 37.
[b] Matched.
[c] $p < 0.01$.
[d] $p < 0.025$ comparing IgM-positive patients with *Chlamydia*-negative patients.
[e] No reported difference of gestational age.

of cervical mucus or by 10 or more polymorphonuclear leukocytes per high power field (hpf) on a cervical Gram stain.[18] About one-half the women with cervicitis had chlamydia; yellow cervical mucus was present in 60% of women in whom *C. trachomatis* was recovered.[18] Ninety-five percent of women with chlamydia had either yellow cervical mucus or 10 or more leukocytes. Although chlamydial cervicitis causes a purulent cervical discharge, symptoms of an abnormal vaginal discharge or other symptoms are usually not present among women with chlamydia, so symptoms are not closely correlated with the recovery of the organism.[16] The relative low sensitivity of symptoms and signs for chlamydial infection makes it difficult to detect the organism using clinical criteria. The presence of *C. trachomatis* infection appears to be even more difficult to discern for pregnant than for nonpregnant women. Most pregnant women have a vaginal discharge and a large proportion of normal pregnant women without *C. trachomatis* have both a cloudy mucus appearance and white blood cells (WBCs) in the cervical mucus. During pregnancy, the presence of *C. trachomatis* has not been related to the presence of a cloudy cervical mucus or to WBCs; the use of these clinical signs to detect women with chlamydia is probably unreliable in pregnant women.

4.1. Perinatal Outcome

Numerous organisms have been associated with an adverse pregnancy outcome such as abortion, stillbirth, premature labor, and premature rupture of the membranes. Group B streptococci,[19] *Ureaplasma urealyticum,*[20,21] *Mycoplasma hominis,*[22] and *Trichomonas vaginalis*[23] have all recently been associated with one or more of these adverse pregnancy outcomes. *C. trachomatis* has also been associated with prematurity and premature rupture of the membranes.[24–26] The impact of *C. trachomatis* is of considerable interest because of the large number of pregnant women with chlamydia. If there is a causal relationship between chlamydia and pregnancy outcome, the mechanism of producing an adverse outcome is not known. *Chlamydia* can attach to and grow in amniotic membrane cells,[27] raising the possibility that an ascent of cervical infection to the amnion could lead to an infection that causes either membrane damage and rupture by producing membrane inflammation and/or the release of prostaglandin precursors.[28]

It is the current hypothesis that women at highest risk for decidual, placental, membrane, or amniotic fluid invasion are those who have recently been exposed to chlamydia. Women with chronic infection have usually manifested an antibody response which may possibly prevent or at least reduce the propensity of chlamydia to infect these sites. Unfortunately, the significance of this potentially important protection is still not fully known. The pregnancy outcome of women with *C. trachomatis* infection is inconsistent from study to study. Some studies have found a marked association between *C. trachomatis* and an adverse outcome[24]; in other investigations prematurity was related only to women with chlamydia who had an IgM antibody,[25] while in many studies there was no apparent relationship between chlamydia and an adverse pregnancy outcome[29–31] (Table II). It is common among all studies of an association between an organism and an adverse pregnancy outcome for the investigators to have focused on a limited number of organisms and for too small a number of women to have been studied for definite conclusions to be reached. We must therefore await large studies in which not only selected organisms but all the organisms associated with an adverse pregnancy outcome are studied simultaneously. In these reports, demographic, social, and other confounding factors of both organism prevalence and pregnancy outcome will also have to be controlled.

However, since new data will not be available for several years, it is important to review the present data linking chlamydia to an adverse pregnancy outcome. It has been demonstrated that experimental human *C. trachomatis* causes abortion and placental infection in cattle.[33] Investigators conducting the early studies on neonatal conjunctivitis since the 1930s have retrospectively found a high rate of prematurity among the infants in whom conjunctivitis developed.[34,35] The first prospective culture studies of chlamydia during pregnancy in the 1970s did not report a difference in the prematurity rate of women with chlamydia compared with women without it.[36–41] However, most of the women in these first prospective culture studies were entered into the study during the third trimester so that second-trimester and early third-trimester pregnancy losses would have occurred before patients were studied (Table II). This potential bias was corrected by Martin *et al.*[24] who enrolled women into their study by the eighteenth week of pregnancy. They found stillbirth, premature delivery, and perinatal death from prematurity to be related to the presence of chlamydia.[24] Most of the adverse pregnancy outcomes occurred during the second or early third trimester. Six of 18 women with and 3% of 238 women without chlamydia had an adverse pregnancy outcome. A markedly premature birth accounted for most of the pregnancy loss. Birth before the thirtieth week of pregnancy occurred in 28% of women with and 2.5% of women without chlamydia.[24] Matching for variables usually present in women with chlamydia did not change the results. However, only 18 women with chlamydia were included in this study and it should also be noted that the women with chlamydia in this study were unusually young. Of those with chlamydia, 60% were under 20 and an additional 33% were under 25 years of age.

In a larger prospective study of chlamydia in more than 1300 women, Harrison et al.[25] found no overall increase in the rate of spontaneous abortion, stillbirth, prematurity, or premature rupture of the membranes among women with chlamydia compared with women without chlamydia. However, these workers further analyzed the pregnancy outcome of the 17 women who had chlamydial IgM antibody. These 17 women represented 24% of the 72 women with C. trachomatis recovered in this study. Women with both chlamydia and an IgM antibody were significantly more likely to have delivered a low-birth-weight infant ($p < 0.025$) and to have premature rupture of the membranes ($p < 0.01$) than either IgM-negative but culture-positive women, or chlamydia culture-negative women. The association between chlamydia and these two outcomes could not be explained by the confounding variables of age, genital mycoplasma infection, vaginal bleeding, or prenatal antibiotic treatment. Recently, Gravett et al.[29] found C. trachomatis to be associated with a premature birth in a case-controlled study of premature labor (case) versus term labor (control). It is of interest that most women in the population studied by Harrison et al.[25] had IgG antibody, and it is probable that most pregnant women with C. trachomatis have chlamydial IgG antibody. The presence of the IgG antibody may protect against decidual or membrane invasion, and these women may not be at risk for an adverse pregnancy outcome. However, women with a recently acquired C. trachomatis infection as determined by the presence of chlamydial IgM antibody may be at risk for an adverse outcome caused by chlamydia. The adolescent women that were studied by Martin et al.[24] may have been at particularly hish risk for an adverse pregnancy outcome from chlamydia because of recently acquired infection.

In contrast to these three studies, there are several other recent prospective studies[29-32] in which there was not even a trend of an increased rate of adverse pregnancy outcome among women wth chlamydia (Table II). Some of these studies are relatively small and many of the patients were enrolled after the time that some of the very early premature births or premature rupture of the membranes would have occurred. However, the inconsistent findings between studies raises uncertainty of whether or not and in what proportion chlamydia is related to an adverse pregnancy outcome. In addition, the relative contribution of chlamydia compared to other organisms must be further studied before more definite conclusions can be reached. If there is an association between chlamydia and these adverse pregnancy outcomes, the relative risk is in the range of 2–3; perhaps the risk exists only among women who recently acquired the infection.

4.2. Postpartum Endometritis

It has become well established that *Chlamydia trachomatis* is a major cause of salpingitis among nonpregnant women. It is therefore not surprising to find an association between chlamydia and postpartum endometritis. In fact, the early retrospective studies made by ophthalmologists as early as the 1930s noted that the mothers of infants with inclusion conjunctivitis had an unusually high rate of postpartum infection.[44-46] Rees *et al.*[47] first confirmed prospectively the presence of chlamydia among mothers in whom postpartum endometritis developed. In many of the infants born of these mothers inclusion conjunctivitis developed. Because of the long latency period of chlamydial infection, the endometritis develops relatively late following delivery, usually between 2 and 6 weeks postpartum.[47] Wager *et al.*[48] differentiated women in whom an early postpartum endometritis developed (within the first 48 hr postpartum) from women in whom postpartum endometritis developed from 2 days to 6 weeks postpartum. A retrospective review of the medical charts was made for a clinical diagnosis of postpartum endometritis among 32 women with antepartum *C. trachomatis* and 359 women without antepartum *C. trachomatis*. This study found that most women in whom early endometritis developed delivered by cesarean section in contrast to the women in whom late endometritis developed, who usually had delivered vaginally. There was no association between chlamydia and early endometritis, a finding subsequently confirmed,[49] but late endometritis developed in 22% of those with and 5% of those without antepartum chlamydia.[48] The association between chlamydia and late postpartum endometritis remained when infected women were compared with controls matched for factors associated with postpartum endometritis. However, the subjects in this retrospective study were not cultured for chlamydia at the time the endometritis developed and other organisms known to be associated with endometritis were not studied.

In the previously mentioned large study conducted by Harrison *et al.*,[25] women with antepartum *M. hominis* had a 7.3 times increased risk of postpartum endometritis compared with women without *M. hominis*, but there was only a weak association between postpartum endometritis and either *C. trachomatis* or *U. urealyticum*. In a smaller study, by Thomp-

Table III. Rate of Postpartum Endometritis or Salpingitis among Vaginally Delivered Women with *Chlamydia* during Pregnancy

| | | Total endometritis rate | | Endometritis among women delivered vaginally | | | | |
| | | | | *Chlamydia* positive | | *Chlamydia* negative | | |
Study	No. studied	N	%	N	%	N	%	p
Wager *et al.*[48]	391	52	13	7/32	22	15/359	5	<0.005
Thompson *et al.*[30]	433	26	6	8/71	11	18/362	5	<0.05
Harrison *et al.*[25]	945	27	3		4	—[a]		0.3 (RR = 2.7)
Ismail *et al.*[32]	201	22	11	6/36	16	6/142	4	<0.01

[a] Data not provided.

son *et al.*,[30] a statistical trend was noted between postpartum endometritis and antepartum chlamydia. In a recent study, *C. trachomatis* was recovered from the cervix or endometrium of 60% and from the endometrium of 23% of the vaginally delivered women with late postpartum endometritis.[50] This is the first direct culture evidence linking chlamydia with this infection. Genital mycoplasma were recovered from the endometrium of 33% of this group. Both chlamydia and genital mycoplasmas may play a role in this clinically mild late postpartum infection. It was noted in the latter study that very few of these individuals were febrile, had a leukocytosis, or were seriously ill. The importance of this late postpartum infection has not been fully established. However, it is interesting to note that from one-third to one-half of infertile women have previously been pregnant. Multiple studies have found an association between distal tubal obstruction and chlamydial antibody titers.[51] Therefore, the possibility exists that a number of the infertile women identified in these studies had developed salpingitis after a normal delivery or following abortion. It is established that in approximately 20% of individuals with chlamydia who recovered from the cervix before abortion a postabortal salpingitis developed.[52] Postabortal salpingitis was confined almost solely to women with chlamydia. Pregnant women who are known to have chlamydia before delivery should receive therapy of the chlamydial infection before discharge from the hospital. In addition, for patients in whom mild signs and symptoms of late postpartum endometritis do develop, cultures for chlamydia are warranted as well as therapy with erythromycin; for nonbreastfeeding women, tetracycline should be considered.

5. Neonatal Infections

At least two neonatal infections have been well documented. *Chlamydia trachomatis* has long been associated with neonatal conjunctivitis; it has recently been established that chlamydia causes neonatal pneumonia. Congenital infection among pregnancies with intact membranes who deliver by cesarean section has not been reported. Neonatal chlamydial infection results when the infant acquires the organism from contact with the infected maternal cervix. The infant born vaginally to a woman with chlamydia frequently becomes infected. From 50 to 70% of infants born to mothers with chlamydia develop either signs or symptoms of infection together with culture and/or antibody evidence of chlamydial infection (Table IV). Given the high rate of maternal chlamydia in some populations, a substantial number of vaginally delivered infants develop one or both of these infections.

5.1. Conjunctivitis

Conjunctivitis develops in 20–50% of infants born of women with chlamydia (Table IV). This wide attack rate is related to the inclusion of infants with minimally symptomatic disease together with infants who are presented for treatment because of overt symptoms. It is estimated that 25% of the infants develop overt symptoms of conjunctivitis and that the other 25% of infants can be detected only by close surveillance. The conjunctivitis usually occurs between 5 and 14 days after birth, a finding that has been used to differentiate chlamydial from gonococcal conjunctivitis.[35] Gonococcal ophthalmia usually occurs within the first 3 days of life. However, there is considerable overlap in the time of onset between the two infections, and *N. gonorrhoeae* cultures must be used to differentiate gonococcal from chlamydial conjunctivitis. Chlamydial conjunctivitis first causes conjunctival hyperemia followed by an inflammatory reaction characterized by a mucopurulent discharge and occasionally a pseudomembrane. Marked eyelid swelling and the purulent discharge can cause difficulty for the infant in opening the eyes after sleep.

Table IV. Development of Infant Infection among Neonates Exposed to Maternal *Chlamydia trachomatis*

Study	No. exposed	Infant chlamydial conjunctivitis		Infection pneumonia		Total infants with C. trachomatis recovered		Infants with seroconversion	
		N	%	N	%	N	%	N	%
Chandler et al.[36]	18	5	28	—		5	28	12	67
Schachter et al.[37]	20	7	35	4	20	10	50	14	70
Frommell et al.[38]	18	7	39	2	11	8	44	11	61
Hammerschlag et al.[39]	6	2	33	1	17	4	67	4	67
Hammerschlag et al.[40]	36[a]	12	33	3	8	25	69	—	
Mårdh et al.[41]	23	0	—	0	—	5	22	—	
Heggie et al.[29]	95	20	21	3	3	27	28	—	
Grossman et al.[31]	89	16	18	16	18	30	34	55	62
Schaefer et al.[53]	61	13	21	14	23	—	—	—	
Ismail et al.[32]	36	11	31	5	14		44–80	—	

[a] Includes only infants who received silver nitrate eye prophylaxis.

The differential diagnosis of neonatal ophthalmia includes the very destructive bacterial infections of gonorrhea and other bacteria such as *Haemophilus influenzae* and *Pseudomonas*. These organisms can be readily diagnosed by Gram stain and culture. Thus, the laboratory workup for neonatal conjunctivitis should include a Gram stain and a bacterial culture to diagnose *N. gonorrhoeae* and other bacteria. Chlamydial conjunctivitis can be rapidly and accurately (80–90% sensitivity) diagnosed by finding inclusions within the Giemsa stain of eye scrapings. A chlamydial culture can also be used.

Chlamydial conjunctivitis is usually a self-limited nondestructive infection. Until recently, it was believed that chlamydial conjunctivitis did not cause permanent eye damage in contrast to adult trachoma, which causes pannus formation (corneal vascularization), cornea scarring and blindness. It has now been demonstrated by careful slit-lamp examination that minimal micropannus formation occurs following neonatal infection.[46] There has been no decrease in visual acuity recognized from chlamydial neonatal eye infection. Nevertheless, early treatment within 12 days of birth prevented the structural changes.

5.2. Pneumonia

In 1977 Beem and Sacon[54] described an interstitial pneumonitis among infants under the age of 6 months, which associated with the recovery of *C. trachomatis.* The pneumonitis usually presents between 4 and 8 weeks after birth,[55] a finding consistent with the long latency period of chlamydial infections. Approximately 30% of all pneumonitis among infants under the age of 6 months is associated with chlamydia.[55]

Infants have the gradual onset of a peculiar repetitive staccato-type cough which has usually persisted for several weeks. Nasal pharangeal congestion and tachypnea are common. Infants are usually afebrile and lack systemic symptoms or signs. Interstitial infiltrates and hyperinflation of the lungs is present on a chest radiograph. Eosinophilia is common and elevated IgM and other immunoglobulin levels are present.[54] Untreated infants have persistent cough and pneumonia for several weeks to months. Sulfasoxazole or erythromycin therapy has reduced the length of cough and has rapidly resolved the pneumonitis in comparison to patients who have received no therapy.[56]

It is not clear whether the pneumonia develops from material that has been aspirated into the lung at the time of delivery or from material that is postnatally aspirated into the lung from infected conjunctival and nasopharangeal sites. Only about half of the infants with pneumonitis have had previous clinically symptomatic conjunctivitis although perhaps an even larger number have nasopharangeal infection consisting of a mucus nasal discharge. Nasopharangeal cultures are the most sensitive culture site. The differential diagnosis includes respiratory syncytial virus infection, adenovirus infection, and a variety of other bacterial pneumonias.[55]

5.3. Other Infections

Infants with pneumonitis commonly have abnormal eardrums. In fact, *Chlamydia trachomatis* has been isolated from the middle ear of infants with chlamydia pneumonia and simultaneous serous otitis media.[57] However, among unselected children who were usually over the age of 1 year, *C. trachomatis* was not isolated from serous otitis fluid.[58] In a retrospective serologic study by Black *et al.,*[59] infants and children aged 1 to 15 years of age with chlamydial antibody had increased rates of pneumonia and conjunctivitis in the first year of life compared with serum-negative children. However, following the first year of age there was no difference between the two groups in episodes of respiratory illness, otitis media, gastroenteritis or other chronic respiratory illness. Thus, there is no clear indication, at present, that a significant proportion of otitis media, gastrointestinal disease, or respiratory illness after the first year of life is attributed to chlamydia.

6. Diagnosis

The possibility of chlamydial infection should always be entertained in those syndromes that have been highly associated with isolation of the organism. Thus, the presence of sterile pyuria in a woman complaining of acute dysuria,[17] the presence of mucopurulent cervicitis in a patient complaining of an abnormal vaginal discharge,[18] and the presence of lower abdominal pain among postpartum women[48] are clinical conditions in which *C. trachomatis* should be suspected on a clinical basis. Chlamydial infection should also be suspected among women with gonorrhea in whom up to 50% will also have *C. trachomatis*. Among neonates, the development of conjunctivitis 5 or more days following delivery and the development of pneumonia, particularly within the first 6 months of life, should also prompt a clinical suspicion of chlamydial infection. If these clinical diagnoses have been made, a presumptive diagnosis of chlamydial infection can be made and appropriate antibiotic therapy instituted.

For individuals with conjunctivitis, chlamydia can usually be found in a Giemsa stain. However, in the remaining syndromes, cultures or fluorescent antibody stains should be used to identify the organism. Infected material for culture should be obtained on Dacron swabs rather than on cotton swabs because of the presence of a cytotoxic agent in the latter. Swabs used to obtain the cultures should be on either aluminum or a plastic shaft. The presence of preservatives in the wood shafts also inhibit the growth of chlamydia. The specimen is collected and temporarily stored in a transport vial containing antibiotics to inhibit other bacteria and yeast. The vial should be refrigerated until the culture is obtained, then refrigerated again until the culture is inoculated. Inoculation should be done within 24 hr.

Chlamydia are inoculated on a monolayer of either McCoy cells or HeLa cells treated with iododeoxyuridine or with cycloheximide. Chlamydial inclusions are identified 2–4 days after the incubation of the cultures. Traditionally, inclusions have been identified by iodine staining, but more recently fluorescent-tagged monoclonal chlamydial antibody has been used to identify chlamydia on the culture plates.[5]

Direct smears of genital secretions have also been recently utilized to make a rapid diagnosis of chlamydial infection without the use of culture.[5] The technique is useful for laboratories that do not have the facilities to culture chlamydia. The direct slide method takes only a few hours to perform. A swab is used to place secretions on a glass slide that is immediately fixed. Specimens can then be easily transported without the concern of bacterial viability. In the laboratory, fluorescene-tagged chlamydial monoclonal antibody is applied to the slide. Fluorescent chlamydial elementary particles appear green under the fluorescent microscope. The sensitivity and specificity (both >90%) of the direct slide identification method appear to be equal to that of the culture among symptomatic individuals with complaints of an abnormal cervical or urethral discharge.[5] However, the sensitivity may be less among asymptomatic individuals, so that the direct method may not be as sensitive as the culture for screening purposes.

Whereas 25–50% of women with these syndromes will have chlamydia, only a proportion of women with chlamydia will be detected by presenting with one or more syndromes. Nevertheless, general screening for *C. trachomatis* even during pregnancy cannot be advocated because of the high cost and general unavailability of the culture. Selected screening of pregnant women at high risk for *C. trachomatis* may be considered. Selection would include women with a purulent cervical discharge, gonorrhea or other sexually transmitted organism, and adolescent women. It is not clear whether patients should be screened with culture or a direct slide test, but the direct slide test may have a reduced sensitivity among asymptomatic women screened compared with the symptomatic patients reported to date.

7. Therapy

Although *in vitro* sensitivity testing of chlamydia has not been well developed, chlamydial eradication *in vivo* has been roughly correlated with *in vitro* inhibition of the organism. Antibiotics that appear to be most active against chlamydia include tetracycline, erythromycin, sulfonamides, and rifampin (see Table V). Clindamycin also appears to have activity against chlamydia with minimal inhibitory concentration <2.0 μg/ml.[60] The sensitivity of chlamydia to penicillin is unclear at the present time. Penicillin is not highly active against chlamydia *in vitro* and, although penicillins inhibit the growth of chlamydia, washing the media and cells free of penicillin permits chlamydia to reinstitute growth. However, ampicillin does appear to exhibit some activity against chlamydia in cervical sites.[62] Cephalosporins and aminoglycosides have virtually no *in vitro* or *in vivo* activity against chlamydia.[64] Therefore, antibiotic reg-

Table V. Summary of Antibiotic Therapy to Treat
Chlamydia trachomatis Cervical Infection among
Nonpregnant Women[a]

Agent	Range of efficacy (%)
Tetracycline/doxycycline	90–100
Erythromycin	76–100
Trimethoprim/sulfamethoxazole	93–100
Rosaramicin	82
Ampicillin[b]	33–80

[a] Modified from ref. 61.
[b] Data from refs. 62 and 63.

imen should include agents which are particularly active against the organism. Among pregnant women and breastfeeding women, erythromycin is the treatment of choice. Sulfonamides or trimethoprim/sulfamethoxazole can be used by asymptomatic patients. Nonbreastfeeding postpartum women could be treated with tetracycline.

7.1. Neonatal Eye Prophylaxis

It is apparent that silver nitrate prophylaxis used for gonococcal ophthalmia does not prevent chlamydia conjunctivitis. In fact, the charge has been made that silver nitrate damage of the conjunctival cells may increase the attack rate of chlamydia over that expected of patients who receive no silver nitrate therapy. Erythromycin and perhaps tetracycline ophthalmic ointments placed in the infant's eye appears to reduce the rate of neonatal chlamydial conjunctivitis. Hammerschlag *et al.*[40] found that neonatal conjunctivitis developed in 33% of individuals randomly treated with silver nitrate and in none of 24 individuals who received erythromycin ointment. However, erythromycin eyedrops did not reduce nasal pharyngeal colonization and eye prophylaxis probably has no effect on the development of subsequent chlamydial pneumonia. In addition, unpublished reports indicate that erythromycin-treated infants can develop conjunctivitis.

7.2. Neonatal Treatment

There still remains a divided opinion on the treatment of neonatal chlamydial conjunctivitis. Traditional therapy has utilized topical sulfanomides, tetracyclines, and erythromycins four times daily for a 3-week course. Frequent recurrent chlamydial conjunctivitis has been noted after topical therapy. Recurrence may be due either to difficulty instilling eyedrops or to noncompliance on the part of the mother. Because of a high failure rate following topical therapy, it is now recommended that oral erythromycin be instituted for 2 weeks. An added advantage of the oral erythromycin therapy is that nasopharyngeal colonization is eliminated and the possibility of pneumonitis is reduced.

Infant pneumonitis has been successfully treated with sulfasoxazole or with erythromycin for 2 weeks.[56] The infants became culture negative and had no clinical relapses. Sulfasoxazole 150 mg/kg per day or erythromycin estolate 40 mg/kg per day has been used.

7.3. Maternal Treatment

Mothers with asymptomatic cervical infection or with mild late postpartum endometritis should be treated with either erythromycin or tetracycline in doses of 500 mg four times daily for 10 days. An alternative regimen is doxycycline 200 mg twice a day for 10 days. Trimethoprim/sulfamethoxazole (160 mg trimethoprim and 80 mg sulfamethoxazole) in two double-strength tablets twice daily for 5 days may also be used for minimally symptomatic or asymptomatic individuals. Pregnant women with chlamydia should not receive tetracycline or erythromycin estolate, which has been associated with liver enzyme elevations during pregnancy.[65]

It is apparent that since chlamydia is a sexually transmitted infection, male contacts of women identified as having chlamydia require examination or treatment, or both. Asymptomatic male chlamydial carriage is common. Male sexual partner therapy is especially indicated if the asymptomatic male is found to have increased number of white blood cells (WBCs) in the urethral discharge. In addition, the physician may be asked to treat female sexual contacts of men with symptomatic nongonococcal urethritis or with proven chlamydial infection. Female contacts of men with chlamydia have a 60–70% prevalence of chlamydia themselves,[66] and the females should be either cultured and/or treated.

In summary, chlamydia is a common infection during pregnancy occurring in 5–30% of individuals. It is particularly related to a young age, perhaps a lower economic status, the presence of other sexually transmitted organisms, and with multiple sexual partners. The organism is also related to mucopurulent cervicitis and to sterile pyuria. There is a controversy as to whether the infection causes prematurity. However, it is well documented that neonatal conjunctivitis and pneumonia frequently occur when infants are born through an infected cervix. Late postpartum maternal endometritis also appears to be a consequence of antenatal infection. Recognition of the possibility of chlamydial infection with these clinical entities and a prompt diagnosis by a combination of clinical criteria, culture, or direct fluorescent antibody stain together with the administration of the appropriate antibiotics should reduce the morbidity caused by this organism.

Acknowledgment

This work was supported by the National Institutes of Health, program project grant AI-12191.

References

1. Halberstaedter, L., and von Prowazek, S., 1907, Über Zelleinschliesse parasitärer Natur beim Trachom, *Arbeit. Kaiserlicken Gesund.* **26**:44.
2. Halberstaedter, L., and von Prowazek, S., 1909, Ueber Chlamydozoen befunde bei Blennorrhoea neonatorum non gonorrhoica, *Berl. Klin. Wochenschr.* **46**:1839.
3. Thygeson, P., and Stone, W., Jr., 1942, Epidemiology of inclusion conjunctivitis, *Arch. Ophthalmol.* **27**:91.
4. Wang, S. P., Grayston, J. T., Kuo, C.-C., *et al.*, 1977, Serodiagnosis of *Chlamydia trachomatis* infections with the microimmunofluorescence test, in: *Nongonococcal Urethritis and Related Infection* (D. Hobson and K. K. Holmes, eds.), p. 237, American Society of Microbiology, Washington, D.C.
5. Tam, M. R., Stamm, W. E., Handsfield, H. H., *et al.*, 1984, Culture-dependent diagnosis of *Chlamydia trachomatis* using monoclonal antibodies, *N. Engl. J. Med.* **310**:1146.
6. Friss, R. R., 1972, Interaction of L cell and *Chlamydia psittaci:* Entry of parasite and host responses to its development, *J. Bacteriol.* **110**:706.
7. Armstrong, J. A., Valentine, R. C., and Fildes, C., 1963, Structure and replication of the trachoma agent in cell cultures as shown by electron microscopy, *J. Gen. Microbiol.* **30**:59.
8. Black, S. B., Grossman, M., Cles, L., and Schachter, J., 1981, Serologic evidence of chlamydial infection in children, *J. Pediatr.* **98**:65.
9. Schachter, J., and Dawson, C. R., 1977, Comparative efficiency of various diagnostic methods for chlamydial infection, in: *Nongonoccal Urethritis and Related Infections* (D. Hobson and K. K. Holmes, eds.), p. 337, American Society of Microbiology, Washington, D.C.
10. Schachter, J., Stoner, E., and Moncada, E., 1983, Screening for chlamydial infections in women attending family planning clinics, *West. J. Med.* **138**:375.
11. Hammerschlag, M. R., Chandler, J. W., Alexander, E. R., *et al.*, 1982, Longitudinal studies on chlamydial infections in the first year of life, *Pediatr. Infect. Dis.* **1**:395.
12. Schachter, J., Grossman, M., Holt, T., *et al.*, 1979, Infection with *Chlamydia trachomatis:* Involvement of multiple anatomic sites in neonates, *J. Infect. Dis.* **139**:232.

13. Shafer, M.-A., Beck, A., Blain, B., et al., 1984, Chlamydia trachomatis: Important relationships to race, contraception, lower genital tract infection and Papanicolaou smear, J. Pediatr. 104:141.
14. Chacko, M. R., and Lovchik, J. C., 1984, Chlamydia trachomatis infection in sexually active adolescents: Prevalence and risk factors, Pediatrics 73:836.
15. Washington, A. E., Gove, S., Schachter, J., and Sweet, R. L., 1985, Oral contraceptive Chlamydia trachomatis infection, and pelvic inflammatory disease, J.A.M.A. 253:2246.
16. Eager, R. M., Beach, R. K., Davidson, A. J., and Judson, F. N., 1985, Epidemiologic and clinical factors of Chlamydia trachomatis in Black, Hispanic and White female adolescents, West. J. Med. 143:37.
17. Stamm, W. E., Wagner, K. F., Amsel, R., et al., 1980, Causes of the acute urethral syndrome in women, N. Engl. J. Med. 303:409.
18. Brunham, R. C., Paavonen, J., Stevens, C., et al., 1984, Mucopurulent cervicitis—The ignored counterpart in women of urethritis in men, N. Engl. J. Med. 311:1.
19. Regan, J. A., Chao, S., and James, L. S., 1981, Premature rupture of membranes, preterm delivery, and Group B streptococcal colonization of mothers, Am. J. Obstet. Gynecol. 141:184.
20. Braun, P., Lee, Y.-H., Klein, J. O., et al., 1971, Birth weight and genital mycoplasmas in pregnancy, N. Engl. J. Med. 284:168.
21. Kass, E. H., McCormack, W. M., Lin, J.-S., et al., 1981, Genital mycoplasmas as a cause of excess premature delivery, Trans. Assoc. Am. Physicians 94:261.
22. Harwick, H. J., Purcell, R. H., Iuppa, J. B., et al., 1970, Mycoplasma hominis and abortion, J. Infect. Dis. 121:260.
23. Hardy, P. H., Hardy, J. B., Nell, E. E., et al., 1984, Prevalence of six sexually transmitted disease agents among pregnant inner city adolescents and pregnancy outcome, Lancet 2:333.
24. Martin, D. H., Koutsky, L., Eschenbach, D. A., et al., 1982, Prematurity and perinatal mortality in pregnancies complicated by maternal Chlamydia trachomatis infections, J.A.M.A. 247:1585.
25. Harrison, H. R., Alexander, E. R., Weinstein, L., et al., 1983, Cervical Chlamydia trachomatis and mycoplasmal infections in pregnancy: Epidemiology and outcomes, J.A.M.A. 250:1721.
26. Gravett, G. G., Hummel, D., Eschenbach, D. A., and Holmes, K. K., 1986, Preterm labor associated with subclinical amniotic fluid infection and with bacterial vaginosis, Obstet. Gynecol. 67:229.
27. Harrison, R. C., and Riggin, R. T., 1979, Infections of untreated human amnion monolayers with Chlamydia trachomatis, J. Infect. Dis. 140:968.
28. McDonald, P. C., Porter, J. C., Schwartz, B. E., et al., 1978, Initiation of parturition in the human female, Semin. Perinatal. 2:273.
29. Heggie, A. D., Lumicao, G. G., Stuart, L. A., and Gyves, M. T., 1981, Chlamydia trachomatis infection in mothers and infants, Am. J. Dis. Child. 135:507.
30. Thompson, S., Lopez, B., Wong, K.-H., et al., 1982, A prospective study of chlamydia and mycoplasma infections during pregnancy: Relation to pregnancy outcome and maternal morbidity, in: Chlamydial Infections (P.-A. Mårdh, K. K. Holmes, J. D. Oriel et al., eds.), p. 155, Elsevier Biomedical Press, New York.
31. Grossman, M., Schachter, J., Sweet, R., et al., 1982, Prospective studies in chlamydia in newborns, in: Chlamydial Infections (P.-A., Mårdh, K. K. Holmes, J. D. Oriel, eds.), p. 213, Elsevier Biomedical Press, New York.
32. Ismail, M. A., Chandler, A. E., Beem, M. O., and Moawad, A. H., 1985, Chlamydial colonization of the cervix in pregnant adolescent, J. Reprod. Med. 30:549.

33. Page, L. A., and Smith, P. C., 1976, Placentitis and abortion in cattle inoculated with chlamydia isolated from aborted human placental tissue, *Proc. Soc. Exp. Med.* **146:**269.

34. Armstrong, J. H., Zacarias, F., and Rein, M. F., 1976, Ophthalmia neonatorum: A chart review, *Pediatrics* **57:**884.

35. Naib, Z. M., 1970, Cytology of TRIC agent infection of the eye of newborn infants and their mother's genital tracts, *Acta Cytol.* **14:**390.

36. Chandler, J. W., Alexander, E. R., Pheiffer, T. A., *et al.*, 1977, Ophthalmia neonatorum associated with maternal chlamydial infections, *Trans. Am. Acad. Ophthalmol. Otolaryngol.* **83:**302.

37. Schachter, J., Grossman, M., Holt, J., *et al.*, 1979, Prospective study of chlamydial infection in neonates, *Lancet* **2:**377.

38. Frommell, G. R., Rothenberg, R., Wang, S.-P., *et al.*, 1979, Chlamydial infection of mothers and their infants, *J. Pediatr.* **95:**28.

39. Hammerschlag, M. R., Anderka, M., Semine, D. Z., *et al.*, 1979, Prospective study of maternal and infantile infection with *Chlamydia trachomatis, Pediatrics* **64:**142.

40. Hammerschlag, M. R., Chandler, J. W., Alexander, E. R., *et al.*, 1980, Erythromycin ointment for ocular prophylaxis of neonatal chlamydial infection, *J.A.M.A.* **244:**2291.

41. Mårdh, P.-A., Helin, I., Bobeck, S., *et al.*, 1980, Colonisation of pregnant and puerperal women and neonates with *Chlamydia trachomatis, Br. J. Vener. Dis.* **56:**96.

42. Harrison, H. R., Boyce, W. T., Haffner, W. H., *et al.*, 1983, The prevalence of genital *Chlamydia trachomatis* and mycoplasmal infections during pregnancy in an American Indian population, *Sex. Trans. Dis.* **10:**184.

43. Khurana, C. M., Deddish, P. A., and delMundo, F., 1985, Prevalence of *Chlamydia trachomatis* in the pregnant cervix, *Obstet. Gynecol.* **66:**241.

44. Thygeson, P., and Mengert, W. F., 1936, The virus of inclusion conjunctivitis: Further observations, *Arch. Ophthalmol.* **15:**377.

45. Dunlop, E. M. C., Harper, I. A., Khalaf Al-Heissaini, M., *et al.*, 1966, Relations of TRIC agent to nonspecific genital infection, *Br. J. Vener. Dis.* **42:**77.

46. Mordhorst, C. H., and Dawson, C. R., 1971, Sequelae of neonatal inclusion conjunctivitis and associated disease in parents, *Am. J. Ophthalmol.* **71:**861.

47. Rees, E., Tait, A. A., Hobson, D., *et al.*, 1977, Chlamydia in relation to cervical infection and pelvic inflammatory disease, in: *Nongonococcal Urethritis and Related Infections* (K. K. Holmes and D. Hobson, eds.), p. 67, American Society for Microbiology, Washington, D.C.

48. Wager, G. P., Martin, D. H., Koutsky, L., *et al.*, 1980, Puerperal infectious morbidity: Relationship to route of delivery and to antepartum *Chlamydia trachomatis* infection, *Am. J. Obstet. Gynecol.* **138:**1028.

49. Blanco, J. D., Diaz, K. C., Lipscomb, K. A., *et al.*, 1985, *Chlamydia trachomatis* isolation in patients with endometritis after cesarean section, *Am. J. Obstet. Gynecol.* **152:**278.

50. Hoyme, U. B., Kiviat, N., and Eschenbach, D. A., 1986, The microbiology and treatment of late postpartum endometritis, *Obstet. Gynecol.*, in press.

51. Moore, D. E., Spadoni, L. R., Foy, H. M., *et al.*, 1982, Increased frequency of serum antibodies to *Chlamydia trachomatis* in infertility due to distal tubal disease, *Lancet* **2:**574.

52. Møller, B. R., Ahrons, S., Laurin, J., and Mårdh, P.-A., 1982, Pelvic infection after elective abortion associated with *Chlamydia trachomatis, Obstet. Gynecol.* **59:**210.

53. Schaefer, C., Harrison, H. R., Boyce, W. T., and Lewis, M.: 1985, Illnesses in infants born to women with *Chlamydia trachomatis* infection, *Am. J. Dis. Child.* **139:**127.

54. Beem, M. O., and Saxon, E. M., 1977, Respiratory tract colonization and a distinctive pneumonia syndrome in infants infected with *Chlamydia trachomatis, N. Engl. J. Med.* **296:**306.

55. Harrison, H. R., English, M. G., Lee, C. K., and Alexander, E. R., 1978, *Chlamydia trachomatis* infant pneumonitis: Comparison with matched controls and other infant pneumonitis, *N. Engl. J. Med.* **298**:702.
56. Beem, M. O., Saxon, E., and Tipple, M. A., 1979, Treatment of chlamydial pneumonia of infancy, *Pediatrics* **63**:198.
57. Tipple, M. A., Beem, M., and Saxon, E., 1979, Clinical characteristics of the afebrile pneumonia associated with *Chlamydia trachomatis* infection in infants less than 6 months of age, *Pediatrics* **63**:192.
58. Hammerschlag, M. R., Hammerschlag, P. E., and Alexander, E. R., 1980, The role of *Chlamydia trachomatis* in middle ear effusions in children, *Pediatrics* **66**:615.
59. Black, S. B., Grossman, M., Cles, L., and Schachter, J., 1981, Serologic evidence of chlamydial infection in children, *J. Pediatr.* **98**:65.
60. Harrison, H. R., Riggins, R. M., Alexander, E. R., and Weinstein, L., 1984, In vitro activity of clindamycin against strains of *Chlamydia trachomatis*, *Mycoplasma hominis* and *Ureaplasma urealyticum* isolated from pregnant women, *Am. J. Obstet. Gynecol.* **149**:477.
61. Stamm, W. E., and Holmes, K. K., 1984, *Chlamydia trachomatis* infection of the adult, in: *Sexually Transmitted Diseases* (K. K. Holmes, P.-A. Mårdh, P. F. Aparling, eds.), p. 258, McGraw-Hill, New York.
62. Bowie, W. R., Manzon, L. M., Barrie-Hume, C. J., *et al.*, 1982, Efficacy of treatment regimens for lower urogenital *Chlamydia trachomatis* infection in women, *Am. J. Obstet. Gynecol.* **142**:125.
63. Brunham, R. C., Kuo, C.-C., Stevens, C. E., and Holmes, K. K., 1982, Treatment of concomitant *Neisseria gonorrhoeae* and *Chlamydia trachomatis* infections in women: Comparison of trimethoprim/sulfamethoxazole with ampicillin-probenecid, *Rev. Infect. Dis.* **4**:491.
64. Sweet, R. L., Schachter, J., and Robbie, M. O., 1983, Failure of β-lactam antibiotics to eradicate *Chlamydia trachomatis* in the endometrium despite apparent clinical cure of acute salpingitis, *J.A.M.A.* **250**:2641.
65. McCormack, W. M., George, H., Donner, A., *et al.*, 1977, Hepatic toxicity of erythromycin estolate during pregnancy, *Antimicrob. Agents Chemother.* **12**:630.
66. Holmes, K. K., Handsfield, H. H., Wang, S.-P., *et al.*, 1975, Etiology of nongonococcal urethritis, *N. Engl. J. Med.* **292**:1199.

Index